Development of Movement Co-ordination in Children

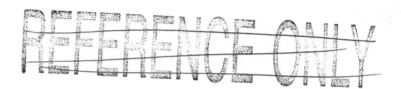
Co-ordination of movement plays a key role in human development and is an active area of study in sport and health sciences. This book looks in detail at how children develop basic skills, such as walking or reaching for objects, and more complex skills, such as throwing and catching a ball accurately or riding a bicycle.

Development of Movement Co-ordination in Children is informed by five major theoretical perspectives – neural maturation, information-processing, direct perception, dynamic systems and constraint theory – and these theories are explained in an introductory chapter.

The international contributions are then brought together under the headings of ergonomics, health sciences and sport. Focusing on practical applications, individual chapters cover many different aspects of movement behaviour and development, ranging from children's overestimation of their physical abilities and the links of injury proneness to the co-ordination of kicking techniques. Both normal and abnormal development is considered.

Development of Movement Co-ordination in Children will be of considerable interest to students, teachers and professionals in the fields of sports science, kinesiology, physical education, ergonomics and developmental psychology.

Geert Savelsbergh is at the Department of Exercise and Sport Science, Manchester Metropolitan University. **Keith Davids** is Dean, School of Physical Education, University of Otago, New Zealand. **John van der Kamp** is at the Faculty of Human Movement Science, Vrije Universiteit of Amsterdam. **Simon J. Bennett** is at the Department of Optometry and Neuroscience, University of Manchester Institute of Science and Technology.

Development of Movement Co-ordination in Children

Applications in the fields of ergonomics, health sciences and sport

Edited by Geert Savelsbergh, Keith Davids, John van der Kamp and Simon J. Bennett

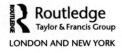

Routledge
Taylor & Francis Group

LONDON AND NEW YORK

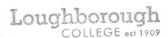

First published 2003
by Routledge
2 Park Square, Milton Park, Abingdon, Oxon, OX14 4RN

Simultaneously published in the USA and Canada
by Routledge
270 Madison Ave, New York NY 10016

Routledge is an imprint of the Taylor & Francis Group

Transferred to Digital Printing 2009

© 2003 Selection and editorial matter Geert Savelsbergh, Keith Davids,
John van der Kamp and Simon J. Bennett; individual chapters,
the contributors

Typeset in Times by
HWA Text and Data Management, Tunbridge Wells

British Library Cataloguing in Publication Data
A catalogue record for this book is available from the British Library

Library of Congress Cataloging in Publication Data
A catalog record for this book has been requested

ISBN 0–415–24736–5 (hbk)
ISBN 0–415–24737–3 (pbk)

Publisher's Note
The publisher has gone to great lengths to ensure the quality of this reprint
but points out that some imperfections in the original may be apparent.

Contents

Illustrations

Tables

Contributors

J. Greg Anson School of Physical Education, University of Otago, New Zealand.

Gregory S. Braswell Department of Psychology, University of California at Santa Cruz, USA.

Simon J. Bennett Department of Optometry and Neuroscience, UMIST, Manchester, UK.

Allen W. Burton* formerly of Division of Kinesiology, University of Minnesota, Minneapolis, USA.

Keith Davids School of Physical Education,University of Otago, New Zealand.

Digby Elliott Department of Kinesiology, McMaster University, Hamilton, Canada.

Robert R. Horn Research Institute for Sport and Exercise Sciences, Liverpool John Moores University, UK.

Idsart Kingma Institute for Fundamental and Clinical Human Movement Sciences, Vrije Universiteit, Amsterdam, Netherlands.

Dawne Larkin School of Human Movement and Exercise Science, The University of Western Australia, Australia.

Annick Ledebt Perceptual–Motor Development and Learning Group, Institute for Fundamental and Clinical Human Movement Sciences, Vrije Universiteit, Amsterdam, Netherlands.

Motohide Miyahara School of Physical Education, University of Otago, New Zealand.

Helen E. Parker School of Health and Physical Education, The University of Notre Dame, Australia.

Jodie M. Plumert Department of Psychology, University of Iowa, USA.

Koop Reynders Institute of Human Movement Sciences, University of Groningen, Netherlands.

*deceased

Annieck Ricken, Centre for Biophysical and Clinical Research into Human Movement, Manchester Metropolitan University, UK.

Richard W. Rodgerson Division of Kinesiology, University of Minnesota, Minneapolis, USA.

Karl S. Rosengren Departments of Kinesiology and Psychology, University of Illinois, Champaign, IL, USA.

Geert Savelsbergh Perceptual–Motor Development and Learning Group, Institute for Fundamental and Clinical Human Movement Sciences, Vrije Universiteit Amsterdam, Netherlands, and Centre for Biophysical and Clinical Research into Human Movement, Manchester Metropolitan University, UK.

Mark A. Scott Research institute for Sport and Exercise Sciences, Liverpool John Moores University, UK.

Dominic A. Simon, Department of Kinesiology, McMaster University, Hamilton, Canada.

Bert Steenbergen Nijmegen Institute for Cognition and Information, University of Nijmegen, Netherlands.

David A. Sugden School of Education, University of Leeds, UK.

Arenda F. te Velde Perceptual–Motor Development and Learning Group, Institute for Fundamental and Clinical Human Movement Sciences, Vrije Universiteit, Amsterdam, Netherlands.

Pauline S. Thiemann Nijmegen Institute for Cognition and Information, University of Nijmegen, Netherlands.

Andrea Utley Centre for Physical Education and Sports Science, University of Leeds, UK.

John van der Kamp Perceptual–Motor Development and Learning Group, Institute for Fundamental and Clinical Human Movement Sciences, Vrije Universiteit, Amsterdam, Netherlands.

Jaap H. van Dieën Institute for Fundamental and Clinical Human Movement Sciences, Vrije Universiteit, Amsterdam, Netherlands.

Dominique van Roon Nijmegen Institute for Cognition and Information, University of Nijmegen, Netherlands.

Martine Verheul Centre for Biophysical and Clinical Research into Human Movement, Manchester Metropolitan University, UK.

Jill Whitall Department of Physical Therapy, University of Maryland, Baltimore, USA.

Mark A. Williams Research Institute for Sport and Exercise Sciences, Liverpool John Moores University, UK.

Preface

The co-ordination of movement at a simple and complex level is one of the key tasks of human development. In their daily activities children demonstrate many different patterns of co-ordinated movement and throughout childhood learn and develop many different skills to perform a variety of tasks. The chapters brought together in this book discuss some of these skills; both very basic skills such as walking, hitting, throwing, catching, kicking and reaching for objects, and more complex skills such as learning to ride a bicycle, crossing the road, using a spoon to eat, drawing and writing.

One of the best known definitions of movement co-ordination is that of the Russian physiologist, Nikolai Bernstein. He saw co-ordination as the mastering of redundant degrees of freedom into a controllable system (Bernstein, 1967, p.127). 'Degrees of freedom' refers to all the possible movements of all the sub-components of the motor apparatus of the human body; for example, joints. There are several different perspectives on how we solve the problem of achieving this mastery and different researchers adopt different perspectives in order to examine the task at hand. These perspectives are discussed in the introductory chapter to the book. Five major paradigms are described: the neural-maturation perspective; information-processing theories; the ecological psychological or direct perception approach; dynamic systems theory; and constraint-led or co-ordinative structure theory. The last three are the more recent approaches and therefore the majority of chapters have been written with these frameworks in mind.

The individual chapters represent the latest research and thinking in the fields of ergonomics, health science and sport and provide the reader with new insights into both theory and practical applications. In all these areas there is an increasing awareness of the importance of understanding the development of movement co-ordination and how this might affect, for example, the design of equipment, the enhancement of everyday activities, rehabilitation practices, or training and practice in sport skills.

For these reasons, we think the book will be of great interest to researchers, teachers, coaches, therapists and students in various fields, including sport sciences, kinesiology, physical education, ergonomics, human movement sciences, health sciences, physical therapy and developmental psychology.

The contributors to the book come from Australia, new Zealand, Canada, Europe and the United States of America. They include those with established reputations and young authors who are just beginning to make their mark. Together, they bring a wide-ranging perspective to bear on this rich and expanding field of study, and we thank them for their contribution to this project.

Geert J.P. Savelsbergh
Keith Davids
John van der Kamp
Simon J. Bennett
Amsterdam, The Netherlands, July 2002

Reference

Bernstein, N. (1967) *The Coordination and Regulation of Movement*. New York: Pergamon Press.

1 Theoretical perspectives on the development of movement co-ordination in children

Geert Savelsbergh, Keith Davids,
John van der Kamp and
Simon J. Bennett

1. Introduction

In a great diversity of daily activities children demonstrate skilled and well co-ordinated movement behaviour. To reach such levels of performance and flexibility takes years of learning and development. This book deals with the development of movement co-ordination of daily activities, like throwing, writing, reaching, walking, catching, kicking and cycling. An important characteristic of skilled performance is the ability to adjust the movement pattern to the (changing) circumstances of the environment.

Nikolai Bernstein (1967) formulated one of the central issues in understanding the development of motor co-ordination: the 'degrees of freedom' problem. The degrees of freedom problem refers to the possible movements of all the components (e.g. muscles, tendons, joints etc.) of the motor apparatus of the human body. Bernstein realised that the non-linear nature of the interactions among these different components of the human body makes their separate regulation impossible and inferred that to be able to control all these components, or degrees of freedom, these movements have to be co-ordinated. Co-ordination, therefore, is the process of mastering the redundant degrees of freedom into a controllable system (see Bernstein, 1967, p. 127).

The issue of mastering the degrees of freedom has been approached in different ways. In this chapter we will discuss five major perspectives, that is, the neural-maturation perspective; information-processing theories, the ecological psycho-logical approach, dynamic systems theory and the constraint theory.

2. Neural-maturation perspective

Achievements in motor behaviour, such as grasping, sitting, crawling and walking, were believed to occur at a predetermined age. This resulted in a perspective of motor development as a rather rigid and gradual unfolding of postures and movements that was mainly attributed to the general process of maturation of the central nervous system. Co-ordinative movement patterns emerge in an orderly genetic sequence; that is, in cephalo-to-caudal and central-to-distal sequences. By an increasing cortical control over lower reflexes the movement patterns became more co-ordinated. For instance Peiper (1963) argued that basic motor skills, like walking, were not learned by experience but simply a result of cerebral maturation. In his book he used the example of a 6-month-old girl with a bilateral congenital hip dislocation. She was put into a plaster cast until 18 months and was unable to stand. At 18 months the cast was replaced by a half cast, and one day later, she started to walk (Peiper ,1963, p. 233). This example illustrates nicely the core idea of this approach.

The major contribution to the understanding of the development of movement co-ordination was the establishment of the so-called 'milestones' of development by Gesell (e.g. Gesell and Amatruda, 1945) and McGraw (1943). Gesell and Amatruda (1945, p. 20) suggested that 'maturation is the net sum of the gene effects operating in a self-limited time cycle'. In the same time period, McGraw argued that motor development is possible if 'a certain amount of neural maturation must take place before any function can be modified by specific stimulation'. This is not a strict neural-maturation point of view and leaves room for environmental influence. In the more recent constraint-led approach, the maturation of the nervous system can be considered as one of the constraints

3. Information-processing approach

The basic idea of the information-processing perspective is that it divides the cognitive system (e.g. the central nervous system) into components and determines the way in which these components process and transform information. In this respect the computer is often used as a model for the brain. The concept of memory is important as the approach emphasises representations for the storage of information. Differences between novices and experts are attributed to differences in stored knowledge with respect to the task at hand, and the associated processing activities. When a skill is learned the suggestion is that the person acquires and stores increasingly complex knowledge about that skill. The differences between experts and novices result from the use of different strategies and informational cues; that is, an expert acquires a variety of problem-solving strategies. From this perspective, children are initially regarded as novices, who then 'move' to expert status as they develop. Thus, development involves improving the strategies for encoding and manipulating information. Two types of model influence and dominate the development of movement co-ordination: the closed- and open-loop models.

The closed- and open-loop models (e.g. Adams, 1971; Miller *et al.*, 1960) had their heydays in the 1960s and 1970s. In these models, feedback loops for error corrections or a feed-forward mechanism, respectively, were invoked for explaining the control and co-ordination of the motor behaviour, but were not often subjected to developmental questions. However, there are a few noticeable exceptions such as Bruner (1970) and Connolly (1970), who promoted closed-loop models. Development was considered as learning to sequence (or programme) the different parts of an action. For instance, when grasping a toy, the infant has to learn that (s)he should reach first. However, at that time, most developmental researchers were primarily concerned with constructing motor tests and gathering normative data (e.g. Cratty, 1970; Wickstrom, 1977; Williams, 1983). As a result most studies were descriptive and a theoretical framework to explain the origin of new motor behaviours was missing, which of course was not very stimulating for the study of motor development (Netelenbos and Koops, 1988; Wade, 1977).

4. The coupling of perception and action: a direct perception perspective

Gibson's (1979) ecological psychology approach to perception is also known as the direct perception perspective. The word 'direct' refers to the fact that objects, places and events in the environment can be perceived without the need for cognitive mediation to make perception meaningful, such as in the information-processing approach. Information in the environment is not static in time and space, but specifies events, places and objects. The child has to learn to pick up and select the appropriate information, not how to interpret or construct meaningful perception from stimuli. Therefore, whenever an infant or child has learned to (actively) pick up the information, (s)he perceives events and not some kind of discrete stimulus. This concept of information is closely related to the concept of affordances.

An affordance expresses the relation between perceiving and acting:

> The affordances of the environment are what it offers the animal, what it provides or furnishes, either for good or ill. The verb to afford is found in the dictionary, but the noun affordance is not. I have made it up. I mean by it something that refers to both the environment and the animal in a way that no existing term does. It implies the complementarity of the animal and the environment.
>
> (Gibson, 1979, p. 127)

Affordances relate to possibilities for action for an organism in a particular environment. Therefore, they relate to the perceiver's own potential action system. For example, for an actor who wants to climb stairs, the co-ordination pattern is specified by the ratio between the tread height (action space) and the actor's leg length (metric of the actor) (Warren, 1984). In more general terms, perceiving and acting are guided by body-scaled ratios, which should be similar over individual differences in body dimensions. Henceforth, developmental changes due to physical growth should not affect the perception of affordances; that is, during development children should remain tuned to similar body-scaled ratios without the need for new learning or reorganisation of the action system (Pufall and Dunbar, 1992; Van der Kamp, Savelsbergh and Davis, 1998).

Within this perspective, Van der Kamp *et al.* (1998) examined how children aged 5, 7 and 9 years reach, grasp and lift cardboard cubes of different sizes (ranging from 2.2 to 16.2 cm in diameter). Recordings were analysed and scored qualitatively for the percentage occurrence of one-handed grasps. The findings showed that the older the child, the higher the occurrence of one-handed grasps (37 per cent, 46 per cent, and 55 per cent for the 5-, 7- and 9-year-olds respectively). Moreover, the older the child, the larger the cubes that were predominantly taken with one hand. From a direct perception approach, it is hypothesised that the detected differences in grasping behaviour between the age groups are due to the increase of hand size with age. Therefore, the observed differences in prehension should disappear when hand size is taken into account. When hand size was scaled to cube size, differences in prehension between the three age groups disappeared and the shift from one-handed to two-handed grasping occurred at the same body-scale ratio between cube size and hand span for all three age groups. In sum, the children perceived the affordances for action.

According to E. Gibson (1988) affordances have to be discovered with the aid of the perceptual systems and exploratory behaviour. Michaels and Carello (1981) stress the active nature of the exploratory behaviour:

> Exploration (attention) is not an unconscious shifting-through and subsequent rejection of most inputs: It is directed control of what will be detected.
>
> (Michaels and Carello, 1981, p. 70)

In the eyes of these authors exploration is an active and directed process which reveals affordances, as illustrated by an experiment carried out by Karen Adolph and co-workers (Adolph *et al.*, 1993). In their study walkers and crawlers were encouraged to ascend and descend a sloping walkway of 10, 20, 30 and 40 degrees. The findings showed a relation between the exploratory activities and locomotion ability. For instance, on descending trials walkers switched from walking to sliding. Also they touched and hesitated most before descending 10- and 20-degree slopes and explored alternative means for descent by testing different sliding positions before leaving the platform. Crawlers hesitated most before descending 30- and 40-degree slopes and did not test alternative sliding positions. The experiment demonstrated the relation between infant locomotion capability, the perception of affordances (traversable by walking or not) and the exploratory activity.

The theory of direct perception offers insights into developmental perceptual–motor processes by studying learning in the context of development. What is learned is the detection of affordances; that is, what action possibilities the environment affords for the child. In this respect, learning to move and to co-ordinate one's actions involves learning to select the appropriate information sources. Moreover, this learning depends on the present action capabilities of the child. These action capabilities may improve by the maturation of the central nervous system, the sensitivity to certain information sources, the growth of body dimensions and the ability to couple information and movements. It is through the active and directed exploration of the environment with his/her own action system that the child learns to detect affordances, pick up the relevant information, and to couple the information to movements.

5. Dynamic systems approach to the development of co-ordination

Within the last decade, there has been an increase in empirical evidence that developmental processes are not smooth and monotonic, but can be characterised by phenomena such as discontinuities, transitions, instabilities, and regressions (Savelsbergh *et al.*, 1999; Van Geert, 1999; Van der Maas, 1993; Wimmers *et al.*, 1998). These phenomena are characteristic of non-linear dynamical processes. The aim of the dynamic systems approach is to characterise spatio-temporal and functional patterns of motor behaviour in terms of their stability properties by formalising the time-evolution of relevant variables into dynamical equations of motion. Stationary, stable states or patterns of activity, as well as abrupt transitions between different states accompanied by loss of stability (induced by changes in external conditions), have been successfully modelled in this way (Kelso, 1995).

The perspective portrays co-ordination as a process that constrains the potentially free variables of a system into a behavioural unit. A collective variable (order parameter) is the parameter that captures the observed behaviour (co-ordination pattern), while a control parameter is the parameter that leads the system through different co-ordination patterns. Within this approach, the behavioural pattern is regarded as a stable collective state attained by the system under certain constraints (boundary conditions) and informational settings (Zanone *et al.*, 1993). When the control parameter passes through a critical point, a co-ordination pattern that was stable becomes unstable, causing a sudden discrete transition to a qualitatively different, stable co-ordination pattern. Such a change appears without any prescription from outside but is acquired by the system itself, i.e. through self-organisation.

From this perspective the development of co-ordination is also seen as a complex, evolving dynamic process. Developmental systems are self-organising in that new behavioural forms emerge in a non-linear fashion at the macroscopic level (e.g. reaching) as a result of interactions between subsystems at more microscopic levels of organisation (e.g. between neurons or between muscles and joints). In this context, self-organisation is defined as the system's ability to acquire a new spatial, temporal or functional structure by itself (i.e. without any prescription of this structure from the outside). The ability of a system to organise itself is most salient when a qualitative change in order occurs. Such a transition is called a non-equilibrium phase transition.

Tools provided by a dynamic systems approach make it possible to detect qualitative changes (i.e. phase transitions) which are induced by quantitative changes in one or more control parameters. The control parameter is not the cause of the change, although its manipulation is instrumental in creating the new order (e.g. walking, reaching and grasping). It controls in the sense of leading the system through its respective states of equilibrium (that is, from one phase to the next); for instance, from reaching to reaching and grasping. A discontinuous phase transition involves an abrupt shift from one stable configuration of behaviour to another without stable intermediate states.

Developmental phases such as reaching, grasping, sitting, crawling etc. can be viewed as stable, preferred configurations of behaviour. When perturbed, the child (the 'system') will return to these configurations in due course; they act as 'attractors' and can be understood and modelled accordingly. During development new attractors will emerge and others will disappear. It may also be the case that the attractors are already present and that a shift from one attractor to another occurs.

Thus, co-ordinated actions such as reaching arise from complex processes of co-operation between subsystems and do not arise from a maturation of prescriptive devices that have been arbitrarily assigned to the system.

The goals of the dynamic systems perspective with respect to motor development are to identify the changes between milestones and search for the underlying mechanism. The significance of the approach is that it provides generally applicable concepts and tools to help gain insights into the trajectories of emerging new behaviours.

6. The constraints model and co-ordinative structure theory

The co-ordinative structure approach tackles the problem of mastering the large number of redundant degrees of freedom involved in a particular movement (Bernstein, 1967; Turvey, 1990). In order to reduce the number of degrees of freedom, task-specific musculo-skeletal organisations emerge from the underlying dynamics of the organism–environment system and lead to task-specific musculo-skeletal organisations or co-ordinative structures. These structures are guided by movement-produced information that is specific to those underlying dynamics (e.g. Kugler and Turvey, 1987; Savelsbergh and Van der Kamp, 1993). Kugler *et al.* (1982) proposed that the development of co-ordination is brought about by changes in the constraints imposed upon the organism–environment system.

Newell (1986) proposed three categories of constraints: organismic (e.g. the central nervous system), task (e.g. reaching with one hand) and environmental (e.g. the size of an object). These different constraints do not operate in isolation, but interact with each other, leading to a task-specific organisation of the co-ordination pattern. Thus co-ordination does not uniquely originate from the central nervous system, as argued by the traditional neuro-maturational theories, but emerges from an interaction between the three categories of constraints.

An experimental example is provided by Newell and co-workers (Newell *et al.*, 1989). In their study, infants of 4 to 8 months old were presented with four object sizes (1.25, 2.5, 2.54 and 8.5 cm in diameter). It was found that the grasping behaviour could be classified primarily by five grips, while 1,023 possible combinations of the ten fingers could be used. Probably, the relation between hand size and object size constrains the grip configuration. Similar observations regarding the constraining effect of velocity on action possibilities were made in a study by Von Hofsten (1983). He demonstrated that infants were able to predict the future location of a moving object. Eight-month-old babies, when presented with objects travelling in a horizontal arc at 60 cm/s, demonstrated considerable catching competence. Some of them even caught objects moving at 90 and 120 cm/s in a variety of positions in front of them. Von Hofsten suggested that the infants used a strategy consisting of an approach component and a tracking component. Both play a role in the control of the movement of the hand in relation to an object. Infants' perception of whether a catch was possible or not was constrained by the approach velocity, with no attempts being made when the object approached with a high velocity.

A necessary requirement in both the Newell *et al.* (1989) and the Von Hofsten (1983) studies was for the infants to detect the information specifying the size and velocity of the object. This information may differ depending on the availability of various sources. For instance, because young infants have no binocular vision until about 5 months, they are dependent on monocular information sources in perceiving object size. The improvement in reaching, grasping and catching during the first half year might therefore be related to the emergence of binocular vision that provides binocular information sources (e.g. disparity). As such, informational constraints (Kugler and Turvey, 1987; Van der Kamp *et al.*, 1996) might prove to be very important in the development of co-ordination.

More generally, the basic idea of the approach is that action-relevant information (the kinematic optical flow field) is generated by and used to control and co-ordinate muscular forces (kinetic force fields). The approach searches for lawful relations between action-relevant information and the generation of forces. These laws of control describe how the change in perceptual flow specifies the changes needed in the (muscular) forces in a way that is consistent with the laws of physics. However, what has remained unclear is how flow and forces are coupled. To answer this question, Kugler and Turvey (1987; Kugler 1986) proposed laws of control which express the lawful relationship between perception and action. Put another way, the laws of control involve the relationship between kinematic optic flow fields (perception) and the kinetics of force fields (movement). The following laws describe the relationships between flow and force:

| Law of ecological optics | $Flow = f(Force)$ |
| Laws of control | $Force = g(Flow)$ |

These general laws identify the parameters of movement in the (kinetic) force field that are uniquely specified by the information in the (kinematic) flow field and vice versa.

An example of such a lawful relation is that between the optic flow pattern and posture. The first experiments that examined the effect of visual information on posture used the 'moving room' paradigm, a room that can be moved above a stable floor (Lee and Lishman, 1974; Lishman and Lee, 1973). Subjects experienced self-motion while they were standing or sitting in the moving room. Lee and co-workers showed that vision has a proprioceptive function in maintaining postural stability.

The constraint-led or co-ordinative structure perspective examines the lawful relationship between information and actions. In a search for these laws, the manipulation of the different constraints will help to identify the laws. When a law is discovered, through a systematic manipulation of the different parameters in the equation the exact effect on the co-ordination pattern can be discovered and the control mechanism involved can be identified. A research strategy to discover such a law is to identify the optical informational constraints, to test the sensitivity for that particular variable, and to examine how the variable is used in the control and co-ordination of motor behaviour. Most of the developmental research in the last fifteen years has taken place within the paradigm of direct perception (e.g. Eppler and Adolph, 1996) and dynamic systems (Thelen and Smith, 1994), and as such has mainly been concerned with the concept of affordances and perceptual learning. With respect to the information used by children and the way this information is coupled to the motor system, much work needs to be done.

7. Structure of the book and topic of the chapters

The chapters presented in the book reflect the different approaches discussed in this introductory chapter. Although it is sometimes difficult to pin down which theoretical approach drives the authors' research, the majority of the chapters can be positioned within a combination of the direct perception and the constraint-led approaches (e.g. chapters 4, 5, 6, 12, 13 and 14). Other chapters use a different approach; for instance, chapter 9 uses an information-processing perspective, chapter 16 a dynamic systems approach, and a combination of dynamic systems and maturation theory is found in chapter 7. The fifteen chapters are divided into three major sections; ergonomics, health sciences, and sport. This division is based on the task at hand in combination with the population studied by the authors.

The ergonomics section starts with an introductory chapter by Jaap van Dieën and Idsart Kingsma. In the first part, the authors introduce the field of ergonomics with its basic aims and objectives. In their opinion, ergonomics deals with optimising the interactions of humans with artefacts in purposeful actions. The authors emphasise the importance of ergonomics for motor development, e.g. the design of artefacts that children interact with during play or activities of daily living. The chapter discusses examples with respect to lifting, which gives some insight into how the use of visual information in anticipatory control of movement develops. Such knowledge might in the future be useful for optimising the design of tools and toys.

In chapter 3 Jodie Plumert discusses the overestimation of children's physical abilities and the relationship with causes of childhood accidents. Despite concern over promoting children's safety, the causes of childhood accidents remain poorly understood. The chapter reviews research showing that children often overestimate their physical abilities and that overestimation of ability may be related to injury risk.

In chapter 4 Arenda te Velde and co-authors examine how road-crossing behaviour in young children develops, and evaluate different training programmes. To this end, training by means of verbal instructions, scale models, roadside judgements, pretend road crossing, and road crossing in real traffic environments are compared. Conflicting outcomes in children's road-crossing abilities at different ages are found, and the beneficial effects of training programmes appear less than one would hope for. The chapter concludes by stressing the need to examine children actually walking across the road both when determining children's ability and when training those abilities.

In chapter 5 Karl Rosengren and Gregory Braswell examine the learning of children's drawing and writing skills. These complex motor skills emerge in the second year of life and exhibit significant changes over the next decade. In their chapter, drawing and writing skills are discussed together because these skills are constrained by similar influences, involve the relatively sophisticated use of some sort of implement for leaving marks on a surface, and involve attempts to communicate information to other individuals. The chapter explores how both of these skills change over the course of learning.

From about one year of age toddlers learn to use a spoon for self-feeding at mealtimes. Newell (1986) argues that learning and development are induced by the changing interaction between the constraints upon action. Based on Newell's framework, chapter 6 by Dominique van Roon, John van der Kamp and Bert Steenbergen discusses the role of constraints on children's learning to use a spoon. The primary emphasis is on the role of task (i.e. the goal of the task, the implement, and non-physical rules) and organismic constraints (i.e. children with cerebral palsy). The chapter concludes with some guidelines for the ergonomic design of spoons for toddlers, and for disabled children and adults.

In the next section, health sciences, the movement co-ordination of different populations, like children with cerebral palsy, developmental movement difficulties and Down syndrome, is discussed. The section starts with the chapter of Motohide Miyahara and Koop Reynders (chapter 7) in which different theoretical perspectives (dynamic systems and neuronal group selection theory) are combined in order to shed new light on reflexes. This chapter also discusses the impact of theoretical transitions on clinical practice for children with movement disorders and conceptual issues from a philosophy of science framework.

In chapter 8, Helen Parker and Dawne Larkin provide an extensive overview on children with co-ordination and developmental movement difficulty. The authors provide a description of the movement difficulties and consequences in terms of psychological and social effects on the developing child. The motor abilities of these children, such as postural control, fitness, reaction speed, timing, and rhythm, are reviewed, in addition to clinical observations on the performance of the functional skills of running, jumping and landing, throwing and catching. The chapter finishes with a section dealing with intervention and the need for intensive physical education directed at specific learning outcomes.

Chapter 9 discusses the perceptual–motor behaviour of children with Down syndrome. Dominic Simon, Digby Elliott and Greg Anson highlight similarities and differences, both in relation to individuals with other developmental disabilities, and in relation to the wider population. Methodologies, evidence, and implications for a variety of findings are presented. The topics covered include movement preparation and perceptual–motor speed, the co-ordination and control of upper limb movements, and structuring practice to optimise motor learning. The authors also review a number of studies on sensory–motor integration and cerebral organisation in children and adults with Down syndrome. At the end of the chapter, consideration is given to whether people with Down syndrome should be considered to be at an earlier developmental stage than their age-matched peers, or to be developing in a qualitatively different and adaptive fashion.

In chapter 10 Bert Steenbergen and collaborators focus on bimanual co-ordination in children with hemiparetic cerebral palsy. First, the authors review research on bimanual upper limb co-ordination in adults and during development, particularly with respect to the temporal and spatial interactions that exist between both hands. It is apparent from this review that strong synchronisation tendencies exist between both hands in the temporal domain, and that they are even stronger during early childhood. Research on spatial interactions between both hands has identified the influence of two types of constraints: egocentric constraints that are defined relative to intrinsic body co-ordinates, and allocentric constraints that are defined relative to extrinsic space co-ordinates. The influence of both constraints on bimanual co-ordination is discussed. In the second part of the chapter, the influence of temporal and spatial constraints on bimanual co-ordination in individuals with hemiparetic cerebral palsy is reviewed. Features of unimanual movement co-ordination in these individuals are discussed. In bimanual tasks, these individuals display a strong tendency for temporal synchronisation. However, spatial interactions have hardly been a subject of study in this group. Therefore, in the third part of the chapter, the authors present preliminary results of a short-term learning experiment in which the role of allocentric and egocentric constraints on the spatial characteristics of drawing semi-circles is examined. The results suggest that the intact hemisphere is reorganised such that it is involved in the control of both the impaired side as well as the unimpaired side. Furthermore, both the allocentric and egocentric constraints have differential effects of the spatial characteristics of the semi-circles. Finally, Steenbergen and collaborators discuss the clinical implications of these findings, such as the necessity to train the unimpaired arm early in rehabilitation.

Whether a young child with cerebral palsy will acquire independent locomotion is a question that quickly arises after the diagnosis has been made. In chapter 11 Annick Ledebt presents studies that have tried to find, during the period of infancy, early predictors that may foresee the ability to walk. When children with cerebral palsy do acquire locomotion it often deviates from normal walking. Gait abnormalities that occur are a combination of primary consequences imposed by the brain damage, and of secondary deviations which result from adaptations to circumvent the primary deficits. Gait analysis might help to disentangle primary consequences and adaptations. This is illustrated by studies on toe walking, one of the most frequent gait deviations in those children.

The sport section starts with a chapter by Savelsbergh and co-workers on the development of interceptive action. The purpose of chapter 12 is to elaborate upon the role of visual information in the co-ordination and control of the development of catching, and focuses on a theoretical perspective based on the work of Gibson (1979), Bernstein (1967) and Newell (1986); that is, constraints on the learning and development of complex motor skills. The role of informational constraints in the control of simple one-handed catching in adults and children is discussed.

The chapter concludes with a model of the different stages in the learning and development of information–movement couplings.

Chapter 13 by Annieck Ricken and co-authors expands on the model presented in chapter 12, to understand and describe the organisation of movement co-ordination of children without and with spastic hemiplegia cerebral palsy during interceptive actions. The authors discuss how movement co-ordination emerges from the multiple degrees of freedom of the biomechanical movement system and the perceptual system and, more importantly, the interaction between them in the form of information–movement couplings.

Throwing behaviour is the topic of chapter 14 by Allen Burton and Richard Rodgerson. The authors take a broad, functionalist approach to the development of throwing behaviour. It is their opinion that throwing can be viewed as the extension of motor behaviour beyond the body and, as such, is most often done with purpose. Such purpose is constrained not only by the task itself but also by person (organismic) and environmental constraints. The authors examine the development of throwing behaviour through the combined perspectives of evolutionary and dynamic systems theory. Burton and Rodgerson begin by asking 'why children throw' and emphasise the links between a wide variety of games and sports and throwing, between throwing and hunting, and ultimately between hunting and evolved anatomy. In their review of the developmental research, the material is organised with an eye toward the functional outcome of accuracy as a dependent variable and the relationship between accuracy and velocity in the requirements of the task. They examine research on changes in throwing outcomes across the elementary-school years, followed by a section in which they consider the research related to changes in throwing form. In addition, further research along two fronts is suggested. First, the importance of observational research of throwing behaviour at its earliest inception during infancy and toddlerhood is emphasised. Second, future experimental research should consider the dynamic relationships between accuracy, velocity and form in the production of functional throwing.

In chapter 15, Mark Scott, Mark Williams and Rob Horn discuss kicking as a common feature of many sports. The authors argue that it is important to understand how the mature kicking action is acquired. Therefore, they provide an overview of our current understanding of how various kicking techniques are acquired and co-ordinated in young performers. In addition, recommendations for future research are highlighted and practical applications identified.

The aim of the final chapter 16 by Jill Whitall is not simply to describe the development of locomotor co-ordination and control across the ages of 4 to 12 years, but rather to apply our knowledge of locomotor co-ordination and control to illustrate current principles of (motor) development. These principles are described, primarily, through a dynamic systems approach. Specifically, childhood is viewed as the time to development skilfulness; in this case, locomotor skilfulness. Using a dynamic systems approach, skilfulness is composed of pattern (co-ordination) and adaptation (control), of which, it is argued, only the former has been studied in detail. The concept of constraints is presented and purported to produce sequences of well-documented species-typical co-ordination changes that are similar between locomotor skills yet are neither universal nor mandatory. Progression to advanced locomotor co-ordination states involves change in control (or rate-limiting) parameters, a process that is not well understood but may be related to gaining postural control and/or bilateral co-ordination. Furthermore, it is argued that the progression of locomotor control, itself, has barely been studied and certainly the interaction with co-ordination is unclear. It is argued that it is essential to incorporate principles and knowledge from perception–action and cognitive/information-processing theories to understanding locomotor control and ultimately locomotor skilfulness.

The chapters of this book form a rich variation on a vibrant and expanding field of study; that is, the development of movement co-ordination in children. The authors provide theoretical insights in combination with implications for practical application.

References

Adams, J.A. (1971) A closed-loop theory of motor learning. *Journal of Motor Behavior*, 3, 111–49.

Adolph, K.E., Eppler, M.A. and Gibson, E.J. (1993) Crawling versus walking infants' perception of affordances for locomotion over sloping surfaces. *Child Development*, 64, 1158–74.

Bernstein, N. (1967) *The Coordination and Regulation of Movement*. New York: Pergamon Press.

Bruner, J. (1970) The growth and structure of skill. In K.J. Connolly (ed.), *Mechanisms of Motor Skill Development*. London: Academic Press.

Connolly, K.J. (1970) Skill development: problems and plans. In K.J. Connolly (ed.), *Mechanisms of Motor Skill Development* (pp. 3–21). London: Academic Press.

Cratty, B.J. (1970) *Perceptual and motor development in infants and children*. London: Macmillan.

Eppler, M.A. and Adolph, K.E. (1996) Towards an ecological approach to perceptual learning and development: commentary on Michaels and Beek. *Ecological Psychology*, 8, 353–5.

Gesell, A. and Amatruda, C.S. (1945) *The Embryology of Behavior*. New York: Harper.

Gibson, E.J. (1988) Exploratory behavior in the development of perceiving, acting, and the acquiring of knowledge. In M.R. Rosenzweig and L.W. Porter (eds), *Annual Review of Psychology* (pp. 1–41). Palo Alto, CA: Annual Review, Inc.

Gibson, J.J. (1979) *The Ecological Approach to Visual Perception*. Boston: Houghton-Mifflin.

Kelso, J.A.S. (1995) *Dynamic Patterns. The Self-organization of Brain and Behavior*. Cambridge: MIT Press.

Kugler, P.N. (1986) A morphological perspective on the origin and evolution of movement patterns. In M.G. Wade and H.T.A. Whiting (eds), *Motor Development in Children: Aspects of Coordination and Control* (pp. 459–525). Dordrecht: Martinus Nijhoff.

Kugler, P.N. and Turvey, M.T. (1987) *Information, Natural Law, and the Self-assembly of Rhythmic Movements*. Hillsdale, NJ: Erlbaum.

Kugler, P.N., Kelso, J.A.S. and Turvey, M.T. (1982) On the control and coordination of naturally developing systems. In J.A.S. Kelso and J.E. Clark (eds), *The Development of Movement Control and Coordination* (pp. 5–78). New York: Wiley.

Lee, D.N. and Lishman, J.R. (1974) Visual proprioceptive control of stance. *Journal of Human Movement Studies*, 1, 87–95.

Lishman, J.R. and Lee, D.N. (1973) The autonomy of visual kinaesthesis. *Perception*, 2, 287–94.

McGraw, M. (1943) *The Neuromuscular Maturation of the Human Infant*. New York: Hafner.

Michaels, C.F. and Carello, C.C. (1981) *Direct Perception*. Englewood Cliffs, NJ: Prentice Hall.

Miller, G.A., Galanter, E. and Pribram, K.H. (1960) *Plans and the Structure of Behavior*. New York: Holt, Rinehart and Winston.

Netelenbos, J.B. and Koops, W. (1988) De ontwikkeling van de motoriek. In W. Koops and J.J. van der Werff (eds), *Overzicht van de Empirische Ontwikkelingspsychologie* 2 (pp. 13–41). Groningen: Wolters Noordhoff.

Newell, K.M. (1986) Constraints on the development of coordination. In M. Wade and H.T.A. Whiting (eds), *Motor Development in Children: Aspects of Coordination and Control* (pp. 341–60). Dordrecht: Martinus Nijhoff.

Newell, K.M., Scully, D.M., McDonald, P.V. and Baillargeon, R. (1989) Task constraints and infant grip configurations. *Developmental Psychobiology*, 22, 817–32.

Peiper, A. (1963) *Cerebral Function in Infancy and Childhood*. New York: Consultants Bureau.

Pufall, P.B. and Dunbar, C. (1992) Perceiving whether or not the world affords stepping onto and over: a developmental study. *Ecological Psychology*, 4, 17–38.

Savelsbergh, G.J.P., Van der Maas, H. and Van Geert, P.C.L. (1999) *Non-linear Analyses of Developmental Processes*. Elsevier: Amsterdam.

Savelsbergh, G.J.P. and Van der Kamp, J. (1993) The development of infants reaching, grasping, catching and posture: a natural physical approach. In G.J.P. Savelsbergh (ed.), *The Development of Coordination in Infancy* (pp. 289–317). Amsterdam: North-Holland.

Thelen, E. and Smith, L.B. (1994) *A Dynamic Systems Approach to the Development of Cognition and Action*. Cambridge, MA: MIT Press.

Turvey, M.T. (1990) Coordination. *American Psychologist*, 45, 938–53.

Van der Kamp, J., Savelsbergh, G.J.P. and Davis, W.E. (1998) Body-scaled ratio as control parameter for prehension in 5 to 9 year old children. *Developmental Psychobiology*, 33, 351–61.

Van der Kamp, J., Vereijken, B. and Savelsbergh, G.J.P. (1996) Physical and informational constraints in the cooridnation and control of human movements. *Corpus, Psyche et Societas*, 3, 102–18.

Van der Maas, H.L.J. (1993) *Catastrophe Analysis of Stepwise Cognitive Development*. Academic thesis, University of Amsterdam.

Van Geert, P.C.L. (1999) *Dynamic Systems of Development. Change Between Complexity and Chaos*. New York: Harvest Wheatsheaf.

Von Hofsten, C. (1983) Catching skills in infancy. *Journal of Experimental Psychology: Human Perception and Performance*, 9, 75–85.

Wade, M.G. (1977) Developmental motor learning. In L.S. Keogh and R. Hutton (eds), *Exercise and Sport Sciences Reviews*. Santa Barbara: Journal Publishing Affiliates.

14   *Savelsbergh, Davids, van der Kamp and Bennett*

Warren, W.H. (1984) Perceiving affordances: visual guidance of stair climbing. *Journal of Experimental Psychology: Human Perception and Performance*, 10, 683–703.

Wickstrom, R.L. (1977) *Fundamental Motor Patterns*. Philadelphia: Lea and Febiger.

Williams, H.G. (1983) *Perceptual and Motor Development*. Englewood Cliffs, NJ: Prentice Hall.

Wimmers, R.H., Savelsbergh, G.J.P., Beek, P.J. and Hopkins, B. (1998) Evidence for a phase transition in the developmental of prehension. *Developmental Psychobiology*, 16, 45–63.

Zanone, P.G., Kelso, J.A.S. and Jeka, J.J. (1993) Concepts and methods for a dynamical approach to behavioral coordination and change. In G.J.P Savelsbergh (ed.), *The Development of Coordination in Infancy* (pp. 89–136). Amsterdam: North-Holland.

Part I
Ergonomics

2 Motor development and ergonomics

Lifting objects as a window on motor control in children

Jaap H. van Dieën and Idsart Kingma

1. Introduction

The present chapter is divided in two parts. The first part introduces the field of ergonomics with its basic aims and objectives and, as such, serves as an introduction to this section of the book where motor co-ordination is discussed within the context of ergonomics. Ergonomics deals with optimising the interactions of humans with artefacts in purposeful actions. On the one hand, ergonomics can be of importance for motor development, when considering the design of artefacts that children interact with during play or activities of daily living. On the other hand, an ergonomic view on motor development (i.e. focusing on interactions with objects, in contrast, for example, to locomotion) can reveal aspects of motor development that otherwise will not be noted. To illustrate this, the development of the co-ordination of lifting will be reviewed. Lifting is probably the most studied motor task in the ergonomics literature. Lifting requires tuning muscle forces produced to the inertial properties of the object to be handled. These properties are, however, unknown to the subject before the object has actually been lifted. Therefore, the control of lifting tasks relies on estimates of these inertial properties based on, for instance, visual information. This example gives some insight into how the use of, especially, visual information in the anticipatory control of movement develops. Such knowledge might in the future be useful for optimising the design of, for instance, tools and toys.

2. Ergonomics: aims and objectives

In a recent ISO document, ergonomics was defined as the discipline 'that produces and integrates knowledge from the human sciences to match jobs, products, and environments to the physical and mental abilities and limitations of people'. In doing so it seeks to safeguard safety, health and well being whilst optimising efficiency and performance (ISO, 1999). An alternative definition given by Wilson (2000) states that 'Ergonomics is the theoretical and fundamental understanding of human behaviour and performance in purposeful interacting socio-technical systems, and the application of that understanding to the design of interactions in the context of real settings'. These definitions stress different aspects of ergonomics and are, in our view, partially conflicting and partially complementary.

Both definitions hint at the traditional application domain of ergonomics, i.e. work tasks. However, ergonomics has never limited itself exclusively to this domain, nor can human behaviour in work tasks, whether mental or physical, be considered in any fundamental way different from that in any other purposeful human activity.

Neither of the two definitions explicitly delineates the type of environments dealt with. Nevertheless, ergonomics clearly deals with man-made environments and objects. Indeed, in the application this is evident since optimal design of the environment is the central goal.

Both definitions imply that ergonomics is a basic science as well as an applied science, though the latter is more explicit in this respect. When considering ergonomics as a basic science, ISO defines ergonomics not as an independent science but rather as an interdisciplinary field of study encompassing contributions from human sciences such as psychology, physiology, and biomechanics. Wilson defines ergonomics explicitly as an independent science focusing on the interactions of humans with the environment in which they operate. In our view, however, declaring the interaction rather then the human him- or herself as the object of study, does not clearly separate ergonomics from other human sciences. For example, in sensory psychology and sensory physiology human environment interactions are central. Hence while the interactions of humans with their environments in the context of a task are the central issue in ergonomics, this does not set ergonomics apart from other human sciences. In this respect, we consider ergonomics not to be a science in its own right, in line with the ISO definition. Ergonomics then defines a field of study partially shared by several human sciences. Its main scientific aims are derived from the field of application, where optimisation through the design of interactions with respect to performance, safety, and health of the human is central. Thus ergonomics as an interdisciplinary field of study integrates knowledge from the human sciences about the interactions of humans with man-made environments, which is pertinent to questions related to health, safety and performance. Ergonomics as an applied science comprises a contribution to the design of such interactions, maximising the capabilities, minimising the limitations and trying to satisfy the needs and desires of humans in the designed environment.

3. Ergonomic issues in motor development

Like adults, children perform tasks within a man-made and often purposefully designed environment. These interactions will affect motor development directly as well as indirectly. Directly, these interactions offer possibilities to practice an important class of motor tasks, such as the manipulation of external objects. Indirectly, these interactions may affect motor development through their effects on health and safety. The nature of these interactions is determined by the stage of the development of the child, in terms of cognition, motor control and anthropometry. If design is to be optimised for children, a thorough knowledge of the mental and physical capabilities of children at the various stages of development is required. In the ergonomics literature there has only been limited attention for these issues.

Optimisation with respect to health effects has been addressed in a number of studies on design for children, most notably the design of school furniture. The criteria for good design in these cases are qualitatively similar to those for adults. In designing school furniture, the prevention of low back pain, which appears to be widely prevalent already in 14-year-olds (Duggleby and Kumar, 1997; Taimela *et al.*, 1997), is usually a specific aim (Jeong and Park, 1990; Prado-Leon *et al.*, 2001) as is the case in studies on office furniture for adults (e.g. Van Dieën *et al.*, 2001). However, quantitatively the criteria will obviously differ. Standards for furniture design need to be set in relation to children's anthropmometry, and simple down-scaling of furniture designed for adults does not suffice (Jeong and Park, 1990; Prado-Leon *et al.*, 2001; Steenbekkers and Molenbroek, 1990). In the design and use of computer equipment, qualitatively similar considerations again apply for children and adults (Macgregor, 2000; Straker *et al.*, 2000). Nevertheless, the quantitative differences of the design criteria can be very substantial, as is obvious for furniture.

When related to health optimisation, criteria are again similar in a qualitative way for adults and children. The quantitative difference in the criteria to be set is not always obvious. Hu *et al.* (1993) analysed injuries that had occurred at home in over 1,500 children. Most injuries occurred in an environment that in all its aspects did appear safe to the parents. The authors suggest that parents fail to identify hazards to their children, because this requires evaluation in the context of the children's psychological and motor development. Thus an environment that is safe for an individual with adult psychological and motor capabilities may be unsafe for a child. Sometimes this is obviously so, but often hazards stemming from a mismatch between the designed environment and the capabilities of the child may be covert even for very cautious parents.

Performance criteria may be relevant for children when considering purposeful action. Of course, children also perform goal-directed tasks, where design optimisation may be aimed at improving performance. For example, the design of school furniture has been shown to affect learning behaviour (Knight and Noyes, 1999; Neill, 1982) and may affect learning performance. Similarly, the design of a pen may affect handwriting and the design of a spoon may facilitate eating (chapter 6 by Van Roon, Van der Kamp and Steenbergen). Such optimisation may be called for especially where impaired physical capabilities can be compensated for by design aimed at improving performance. However, qualitatively different criteria for design often hold when considering children instead of adults. This difference is directly related to the task goal. In the usual context of ergonomics (i.e. working life), the goal is producing something, whereas in children it is often performing the task itself. When considering play, performance criteria would not hold. A valid criterion could be to promote physical activity and exploration and thus to support motor development. Many ergonomic studies have dealt with redesigning work tasks such that a lower level of physical exertion is required, allowing higher productivity. In contrast, where children are concerned, a design that is challenging the child to become physically active would often be preferable. For example, electrically driven carts may be considered ergonomically sound when used for transporting goods and people in warehouses. From the point of view of the physical and motor development of a child, however, replacing a bicycle by an electrically driven cart is evidently not a sound measure. Stratton (2000) describes an interesting example of a study in which physical activity of children was promoted through the design of the environment. Fluorescent markings applied on the pavement of a playground were shown to increase the time spent on physically exerting activities in 5- to 7-year-olds. The concomitant increase in heart rate, which in many ergonomic studies would be interpreted as a negative outcome, was in this case considered a positive outcome. In similar vein, Yamada (1998), interpreted EEG changes and eye blink inhibition, which are usually interpreted as negative signs of increased mental load, as positive indications of the attractiveness of a computer game.

As stated above, ergonomics applications for children would require adequate knowledge of the capabilities of children. Hence the study of motor development is of relevance to ergonomics. Questions on motor development of interest for ergonomics should focus on interactions of children with environments, or specific objects in the environment such as tools or toys. Handling tools or navigating in an environment requires the integration of information obtained about external objects in the control of the movements to be performed. The most important source of information is the visual system. In many instances the information obtained about the external objects is incomplete, noisy, or otherwise inexact. Nevertheless, when anticipatory control is required, such as when picking up objects or when moving fast through a restricted space, adequate matching of the muscle forces produced to the properties of the environment is crucial. It can be expected that studying such tasks will, in view of these demands, yield unique information on motor development and, in fact, many every day actions comprise this class of movements. Below we will briefly review the literature to provide two examples of the development of the use of visual and haptic information in the control of movements.

4. Motor control of lifting in children

When a child uses a toy or a tool, this action generally starts with picking up the object. It is not evident that picking up an object occurs in a smooth, well co-ordinated way without dropping the object. Smoothly picking up the object requires adequate application of grip forces (i.e. forces to prevent slipping of the object) and load forces (i.e. vertical forces to lift the object). Information concerning the weight of the object, the slipperiness of its surface, and the fragility of the object are needed to scale these forces accurately. The information needs to be taken into account prior to the lifting movement in order to scale force during the loading phase (i.e. the period during which force is exerted on the object before it leaves the support surface). The problem is that most information becomes manifest only after the loading phase. Therefore, it is unavailable at the instant when grip and load forces are to be applied.

When adults do not know the precise weight of an object, but do know its possible range, some of them apply a 'target strategy', meaning that they scale their load and grip forces to an object weight in the middle of the range that they expect to be possible. This was found in precision grip lifting (Gordon *et al.*, 1991a) as well as in whole body lifting tasks (de Looze *et al.*, 2000). Others apply a 'probing strategy', meaning that they increase their load and grip force stepwise until the object is lifted (Gordon *et al.*, 1991a). For novel, unusually dense objects, adults primarily scale their forces for a lower weight, but they learn to scale their forces for the actual weight within a few lifting movements (Gordon *et al.*, 1993). For scaling of forces, adults use not only experienced weight from previous lifts, but also haptically (Gordon *et al.*, 1991a) as well as visually (Gordon *et al.*, 1991b) acquired size information, apparent fragility information (Savelsbergh *et al.*, 1996) and information about the type of material (Ellis and Lederman, 1999). Most likely, other aspects from daily life related to the forces required to manipulate an object are also taken into account. Some of these aspects might be apparent roughness, shape, etc.

Children may learn to use some of this information for force scaling quite early, whereas other information is only used in later years. What follows is an overview of the current knowledge about the development of the scaling of grip and load forces in children. This knowledge is important for understanding motor development and may potentially contribute to optimising the design of tools and toys used by children.

Learning to co-ordinate load and grip forces

In adults, load forces and grip forces are tightly coupled, in that when during cyclic or point-to-point movements the load force changes to accelerate or decelerate an object, the grip force changes in phase (Flanagan *et al.*, 1993). Even when the arm joints do not move and the acceleration is caused by jumping while holding an object, or when the grip is inverted (the finger and thumb have to be pushed apart to hold an object), this tight coupling between load and grip forces persists. This suggests a feedforward coupling between load and grip forces. In contrast, small children lift an object using mainly a feedback strategy, as evidenced by a sequential rise of grip and load force and a stepwise increase of load force (Forssberg *et al.*, 1991). From two years on, grip and load forces start to be generated in parallel, and single-peaked force rate profiles begin to occur. This is thought to reflect a gradual transition from feedback to feedforward control (Forssberg *et al.*, 1991).

Not only does the co-ordination between load and grip forces take several years to develop, but so does the optimal scaling of these forces themselves. Force and movement patterns are much more variable in young children (Forssberg *et al.*, 1995). Furthermore, grip forces are relatively high in young children: a 150 per cent safety margin was found in 1- to 2-year-old children against a 40 per cent safety margin in adults. This safety margin is defined as the actual grip force in excess of the grip forces that is precisely needed to prevent slipping of the object. At 5 years of age differences in safety margin between children and adults have disappeared (Forssberg *et al.*, 1995). The large grip forces in young children are functional since those children still have a large variability in grip force. Therefore, a large safety margin may be needed. In fact, parents allowing small children help to set the table may be aware that this safety margin is at times insufficient. With increasing age, the variability in grip forces decreases and the safety margin decreases in parallel (Forssberg *et al.*, 1995). The grip force required to prevent the slipping of an object depends not only on the weight and acceleration of the object, but also on the texture of the grip surface. Small children adapt grip forces to the surface friction of an object after a number of lifts. However, they do not take full account of surface friction, since their grip safety margin is larger when handling objects with rough surfaces, as compared to smooth surfaces (Forssberg *et al.*, 1995). In addition, they appear not to be able to memorise what they have learned over a few trials, since random changes between surfaces cause surface effects to disappear completely. After the age of 3, children start to respond to surface texture differences in random trials, but only later during the lifting movement. Initial, and thus really anticipated, differences are only seen from 12 to 13 years onward (Forssberg *et al.*, 1995). Still, the anticipation in this group is not yet the same as in adults. The influence of a previous lift remains over the whole lift in 12- to 13-year-old children, whereas it is restricted to the first 200 ms in adults.

Learning to use weight information from previous lifts

When objects of equal appearance but different weight are lifted several times, the smallest children do not seem to anticipate on the basis of previous lifts (Forssberg *et al.*, 1992). For heavier objects, they simply prolong the duration of the loading phase until the force is sufficient to lift the object. However, some children between 1 and 2 years already do use information from previous lifts, as evidenced by higher peak force rates when lifting heavier objects. Control over the acceleration of the objects, comparable to adults, is achieved at 6 to 8 years and smooth adult-like force profiles including mature anticipation is found at 8 to 11 years of age (Forssberg *et al.*, 1992). In a more difficult task, with random variation of the order of weights, again some influence of the previous lift is already seen in 1- to 2-year-old children. This influence gradually increases with age up to 11 to 15 years (Forssberg *et al.*, 1992).

Learning to use size information

Preparation for grasping by scaling hand aperture to object size develops quite early, mainly in the first year (Forssberg *et al.*, 1992). However, during the grasping phase there is continuous visible information, and children do not have to rely on sensori-motor memory formed prior to the movement. In contrast, anticipatory scaling of load and grip forces in response to object size changes requires memory representation of the relation between size and weight. It can thus be expected that the ability to use size information for force scaling develops later and more slowly, as compared to the scaling of hand aperture.

When the size and weight of an object change in parallel, participants can theoretically predict the required force for the next weight. Gachoud and co-workers (Gachoud *et al.*, 1983) compared kinematics and EMG patterns between adults and 6- to 9-year-old children in a simple mono-articular lifting task, using a series of objects with a parallel increase of volume and weight. They showed that 6- to 9-year-old children, like adults, were able to compensate lifting forces for weight increase, such that the kinematic pattern was relatively unaffected by weight increase. However, adults lifted objects using only agonist muscles and compensated for weight increase by increasing agonistic muscle force. In contrast, 6- to 9-year-old children used both agonist and antagonist muscles, and compensated for weight increase by decreasing antagonistic muscle force. This shows that in a certain stage of motor development overt kinematics can have a mature appearance, but the underlying motor commands do not necessarily have to be as efficient as in adults. Gachoud *et al.* (1983) concluded that children up to 9 years of age still lack a trustworthy representation of size/weight co-variation, and therefore apply a standard lifting force and a reactive breaking force by antagonists. However, the absence of a primary (anticipated) response to size changes in children up to 6 to 9 years of age is not corroborated by more recent experiments, as will be shown below. Possibly, the findings of Gachoud *et al.* (1983) must be attributed to the restricted way of lifting applied in that study.

In lifting two objects of equal weight but different volume, Gordon *et al.* (1992) showed that children from 2½ years of age start scaling load forces and grip forces in response to a change of object size. In fact, 3- to 7-year-old children responded more strongly and consistently to a change in object size than adults did. The children often applied a much larger force in lifting the large box, resulting in a 50 per cent overshoot of the peak acceleration of the object. The majority of adults did show a load force overshoot, but those overshoots were generally small and did not reach significance.

Development of the size–weight illusion

The overshoot in load forces when a large object is lifted in comparison to a small object of equal weight has been related to the so-called size–weight illusion (Davis and Roberts, 1976; Gordon *et al.*, 1991c; Granit, 1972). This illusion, first described by Charpentier (1891), means that participants, after lifting a small and a large object of equal weight, report the large box to feel lighter. The leading hypothesis is that the illusion stems from a mismatch between expected and actual feedback related to object weight (Flanagan and Beltzner, 2000). The idea is that subjects (unconsciously) apply a larger load force to the larger object because they expect it to be heavier. Subsequently, the larger load force causes an unanticipated larger acceleration of the large object, causing it to feel lighter. In some recent publications the direct connection between load force overshoot and the size–weight illusion has been disputed, because the illusion is more consistent than the force overshoot (Mon-Williams and Murray, 2000), and the force overshoot disappears after a number of lifts, whereas the illusion does not (Flanagan and Beltzner, 2000).

Children of 6 to 7 years of age were reported to experience the size–weight illusion as well (Gordon *et al.*, 1992). Considering the fact that their force overshoot is much larger compared to adults, the sensory mismatch hypothesis would predict that the illusion would also be larger in 6- to 7-year-old children compared to adults. To date, no data are available to verify (or falsify) this prediction.

It should be noted that the size of an object is not the only property that has been related to weight illusion. Its material appearance (e.g. wood or metal look) can also cause a weight illusion (Ellis and Lederman, 1999). Furthermore, the load force is not the only force that has been used to explain the weight illusion. In precision grip experiments, larger objects are lifted not only with a larger load force, but also with a larger grip force (e.g. Gordon *et al.*, 1991c). This grip force can be manipulated separately from load force, since it increases when the grip surface is more slippery. Flanagan *et al.* (1995) used objects of equal weight and size (small film canisters filled with loads), but differing in surface. One object was covered with silk, the other with sandpaper. Participants judged objects covered with silk to be heavier. This was not an effect of the surface per se, because it disappeared when the participants lifted the film canisters with the thumb below the object instead of with the thumb and index finger on both sides. With the thumb below, no additional grip force is needed for the sandpaper object compared to the silk object.

Since children have a weaker response to surface changes with respect to their applied grip force (Forssberg *et al.*, 1995), it might be anticipated (but remains to be proven) that children show a weaker surface–weight illusion as compared to adults. This contrasts with the effect of size, which we predicted to be stronger in children compared to adults.

Learning to respond to perturbations

Successfully lifting and manipulating an object requires the ability to respond quickly and with adequate forces to sudden perturbations. In daily life this occurs, for instance, when an object hits something or when a part falls from the object. When perturbations were applied by the (experimenter-induced) dropping of weights in a hand-held object, 2-year-old children already responded with an increase of grip forces (Eliasson *et al.*, 1995). However, up to 5 years of age the response was delayed in comparison to adults. Up to 10 years of age the amplitude of the grip response was reduced. Therefore, it appears that mature responses to external perturbations are not yet fully developed at 10 years of age (Eliasson *et al.*, 1995).

In self-imposed perturbations (by dropping weights), mature responses appear to develop slightly earlier. The timing of responses was incorrect in children up to 5 years of age. The magnitude of responses was reduced in comparison with adults up to 7 years. At 9 to 10 years of age, both the timing and the magnitude of grip responses to self-imposed perturbations were at an adult level.

5. Children and ergonomics

The review of the development of the control of lifting should make clear that it is to be expected that children drop objects lifted or carried more often than adults do. From an ergonomics perspective one might, on the basis of performance criteria, consider designing objects like glasses and beakers to be used by children with a non-slippery surface, to minimise the risk that children will drop them and spill the contents. However, when designing toys, the motor development criterion should prevail, and a better option would be to design toys such that children experience handling objects with rough as well as slippery surfaces.

The work on the development of lifting illustrates that children handle objects in a different way, and knowledge of these differences might be required in designing for children. However, it also illustrates that there still is a wide gap between basic science efforts in studying motor development on one hand and useful ergonomics applications of such knowledge on the other hand. This can be further illustrated by a second example.

There is abundant literature on the estimation of the time to contact with a moving object, and the development of such estimates has also been studied (see chapter 12 by Savelsbergh, Rosengren, Van der Kamp and Verheul). Time-to-contact estimates form the basis for interceptive actions, e.g. catching a ball, but they are also important when crossing a street. In this case, these estimates will be used in deciding whether or not to cross in front of an oncoming vehicle. It has been shown that adults integrate velocity and distance information about an oncoming vehicle to estimate its arrival time. The estimates made by children up to 12 years clearly differ from those in adults. Importantly, the underestimates they make are larger (Hoffmann *et al.*, 1980), which causes an increased risk. Furthermore, they have been shown to use distance information only up to the age of 7 to 8 years of age (Hoffmann, 1994; Connelly *et al.*, 1998; see also chapter 4 by Te Velde, Van der Kamp and Savelsbergh). Thereafter, velocity information is used, although at 9 to 10 years the integration of information appears incomplete and velocity information is used predominantly (Hoffmann, 1994). From an ergonomics perspective, generalising these results to a real-life context is an important issue. Unfortunately, the ecological validity of these laboratory-based studies can be questioned, since there are strong arguments to assume, for instance, that judgements that a road could be crossed differ from judgements actually to cross a road (Ebbessen *et al.*, 1977). Actually, it turns out that children opt for larger safety margins when crossing than adults (Lee *et al.*,1984; Connelly *et al.*, 1998), which could compensate for their underestimates of arrival times. Furthermore, the visual environment (e.g. distracting information) could strongly affect judgements and these effects may differ between children and adults. Finally, in spite of the clear relevance of this problem, we are not aware of any studies in which, for instance, the effect of the design of a pedestrian crossing on children's judgements is investigated. This type of study would be necessary to bridge the gap between, in this case, perceptual psychology and ergonomics.

In our view there are clear areas of application of ergonomics in relation to design for children. Such applications can promote the health and safety of children, optimise performance in some cases and support motor development in other cases. As the above examples illustrate, knowledge of children's development is a prerequisite for the adequate application of ergonomics in these areas. Ergonomists and basic scientists working in these areas need to communicate more in order to achieve these goals.

References

Charpentier, A. (1891) Analyse experimentale de quelques elements de la sensation de poids [Experimental study of some aspects of weight perception]. *Archives de Physiologie Normales et Pathologiques*, 3, 122–35.

Connelly, M.L., Conaglen, H.M., Parsonon, B.S. and Isler, R.B. (1998) Child pedestrians' crossing gap thresholds. *Accident Analysis and Prevention*, 30, 443–53.

Davis, C.M. and Roberts, W. (1976) Lifting movements in the size-weight illusion. *Perception and Psychophysics*, 20, 33–6.

De Looze, M.P., Boeken-Kruger, M.C., Steenhuizen, S., Baten, C.T., Kingma, I. and Van Dieën, J.H. (2000) Trunk muscle activation and low back loading in lifting in the absence of load knowledge. *Ergonomics*, 43, 333–44.

Duggleby, T., and Kumar, S. (1997) Epidemiology of juvenile low back pain: a review. *Disability and Rehabilitation*, 19, 505–12.

Ebbessen, E.B., Parker, S. and Konecni, V.J. (1977) Laboratory and field analyses of decision involving risk. *Journal of Experimental Psychology: Human Perception and Performance*, 3, 576–89.

Eliasson, A.C., Forssberg, H., Ikuta, K., Apel, I., Westling, G. and Johansson, R. (1995) Development of human precision grip. V. Anticipatory and triggered grip actions during sudden loading. *Experimental Brain Research*, 106, 425–33.

Ellis, R.R. and Lederman, S.J. (1999) The material–weight illusion revisited. *Perception and Psychophysics*, 61, 1564–76.

Flanagan, J.R. and Beltzner, M.A. (2000) Independence of perceptual and sensorimotor predictions in the size–weight illusion. *Nature Neuroscience*, 3, 737–41.

Flanagan, J.R., Tresilian, J. and Wing, A.M. (1993) Coupling of grip force and load force during arm movements with grasped objects. *Neuroscience Letters*, 152, 53–6.

Flanagan, J.R., Wing, A.M., Allison, S. and Spenceley, A. (1995) Effects of surface texture on weight perception when lifting objects with a precision grip. *Perception and Psychophysics*, 57, 282–90.

Forssberg, H., Eliasson, A.C., Kinoshita, H., Johansson, R.S. and Westling, G. (1991) Development of human precision grip I. Basic coordination of force. *Experimental Brain Research*, 85, 451–7.

Forssberg, H., Eliasson, A.C., Kinoshita, H., Westling, G. and Johansson, R.S. (1995) Development of human precision grip. IV. Tactile adaptation of isometric finger forces to the frictional condition. *Experimental Brain Research*, 104, 323–30.

Forssberg, H., Kinoshita, H., Eliasson, A.C., Johansson, R.S., Westling, G. and Gordon, A.M. (1992) Development of human precision grip II. Anticipatory control of isometric forces targeted for object's weight. *Experimental Brain Research*, 90, 393–8.

Gachoud, J.P., Mounoud, P., Hauert, C.A. and Viviani, P. (1983) Motor strategies in lifting movements: a comparison of adult and child performance. *Journal of Motor Behavior*, 15, 202–16.

Gordon, A.M., Forssberg, H., Johansson, R.S., Eliasson, A.C. and Westling, G. (1992) Development of human precision grip. III. Integration of visual size cues during the programming of isometric forces. *Experimental Brain Research*, 90, 399–403.

Gordon, A.M., Forssberg, H., Johansson, R.S. and Westling, G. (1991a) The integration of haptically acquired size information in the programming of precision grip. *Experimental Brain Research*, 83, 483–8.

Gordon, A.M., Forssberg, H., Johansson, R.S. and Westling, G. (1991b) Integration of sensory information during the programming of precision grip: comments on the contributions of size cues. *Experimental Brain Research*, 85, 226–9.

Gordon, A.M., Forssberg, H., Johansson, R.S. and Westling, G. (1991c) Visual size cues in the programming of manipulative forces during precision grip. *Experimental Brain Research*, 83, 477–82.

Gordon, A.M., Westling, G., Cole, K.J. and Johansson, R.S. (1993) Memory representations underlying motor commands used during manipulation of common and novel objects. *Journal of Neurophysiology*, 69, 1789–96.

Granit, R. (1972) Constant errors in the execution and appreciation of movement. Brain, 95, 451–60.

Hoffmann, E.R. (1994) Estimation of time to vehicle arrival. *Perception*, 23, 947–55.

Hoffmann, E.R., Payne, A. and Prescott, S. (1980) Children's estimates of vehicle approach times. *Human Factors*, 22, 235–40.

Hu, X., Wesson, D. and Kenney, B. (1993) Home injuries to children. *Canadian Journal of Public Health*, 84, 155–8.

ISO (1999) ISO Working draft. Ergonomics principles in the design of work systems. TC/159/SC 1, ISO/CD6385.

Jeong, B.Y. and Park, K.S. (1990) Sex differences in anthropometry for school furniture design. *Ergonomics*, 33, 1511–21.

Knight, G. and Noyes, J. (1999) Children's behaviour and the design of school furniture. *Ergonomics*, 42, 747–60.

Lee, D.N., Young, D.S. and McLaughlin, C.M. (1984) A roadside simulation of road crossing for children. *Ergonomics*, 27, 1271–81.

Macgregor, D.M. (2000). Nintendonitis? A case report of repetitive strain injury in a child as a result of playing computer games. *Scott Medicine Journal*, 45, 150.

Mon-Williams, M. and Murray, A.H. (2000) The size of the visual size cue used for programming manipulative forces during precision grip. *Experimental Brain Research*, 135, 405–10.

Neill, S.R. (1982) Preschool design and child behaviour. *Journal of Child Psychology Psychiatry*, 23, 309–18.

Prado-Leon, L.R., Avila-Chaurand, R. and Gonzalez-Munoz, E.L. (2001) Anthropometric study of Mexican primary school children. *Applied Ergonomics*, 32, 339–45.

Savelsbergh, G.J.P., Steenbergen, B. and Van der Kamp, J. (1996) The role of fragility information in the guidance of the precision grip. *Human Movement Science*, 15, 115–27.

Steenbekkers, L.P. and Molenbroek, J.F. (1990) Anthropometric data of children for non-specialist users. *Ergonomics*, 33, 421–9.

Stratton, G. (2000) Promoting children's physical activity in primary school: an intervention study using playground markings. *Ergonomics*, 43, 1538–46.

Taimela, S., Kujala, U.M., Salminen, J.J. and Viljanen, T. (1997) The prevalence of low-back-pain among children and adolescents: a nationwide, cohort-based questionnaire survey in Finland. *Spine*, 22, 1132–6.

Van Dieën, J.H., de Looze, M.P. and Hermans, V. (2001) Effects of dynamic office chairs on trunk kinematics, trunk extensor EMG, and spinal shrinkage. *Ergonomics*, 44, 739–50.

Wilson, J.R. (2000) Fundamentals of ergonomics in theory and practice. *Applied Ergonomics*, 31, 557–67.

Yamada, F. (1998) Frontal midline theta rhythm and eye blinking activity during a VDT task and a video game: useful tools for psychophysiology in ergonomics. *Ergonomics*, 41, 678–88.

3 Children's overestimation of their physical abilities

Links to injury proneness

Jodie M. Plumert

1. Introduction

Promoting children's safety and health are concerns shared by paediatricians, developmental psychologists, and educators. Injury prevention clearly plays an integral role in children's health, as unintentional injuries are the leading cause of death in children under age 18 (Rodriguez and Brown, 1990; Singh and Yu, 1996). Approximately 22,000 children die each year in the U.S. as a result of drowning, poisoning, choking on foreign objects, automobile and bicycle collisions, pedestrian injuries, electrocutions, burns, or falls. The alarming statistics on children's injuries have led to a number of investigations by researchers in a variety of fields on issues such as pedestrian safety (Christoffel *et al.*, 1986; Connelly *et al.*, 1998; Dunne, Asher, and Rivara, 1992; Lee *et al.*, 1984), childhood drowning (Nixon *et al.*, 1986), bicycling safety (Langley *et al.*, 1983), and children's ability to operate motorised vehicles (Pick *et al.*, 1987). Although overviews of strategies for reducing childhood injury have called for a better understanding of the underlying factors that contribute to the occurrence of injuries (Brooks and Roberts, 1990; Peterson and Mori, 1985; Roberts, 1986), little is yet known about how developmental changes in cognitive and perceptual skills contribute to unsafe behaviour.

One perceptual–cognitive skill that may play an important role in children's safety is the ability to evaluate one's level of skill in relation to the demands of the task (see also Lee *et al.*, 1984). When deciding whether it is safe to cross a street, for example, children must take into account both the speed of oncoming cars and how quickly they can walk or run. According to J.J. Gibson (1979), adaptive behaviour within the environment depends upon perceiving affordances, or the fit between one's own physical characteristics and the properties of the environment in which actions take place. Although accidents are complex phenomena and undoubtedly have several root causes, errors in judging the relation between one's physical abilities and the demands of the situation may be one important factor contributing to accident risk. For example, although some pedestrian accidents may result when children fail to follow simple rules like looking both ways when crossing a street, others may result when children make errors in judgement about their ability to run through traffic gaps.

Studies of the ability to make judgements about the fit between one's own skills and the characteristics of the environment have shown that even infants adjust their actions in response to changing environmental circumstances. For example, visual cliff studies showed that crawlers refuse to cross over the deep side, but readily venture out over the shallow side (Gibson and Walk, 1960). Later studies demonstrated that walking infants shift from walking to crawling when presented with a non-rigid surface such as a waterbed (Gibson *et al.*, 1987). Adolph *et al.* (1993) also found that walking infants changed their means of locomotion from walking to climbing or sliding as the slope of the surface increased. Likewise, McKenzie *et al.* (1993) found that infants exhibited progressively more leaning during their reaches as objects became increasingly distant. Thus, when environmental circumstances change, it appears that even infants readily modify their actions to reach a goal.

Despite the fact that infants and children show remarkable skill in adjusting their actions to provide a better fit with the demands of the situation, studies also have shown that they often overestimate what they can accomplish with those actions (Adolph, 1995; Adolph *et al.*, 1993; McKenzie and Forbes, 1992). For example, Adolph *et al.* (1993) and Adolph (1995) found that although toddlers were less likely to go down than up slopes, they consistently overestimated their ability to ascend and descend slopes that were beyond their ability. Likewise, McKenzie *et al.* (1993) found that even when objects were well out of reach, infants attempted to grasp the objects. They noted, in fact, that many infants would have fallen while trying to grasp objects that were well out of reach had they not been restrained in their infant seats. McKenzie and Forbes (1992) also found that 9- and 12-year-old boys consistently overestimated the height of steps that they could climb (for another viewpoint see Pufall and Dunbar, 1992). Moreover, although adults generally are quite accurate at judging reachability or climbability, studies have shown that they too have a tendency to overestimate their abilities. For example, Carello *et al.* (1989) found that adults overestimated their ability to reach objects across a variety of postures. Thus, it appears that even adults do not always accurately perceive the boundary between actions that are within and beyond their ability.

Taken together, these results suggest that children may perceive the boundary between actions that are within and beyond their ability as fuzzy. Moreover, when faced with uncertainty, it appears that children are more likely to overestimate than underestimate their abilities. One hypothesis this suggests about unintentional injuries is that children are most likely to make errors in judgement when confronted with activities that are just beyond their ability. For example, children may be more likely to run out in front of cars when gaps between cars are intermediate in size and hence more ambiguous than when gaps are fairly large or quite small and presumably less ambiguous. Thus, when children are confronted with situations that are beyond their ability, injury risk should peak in the range just beyond their ability. Rivara and Aitken (1998) make a similar point in their review of childhood injury prevention strategies. They suggest that children and adolescents are particularly vulnerable to injury when they are first mastering a new task and do not have all of the skills necessary to accomplish the task successfully every time. In other words, they contend that injuries can occur in this window of vulnerability because there is a mismatch between the child's skills and the task demands.

Over the last several years, we have been examining the links between ability overestimation and unintentional injuries (Plumert, 1995; Plumert and Schwebel, 1997; Schwebel and Plumert, 1999; Schwebel *et al.*, 2000). The goals of this research are twofold: (a) to determine whether children who overestimate their physical abilities have a history of injuries requiring medical attention; and (b) to determine what factors play a role in overestimation of physical ability. Ultimately, the goal of this work is to build a comprehensive model of the underlying causes of unintentional childhood injuries.

All of our studies involve a laboratory assessment in which 6- and 8-year-old children are asked to judge whether or not they can perform activities of varying levels of difficulty before they attempt to perform each activity. There are four tasks:

a   The *vertical reach* task involves removing a toy from a shelf standing on tip toes.
b   The *horizontal reach* task involves reaching out from a squatting position for a toy duck on a wooden block without touching hands or knees on the floor.
c   The *stepping* task involves stepping across two sticks placed parallel to each other.
d   The *clearance* task involves getting under a wooden bar attached to two posts without knocking the bar off or putting hands or knees on the floor.

Children make judgements about their ability to perform each of these activities at four levels of difficulty, resulting in 16 test trials. The *well within* version is 13 per cent below the child's maximum level of ability; the *just within* version is at the child's maximum level of ability; the *just beyond* version is 8 per cent above the child's maximum level; and the well beyond version is 13 per cent above the child's maximum level. For all tasks, levels of difficulty are scaled to the abilities of the individual children. Before making each judgement, children are instructed to put themselves in the starting position for each activity. To make their judgement about the vertical reach, for example, children first step up to a line on the floor positioned directly below the shelf. With hands at their sides, children then judge whether they can perform the task successfully. We assess the accuracy of children's judgements by comparing children's judgements of their ability to perform the tasks with their actual ability to perform the tasks.

The goal of the first investigation was to determine whether children and adults overestimate their physical abilities and whether overestimation of ability is related to childhood injury risk (Plumert, 1995). The first experiment in this investigation revealed that 6- and 8-year-olds often overestimated their ability to perform tasks that were beyond their ability (see figure 3.1). Adults also had difficulty making judgements about tasks that were just beyond their ability, but had less difficulty than children in making judgements about tasks that were well beyond their ability.

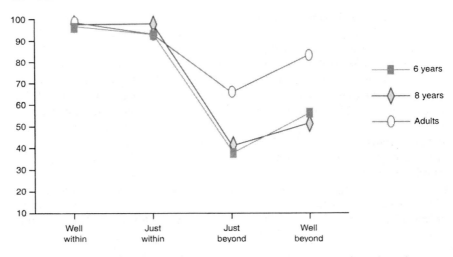

Figure 3.1 Children and adults' judgements about their ability to perform the task as a function of level of difficulty (see text for explanation)

In addition, children and adults made the fastest decisions about tasks that were easy for them to perform, followed by tasks that were just within their ability, followed finally by tasks that were just beyond and well beyond their ability. Moreover, 6-year-olds, but not 8-year-olds, who were less accurate in judging their physical abilities had experienced more accidents requiring medical attention ($r = -0.44$).

What factors might influence children's judgements about their physical abilities? One factor that may play an important role is feedback about physical skills. Presumably, one way children learn about the relation between their abilities and the demands of the situation is by attempting to perform physical activities. I examined this issue by giving 6- and 8-year-olds experience with each of the activities before the test trials (Plumert, 1995). Analyses revealed that 8-year-olds, but not 6-year-olds, benefited from prior experience with performing the tasks. That is, 8-year-olds' judgements about their ability to perform tasks well beyond their ability ($M = 77$ per cent) were more accurate than their judgements about tasks just beyond their ability ($M = 45$ per cent). Six-year-olds' judgements about their ability to perform tasks well beyond ($M = 37$ per cent) and just beyond their ability did not differ (38 per cent). As before, 6-year-olds who were less accurate in judging their abilities in the laboratory setting had experienced more accidents requiring medical attention ($r = -0.48$).

2. Peer influences

Another factor that may play a role in children's overestimation of their physical abilities is peer influence. That is, children may use the performance of other children to inform them about their own abilities. For example, a child who sees another child successfully ride her bike down a steep bumpy hill may think that she also can successfully ride her bike down the hill. Festinger (1954) suggested that such comparisons are useful for making accurate assessments about what one is capable of doing, particularly under conditions of uncertainty. Thus, when children are confronted with situations in which they are not sure whether they are capable of performing an activity, they may look to the performance of peers to inform them about their own ability.

We assessed the influence of social comparison information on children's judgements about their physical abilities by having children view a videotape of a same-age and same-sex peer either succeeding or failing on the four tasks (Schwebel and Plumert, 1997). Children watched the videotape just before they played the game so that they could use the other child's performance to assess the difficulty of the tasks. We expected that children who watched the peer fail on all the tasks would be more conservative in their judgements about their own abilities than would children who watched the peer succeed on all the tasks. Our results revealed that when children observed the peer in the video fail on all of the activities, they were more conservative about their own abilities than when they observed the peer succeed. Thus, both 6- and 8-year-olds used the peer's performance to inform them about their own abilities. This study also revealed that 6-year-old boys who were less accurate in judging their physical abilities experienced more severe day-to-day injuries ($r = -0.51$).

3. Influence of temperament

A third factor that may influence children's ability to make accurate judgements about their physical abilities is temperament. Temperament is defined as a set of individual differences expressed as generally stable behavioural tendencies throughout childhood and into adulthood. Temperament reflects both reactivity to external stimuli as well as internal self-regulation (Goldsmith *et al.*, 1987; Rothbart, 1989). Conceptually, temperament is viewed as a mediator of the child's experience (Rothbart and Bates, 1997). That is, temperamental characteristics such as activity level and approach tendencies may lead children to seek out some situations and avoid others (Scarr and McCartney, 1983). For example, highly active and approach-oriented children may seek out new and unfamiliar situations. Novel situations may lead to injuries because such situations force children to react to potentially unforeseen, dangerous problems. Moreover, highly active and impulsive children are quick to respond and often rush into activities without thinking about them (Rothbart *et al.*, 1994). Children who make decisions impulsively may be more prone to errors in judgement than children who make decisions more carefully. As a result, impulsive and overactive children may be at greater risk of injury.

Thus far, we have conducted two studies to address the question of whether impulsive children are more likely to overestimate their physical abilities than are their non-impulsive counterparts (Plumert and Schwebel, 1997; Schwebel and Plumert, 1999). In the first study, we asked 6- and 8-year-old children to make judgements about their ability to perform tasks that were within and beyond their ability using the laboratory assessment developed in our previous studies (Plumert and Schwebel, 1997). We also asked the parents of these children (usually the mother) to complete the Child Behavior Questionnaire (CBQ), a widely used measure of children's temperament (Rothbar *et al.*, 1993). We found that highly active and undercontrolled 6-year-olds were more likely to overestimate their ability than were less active and more controlled counterparts. Interestingly, we also found that highly active and undercontrolled 8-year-olds made faster judgements about their abilities than did less active and more controlled 8-year-olds. Thus, it appears that temperamental characteristics are related to ability overestimation, particularly for younger children.

In our second investigation, we examined the longitudinal links between temperamental characteristics and ability overestimation (Schwebel and Plumert, 1999). In other words, is impulsivity during the pre-school years related to ability overestimation at age 6? We found that behavioural measures of inhibitory control during toddlerhood were related to ability overestimation measures during the early elementary school years. In other words, children who exhibited less inhibitory control as toddlers overestimated their ability more frequently as 6-year-olds. Likewise, children who were rated by their mothers as impulsive and highly active as pre-schoolers overestimated their ability more frequently as 6-year-olds. Thus, it appears that children who are more impulsive and less controlled at young ages are more likely to overestimate their physical abilities at older ages.

Together, these findings indicate that children have difficulty making judgements about the fit between their physical abilities and the demands of the situation, particularly when the situation is ambiguous. Not surprisingly, younger children (i.e. 6-year-olds) were more likely to overestimate their physical abilities in our tasks than were older children (i.e. 8-year-olds). Moreover, ability overestimation was related to injury proneness in 6-year-olds, but not 8-year-olds. Why might this be the case? One explanation for this discrepancy is that the factors that contribute to errors in the laboratory differ for the two age groups. More specifically, although the factors that cause 6-year-olds to make more errors in judging their physical abilities in the laboratory may be similar to the ones that resulted in injuries in early childhood, the same may not be true for 8-year-olds. Further research, however, is necessary before any definitive conclusions can be drawn about developmental differences concerning the relation between ability over-estimation and injury proneness.

4. Future directions: children's bicycling behaviour

Over the past two years, we have begun to study how ability overestimation may put children at risk of injuries in the context of children's bicycling safety. Bicycle crashes are among the most common causes of severe injuries in childhood (Rivara, 1985). Approximately 500,000 bicycle-related injuries are treated in hospital emergency rooms each year in the US (Baker *et al.*, 1993). Children between the ages of 5 and 15 represent a particularly vulnerable segment of the population, having the highest rate of injury per million cycling trips (Rivara and Aitken,

1998). Despite growing national concern over promoting children's bicycling safety, however, the underlying causes of bicycle crashes remain poorly understood. Clearly, understanding the causes of car–bicycle collisions is important for designing interventions to prevent such events from occurring.

How good are children at judging whether a traffic gap affords crossing? Although nothing is yet known about children's road-crossing behaviour while bicycling, several studies have addressed children's road-crossing while walking (Connelly *et al.*, 1998; Demetre *et al.*, 1992; Dunne *et al.*, 1992; Lee *et al.*, 1984). Lee *et al.* (1984), for example, devised an analogue road-crossing task to assess developmental changes in children's ability to accurately judge whether traffic gaps afford crossing. Five- to 10-year-old children crossed a 'pretend' road set up directly parallel to an actual road. Children were instructed to watch the cars on the actual road and to cross the pretend road when they felt that they could safely reach the other side. The time at which the car reached the crossing line and the distance between the child and the pretend curb at the time that the car reached the crossing line were recorded. Their findings indicated that although children generally were cautious, they occasionally accepted gaps that were too short. Had children been crossing the actual road, they would have been hit on approximately 6 per cent of their crossings. In addition, a higher proportion of younger children than older children made such errors. Approximately 75 per cent of the 5-year-olds made at least one road-crossing error, whereas only 58 per cent of 9-year-olds did so. These findings suggest that younger children are more likely than older children to overestimate their ability to walk through traffic gaps.

A similar study conducted in New Zealand by Connelly *et al.* (1998) revealed that children sometimes choose gaps that are unsafe, particularly when cars are travelling at high speeds. In this study, 5- to 6-year-olds, 8- to 9-year-olds, and 11- to 12-year-olds stood at the side of an actual road and made judgements about traffic gaps. Their task was to indicate the last possible moment that they would cross in front of an oncoming car. Two results are of particular interest. First, although the test site was in a 50-kph speed zone, over two-thirds of the vehicles exceeded the posted speed limit. In fact, 39 per cent of the vehicles exceeded the speed limit by 6 kph or more. Second, children often chose unsafe gaps when cars were travelling at speeds of 60 kph or more. This was particularly true of the boys in the 8- to 9-year-old group. One implication of this work is that children rely primarily on distance when making judgements about traffic gaps.

Currently, very little is known about children's ability to judge traffic gaps while bicycling. One reason why we know so little about children's road-crossing behaviour while bicycling is that it is difficult to study bicycling behaviour without putting research participants at risk of injury. For example, one cannot study whether impulsive children are more likely to make errors in judging the size of traffic gaps by asking them to bicycle across busy roads in the real environment. Another reason we know so little about the causes of bicycling crashes is that it is difficult to study bicycling behaviour in a controlled environment. Without control over the timing and nature of events in an experiment, it is difficult to draw valid conclusions about how these events influence children's bicycling behaviour.

Advances in virtual environment technology, however, offer a way of studying the problem of bicycling safety in a controlled manner without putting children at risk of injury (e.g. Cremer *et al.*, 1995). Using a high-fidelity, interactive bicycling simulator, we can safely present children with the same kinds of bicycling challenges as they confront in the real environment. We can then use their performance in the simulated environment to make inferences about their performance in the real environment.

We have begun to investigate children's ability to make road-crossing judgements using an immersive, interactive bicycling simulator. In our initial pilot study, thirty-two 12- and 14-year-old children rode a bicycle mounted on a stationary trainer through a simulated environment. The bicycle was instrumented to provide information to the simulator about steering angle, hand braking, and the speed of the rear wheel's rotation that was used to determine the apparent motion of the bicycle through the virtual environment. High-resolution, textured graphics were projected onto an array of three 21-inch computer monitors providing children with a clear view of the approaching cross traffic at the intersections.

The session began with a 3-minute warm-up session on the simulator designed to familiarise children with the characteristics of the bicycle and the simulated environment. The simulated environment used for the warm-up session was a straight, residential street with three intersections. During the warm-up period, there was no traffic on the street with the child and no cross-traffic at any of the intersections. Children were instructed to stay on the street and to stop at each intersection. The practice session provided children with the opportunity to learn how to steer, pedal, and stop the bicycle. Following the warm-up session, children participated in an approximately 10- to 15-minute test session on the simulator. The test section of the simulated environment was a straight, residential street with 12 intersections. There was no traffic on the street with the child, but there was moving cross-traffic at each intersection. The cross-traffic always moved from left to right and was restricted to the lane closest to the participant. There were five different distances between the cars (100 ft, 150 ft, 200 ft, 250 ft and 300 ft). The distances between the passing cars were randomly ordered. (It is important to note that all of these distances represented crossable gaps.) For half of the participants, all cars on the road were travelling at a rate of 25 mph. For the other half, the cars travelled at a rate of 35 mph. Children were instructed to stop at each intersection and to cross when they felt it was acceptable to cross.

Two issues were of particular interest. First, are there developmental differences in children's road-crossing judgements? That is, are older children more cautious than younger children? Second, are children more cautious when cross-traffic is moving at a faster speed? In the real environment, one would expect to see more cautious behaviour with faster traffic because the consequences of getting hit are more severe. However, because there are no real consequences of getting hit in the simulated environment, children may not respond in the same way to faster rates of traffic. In fact, children may be less cautious with the faster traffic because it may be more fun to try to cross recklessly in front of fast-moving traffic.

The results of the study suggest that children understood the task quite well and found the simulated environment quite realistic. As expected, older children were more cautious than younger children. Interestingly, the distance between the bike and the approaching car did not differ for 12-year-olds ($M = 84$ ft, $SD = 9.0$) and 14-year-olds ($M = 85$ ft, $SD = 7.0$) when they started bicycling across the intersection, $F(1, 28) = 0.28$, *ns*. However, the distance between the bike and the approaching car was greater for 14-year-olds ($M = 53$ ft, $SD = 7.1$) than for 12-year-olds ($M = 48$ ft, $SD = 10.1$) at the point at which the bike cleared the path of the approaching car, $F(1, 28) = 3.53, p = 0.07$. This suggests that the older children increased their speed as they crossed the intersection.

Unexpectedly, there were few indications that children were more cautious when the cross traffic was moving faster. Although children who faced cross traffic moving at 35 mph ($M = 4.5$ ft, $SD = 2.4$) allowed more cars to pass before crossing the road in the first block of trials (i.e. intersections 1 to 3) than did their counterparts in the 25 mph ($M = 2.9$ ft, $SD = 1.2$) group, $F(1, 30) = 5.70, p < 0.05$, there were no significant differences between the two speed conditions for the other three blocks of trials (i.e. intersections 4 to 6, 7 to 9, and 10 to 12). Moreover, the distance between the bike and the approaching car did not differ for children in the 25 mph ($M = 83$ ft, $SD = 8.6$) and 35 mph ($M = 86$ ft, $SD = 7.2$) conditions when they started bicycling across the intersection, $F(1, 28) = 0.96$, *ns*. Interestingly, by the time the bike cleared the path of the approaching car, however, children in the 35 mph ($M = 48$ ft, $SD = 8.6$) condition left *less* distance between themselves and the approaching car than did children in the 25 mph condition ($M = 53$ ft, $SD = 8.6$), $F(1, 28) = 3.90, p = 0.06$. Thus, consistent with the findings of Connelly *et al.* (1998), it appears that children used distance rather than a combination of distance and speed to judge the acceptability of traffic gaps.

Together, these results indicate that using a bicycling simulator to study children's bicycling behaviour is a promising approach for understanding and preventing bicycle crashes. Several questions remain unanswered, however. For example, why might children misjudge traffic gaps? Several possibilities exist. One that has been discussed throughout this chapter is children overestimate how quickly they can cross the road. If children overestimate their road-crossing ability, they may choose traffic gaps that are too small for safe crossing. However, another possible reason why children make errors in judging traffic gap affordances is that they have difficulty judging time to contact, or how long it will take a vehicle to reach the crossing line. Clearly, distinguishing between these two alternatives is an important step in understanding the underlying causes of road-crossing errors. Future work will focus on answering these and other questions related to bicycling safety.

5. Conclusions

From a general standpoint, the observation that children have a tendency to over-estimate their physical abilities raises an interesting developmental issue. Namely, by its very nature, development involves aspiring to do things that are beyond one's current level of ability. Without such motivation, it seems unlikely that development would move forward. As others have pointed out (e.g. Bjorklund and Green, 1992), there may be a beneficial component to a general bias to overestimate one's ability that offsets some of the potential hazards in doing so. The developmental dilemma, therefore, is continually to aspire to try new and difficult things but not to try things that might have disastrous consequences. Children who have difficulty making this distinction are likely to be at risk of serious unintentional injuries. The research presented here provides an initial starting point for understanding developmental changes in judgements about physical abilities during middle childhood and in unravelling possible factors contributing to childhood injuries.

References

Adolph, K.E. (1995) Psychophysical assessment of toddlers' ability to cope with slopes. *Journal of Experimental Psychology: Human Perception and Performance*, 21, 734–50.

Adolph, K.E., Eppler, M.A. and Gibson, E.J. (1993) Crawling versus walking infants' perception of affordances for locomotion over sloping surfaces. *Child Development*, 64, 1158–74.

Baker, S.P., Li, G., Fowler, C. and Dannenberg, A.L. (1993) *Injuries to Bicyclists: A National Perspective*. Baltimore, MD: The Johns Hopkins University Injury Prevention Center.

Bjorklund, D. and Green, B.L. (1992) The adaptive nature of cognitive immaturity. *American Psychologist*, 47, 46–54.

Brooks, P.H. and Roberts, M.C. (1990) Social science and the prevention of children's injuries. *Social Policy Report of the Society for Research in Child Development*, 4, 1–11.

Carello, C., Grosofsky, A. Reichel, F.D., Solomon, H.Y. and Turvey, M.T. (1989) Visually perceiving what is reachable. *Ecological Psychology*, 1, 27–54.

Christoffel, K.K., Schofer, J.L., Jovanis, P.P., Brandt, B., White, B. and Tanz, R. (1986) Childhood pedestrian injury: a pilot study concerning etiology. *Accident Analysis and Prevention*, 18, 25–35.

Connelly, M.L., Conaglen, H.M., Parsonson, B.S. and Isler, R.B. (1998) Child pedestrians' crossing gap thresholds. *Accident Analysis and Prevention*, 30, 443–53.

Cremer, J., Kearney, J. and Papelis, Y. (1995) HCSM: a framework for behavior and scenario control in virtual environments. *ACM Transactions on Modeling and Computer Simulation*, 5, 242–67.

Demetre, J.D., Lee, D.N., Pitcairn, T.K., Grieve, R., Thomson, J.A. and Ampofo-Boateng, K. (1992) Errors in young children's decisions about traffic gaps: experiments with roadside simulations. *British Journal of Psychology*, 83, 189–202.

Dunne, R.G., Asher, K.N. and Rivara, F.P. (1992) Behavior and parental expectations of child pedestrians. *Pediatrics*, 89, 486–90.

Festinger, L. (1954) A theory of social comparison. *Human Relations*, 7, 117–40.

Gibson, E.J., Riccio, G. Schmuckler, M.A., Stoffregen, T.A., Rosenberg, D. and Taormina, J. (1987) Detection of the traversability of surfaces by crawling and walking infants. *Journal of Experimental Psychology: Human Perception and Performance*, 13, 533–44.

Gibson, E.J. and Walk, R.D. (1960) The 'visual cliff'. *Scientific American*, 202, 64–71.

Gibson, J.J. (1979) *The Ecological Approach to Visual Perception*. Hillsdale, NJ: Erlbaum.

Goldsmith, H.H., Buss, A.H., Plomin, R., Rothbart, M.K., Thomas, A., Chess, S., Hinde, R.A. and McCall, R.B. (1987) Roundtable: what is temperament? Four approaches. *Child Development*, 58, 505–29.

Langley, J., McGee, R., Silva, P. and Williams, S. (1983) Child behavior and accidents. *Journal of Pediatric Psychology*, 8, 181–9.

Lee, D.N., Young, D.S. and McLaughlin, C.M. (1984) A roadside simulation of road crossing for children. *Ergonomics*, 12, 1271–81.

McKenzie, B.E. and Forbes, C. (1992) Does vision guide stair climbing? A developmental study. *Australian Journal of Psychology*, 44, 177–83.

McKenzie, B.E., Skouteris, H., Day, R.H., Hartman, B. and Yonas, A. (1993) Effective action by infants to contact objects by reaching and leaning. *Child Development*, 64, 415–29.

Nixon, J., Pearn, J., Wilkey, I. and Corcoran, A. (1986) Fifteen years of child drowning: a 1967–1981 analysis of all fatal cases from the Brisbane drowning study and an 11 year study of consecutive near-drowning cases. *Accident Analysis and Prevention*, 18, 199–203.

Peterson, L. and Mori, L. (1985) Prevention of child injury: an overview of targets, methods, and tactics for psychologists. *Journal of Consulting and Clinical Psychology*, 53, 586–95.

Pick, H.L. Jr., Plumert, J.M. and Arterberry, M.E. (1987) *All-terrain Vehicles and Children: Perceptual-motor, Cognitive, and Social Risk Factors*. Report prepared for the Consumer Product Safety Commission (Contract No. CPSC-C-87-1289).

Plumert, J.M. (1995) Relations between children's overestimation of their physical abilities and accident proneness. *Developmental Psychology*, 31, 866–76.

Plumert, J.M. and Schwebel, D.C. (1997) Social and temperamental influences on children's overestimation of their physical abilities: links to accident proneness. *Journal of Experimental Child Psychology*, 67, 317–37.

Pufall, P.B. and Dunbar, C. (1992) Perceiving whether or not the world affords stepping onto and over: A developmental study. *Ecological Psychology*, 4, 17–38.

Rivara, F.P. (1985) Traumatic deaths of children in the United States: currently available prevention strategies. *Pediatrics*, 75, 456–62.

Rivara, F.P. and Aitken, M. (1998) Prevention of injuries to children and adolescents. *Advances in Pediatrics*, 45, 37–72.

Roberts, M.C. (1986) Health promotion and problem prevention in pediatric psychology: an overview. *Journal of Pediatric Psychology*, 11, 147–61.

Rodriguez, J.G. and Brown, S.T. (1990) Childhood injuries in the United States. *American Journal of Disease Control*, 144, 627–46.

Rothbart, M.K. (1989) Temperament in childhood: a framework. In G.A. Kohnstamm, J.A. Bates, and M.K. Rothbart (eds), *Temperament in Childhood* (pp. 59–73). New York: Wiley.

Rothbart, M.K., Ahadi, S. and Hershey, K.L. (1994) Temperament and social behavior in children. *Merrill-Palmer Quarterly*, 40, 21–39.

Rothbart, M.K. and Bates, J.E. (1997) Temperament. In W. Damon and N. Eisenberg (eds), *Handbook of Child Psychology: Vol. 3: Social, Emotional, and Personality Development*. New York: Wiley.

Scarr, S. and McCartney, K. (1983) How people make their own environments: a theory of genotype-environment effects. *Child Development*, 54, 424–35.

Schwebel, D.C. and Plumert, J.M. (1999) Longitudinal and concurrent relations between temperament, ability estimation, and injury proneness. *Child Development*, 70, 700–12.

Schwebel, D.C., Plumert, J.M. and Pick, H.L. (2000) Integrating basic and applied developmental research: a new model for the twenty-first century. *Child Development*, 71, 222–30.

Singh, G.K. and Yu, S.M. (1996) U.S. childhood mortality, 1950–1993: trends and socioeconomic differentials. *American Journal of Public Health*, 86, 505–12.

4 Road-crossing behaviour in young children

Arenda F. te Velde, John van der Kamp and Geert Savelsbergh

1. Introduction

It is widely acknowledged that young children are over-represented in traffic accidents. It is therefore obvious that reducing the number of child pedestrian accidents is an important research aim. Through the introduction of (additional) pedestrian facilities, specific traffic regulation and other improvements to roadway situations, the problem of children's traffic safety may be reduced. In the end, however, such measures will only be beneficial if children's road-crossing skills are taken into account. To this end, not only is an analysis of the pedestrian task indispensable, but it also needs to be established how the (component) skill(s) of road-crossing change with age. The present chapter therefore aims to describe the age-related changes in road crossing and its component skills in 4- to 12-year-old children. Furthermore, training programmes that are directed at improving the component skills of road crossing, and that may reduce child pedestrian casualties, are reviewed. The improvements appear to be less than one would hope for, and as such we discus whether the results from simulated environments should be generalised to actual traffic situations. We will dwell on some of the more important methodological aspects (e.g. the practice environment). Although characteristics like temperament and socialisation might explain a substantial proportion of safe or unsafe road-crossing behaviour (Plumert and Schwebel, 1997; Schwebel and Plumert, 1999; West *et al.*, 1999), these will not be taken into account. Likewise, socio-economic and environmental characteristics are beyond the scope of this chapter. Before turning to children's road-crossing skills, however, we start with an assessment of children's exposure to risk situations.

2. Risk and exposure

Recent statistics show that child pedestrians up to 15 years of age are three times more at risk than older children and adults to be involved in a fatal accident (Road Accidents Great Britain, 2000), the risk being dependent on country, socio-economic status, age and gender (Chapman and O'Reilly, 1999). Rivara (1990) reported that casualty rates in the United States varied from 1.9 to 5.4 fatalities per 100,000 children between 5 and 9 years of age, and from 0.9 to 2.0 per 100,000 for children between 10 and 14 years of age (cf. Dhillon *et al.*, 2001; Howarth *et al.*, 1974; Routledge *et al.*, 1974). Obviously, reported injury rates are higher: respectively 111 and 79 per 100,000 children between 5 and 9 years and 10 and 14 years of age (Rivara, 1990). However, in the past few decades there has been a decrease in casualty rates in 5- to 9-year-olds. Nowadays, it is at a somewhat older age that children appear particularly at risk (Chapman and O'Reilly, 1999). This shift may be due to a decline in children's traffic exposure. Parents have become more reluctant to allow their children to walk unaccompanied, and there has been a concomitant increase in age at which children are allowed to cross roads unaccompanied (Roberts, 1993).

Nevertheless, a consideration of children's traffic exposure emphasises the vulnerability of young children to traffic. In most definitions exposure relates to the number of children playing in the street without supervision, frequency of encounters with a car, frequency of crossing roads each day, and mode of travel to school (e.g. Van der Molen, 1981). It appears that, dependent on country and socio-economic status (e.g. owning a car), primary school children cross between one and ten roads each day (Macpherson *et al.*, 1998; Rao *et al.*, 1997; Roberts *et al.*, 1997). The number of road-crossings increases with age, and this contributes to the increasing exposure to traffic (Demetre and Gaffin, 1994; Howarth *et al.*, 1974; Routledge *et al.*, 1974; Rao *et al.*, 1997; Stevenson, 1996). For instance, Rivara and co-workers (Rivara *et al.*, 1989) report that 3 per cent to 33 per cent of kindergarten school children walk to school unaccompanied, whereas this increases to 15 per cent to 69 per cent of children in the fourth grade. On their way to school, the younger children in particular are accompanied by a parent, whereas on their way back home, children tend to walk with peers. When children play outdoors, they are more likely to walk than when going to school (Towner *et al.*, 1994). Importantly, it has been found that, within an age group, increased exposure is accompanied by increased risk, whereas with age groups, the risk relative to exposure decreases (Howarth *et al.*, 1974; Macpherson *et al.*, 1998; Routledge *et al.*, 1974). The decline in the relative rate of children's traffic accidents suggests, among other things, an increase in road-crossing skill with age. These age-related changes will be considered in the next section.

3. Road-crossing skills

The pedestrian road-crossing task can be divided into many component skills (Foot *et al.*, 1999; Thomson *et al.*, 1996; Van der Molen *et al.*, 1981; Vinjé, 1981). In the present chapter we restrict ourselves to only four of these component skills. First, pedestrians have to find a safe site and a safe route to cross. Before they actually cross the road, pedestrians have to detect the presence of traffic, which involves strategic looking behaviour. Subsequently, the pedestrian requires information about the time available to cross the road; that is, the pedestrian must visually judge whether a traffic gap is 'crossable'. Finally, after having judged that a traffic gap is safe, pedestrians' crossing behaviour (e.g. movement time and path) should be consistent and adapted to the situation. In order to determine at what age these component skills are properly developed, the remainder of this section reviews the development of these four component skills of the road-crossing task. It needs to be emphasised beforehand that possessing well-developed component skills does not guarantee safe road-crossing behaviour, although it may provide an indication of what may be expected of a child at a particular age (cf. West *et al.*, 1999).

Select a safe site and a safe route

A child must select a safe site and route to cross. That is, a child should be able to distinguish safe places from dangerous places and situations where crossing should not be attempted. A safe site to cross is usually considered a place that provides an unobstructed view of oncoming vehicles. In contrast, locations where visibility is restricted, such as at bends or near parked cars, and complex situations, such as junctions where traffic might arrive from a number of directions, are considered dangerous.[1]

At what age are children able to select a safe site to cross a road? To answer this question, Ampofo-Boateng and Thomson (1991) presented children between 5 and 11 years of age with a tabletop traffic simulation and photographs of road situations, and took the children to real-world sites. They found that, on the one hand, in all the three testing situations the 5- to 7-year-olds frequently recognised dangerous situations (e.g. crossing between parked cars, at junction, or near a hedge) to be safe ones. Identifying safe places, on the other hand, was much better. Their judgements appeared to rely almost exclusively on the visible presence of vehicles that were nearby. Their judgements were based on a rule of thumb 'don't cross if you see cars, do cross if you don't', whether the view was blocked or not. The young children also tended to prefer the shortest route to the destination as the safest (see also Ampofo-Boateng *et al.*, 1993; Thomson *et al.*, 1998; Thomson *et al.*, 1992). Only at 9 years of age did children start to correctly recognise the dangerous sites; for example, those where vehicles might be hidden from view. These findings thus confirmed earlier observations of Demetre and Gaffin (1994), who took children to a real-world site and found that 8-year-olds, but not 6-year-olds, identified the place with a clear view (i.e. without parked cars) as the safest site to cross. Moreover, children who had experience with crossing a road unaccompanied were much more likely to select a site that provided a clear view.

In short, these findings and others (e.g. Whitebread and Neilson, 2000) strongly suggest that children's ability to select safe sites to cross a road is not appropriately developed before 9 years of age. The ability appears strongly related to experience. These findings are consistent with figures that about 40 to 70 per cent of 5- to 6-year-old children's accidents involve attempts to cross near parked cars, compared with about 20 per cent of 13- to 14-year-olds' accidents (Van der Molen, 1981). It appears that at the age of 9 years children are increasingly aware that the visibility of oncoming traffic may be obstructed. It is important to note, however, that in none of these studies children were actually required to cross the road.

Looking behaviour

After having selected a place to cross, the child, before making a decision to cross, has to detect whether any traffic is approaching. Obviously, visual search strategies are highly dependent on the road traffic situation and the moment-to-moment changes of that situation. However, when standing (or walking and running) at the kerbside, every visual search strategy should contain looking left–right–left before crossing the road. Limbourg and Gerber (1981) found in an actual road-crossing task that only about 10 per cent of the 3- to 7-year-old children stopped at the kerb before crossing the road, and that about 20 per cent of these children looked left and right before crossing. In a recent study, Zeedyk *et al.* (2002) confirmed these observations. Five- and 6-year-olds were asked to cross a road at a T-junction at which there was an approaching car, and between parked cars. Road-crossing behaviour was extremely poor. More than half of the children failed to stop before proceeding from the kerb onto the road. Looking before proceeding was exhibited by no more than about 30 per cent of the children, and when looking did occur it was as likely to be in the inappropriate as in the appropriate direction. Strikingly, at the T-junction only 7 per cent of the children looked for oncoming traffic. Also, looking whilst crossing the road occurred more often when crossing from between parked cars. Rivara *et al.* (1991) also examined somewhat older children. Remarkably, they found that at 7 to 9 years of age children stopped even less often at the kerb than children of 5 and 6 years of age (25 per cent and 50 per cent respectively). Looking left–right–left before crossing the road was observed in about 25 per cent of the children and did not change with age. Likewise, the percentage of children (15 per cent) who kept looking for traffic while crossing did not change with age. From these studies, all of which observed children actually crossing a road,[2] it can be concluded that looking behaviour is poor in 3- to 6-year-old children. They do not stop at the kerb, they do not look left–right–left to detect traffic, and looking during crossing is virtually absent. Moreover, it appears that even at 9 years of age, children do not perform much better. At what age children do, or whether they should, consistently stop at the kerb and look left–right–left before proceeding onto the road remains to be established. Nevertheless, one recent study (Whitebread and Neilson, 2000), which used three television screens that showed the views to the left, centre and right along a road, suggests that even 11-year-old children have not fully attained adult looking performance. The authors investigated the visual search strategies adopted by children of primary school age and their relation to the development of general performance as a pedestrian. Children were required to detect information from video presentations and make a decision about when it was safe to cross the road. Eye and head movements were measured. It was found that 4- and 5-year-old children had less but longer fixations, and often had problems of keeping attention on one of the screens. The oldest children fixated more frequently and for shorter durations, but did not reach the frequency of switching attention demonstrated by the adults. Children at 10 and 11 years of age and adults performed a 'last-minute' check of all three directions before deciding the road was safe to cross. Whitebread and

Neilson showed that the visual search characteristics were related (within age groups) with component road-crossing skills (i.e. selecting a safe site, detecting dangerous vehicles, and identifying safe crossing times). While there were large individual differences, perhaps implying that exposure is an important determinant, this study suggests that a shift in visual search strategy occurs certainly not before the age of 7–8 years, and even at the age of 11 adult looking behaviour is not yet fully acquired.

Visually judging 'crossable' traffic gaps

When a child has detected an oncoming vehicle, it must judge whether, and if so when, it is safe to cross the road in front of the vehicle. That is, the child must visually judge whether a traffic gap is 'crossable'. Only when the time to arrival of an approaching vehicle is longer than the time needed to reach the far kerb can the child cross the road safely. Hence, the child must perceive the size of gaps not in any abstract or absolute terms but in terms of the time it will take to walk across the road (Lee *et al.*, 1984). In this respect, a consideration of the child's conception of speed (Cross and Mehegan, 1988) may distort the investigator's view of young children's difficulties in judging whether a traffic gap is crossable. A prediction motion task, as used by Hoffmann *et al.* (1980), may be the more suitable methodology. In this study, 5- to 10-year-old children were shown movie film clips of vehicles approaching with speeds between 27 and 55 kph. The clips terminated when the vehicle was at a distance of 20, 60 or 100m from the camera position. The children's task was to press a key when they thought that the vehicle would have passed their location beside the road. It was found that all children underestimated time to arrival, but this underestimation decreased with age, and performance comparable to adults was reached at about 12 years of age. Nevertheless, there were large variations within each age group, and even among the 5- to 6-year-olds there were children who performed in the adult range. Underestimating a vehicle's time to arrival does not necessarily mean, however, that children's crossability judgements are cautious, because it remains unknown from this study how they estimate the time to cross the road.

Lee and co-workers (Demetre *et al.*, 1992; Lee *et al.*, 1984: Young and Lee, 1987) described a simple, safe method involving normal traffic where 5- to 10-year-old children's road crossing was investigated in a roadside simulation task. The method comprised a pretend road, which the child was told to cross as if crossing the adjacent road in the face of oncoming vehicles. The children were generally more cautious than the adults, which may indicate that adults accepted smaller gaps (cf. Pitcairn and Edlmann, 2000). For instance, 5-year-olds rejected almost half of the gaps of adequate duration. The number of missed opportunities decreased with age (see also Whitebread and Neilson, 2000; but see Pitcairn and Edlmann, 2000). Though children were overcautious, they did occasionally accept unsafe, too short gaps. The proportion of children that accepted tight fits was sometimes (Lee *et al.*, 1984), but not always (Demetre *et al.*, 1992; Young and Lee, 1987; see also Pitcairn and Edlmann, 2000) found to decrease with age. Finally, it was stressed that, with an increase in age, an increasing number of children performed in the adult range, suggesting that even the youngest children could be trained to an adequate level (see section 4). These findings suggest that young children are not as accurate as adults in judging whether or not a road is crossable. Rather than a general inability in visually timing *per se*, the relative inaccuracy may reflect a compensatory strategy of setting a wider safety margin (Demetre *et al.*, 1992; Lee *et al.*, 1984).

Because the oncoming vehicle's speed was not controlled, it cannot be excluded that younger children were using distance instead of time to arrival, as was assumed by Lee and co-workers, to decide whether a traffic gap was crossable. Assuming that traffic speeds under 30 mph were overrepresented (see Connelly *et al.*, 1998), a decision based on distance would also lead to rejecting larger (in time) gaps, and consequently rejecting more gaps. In their study, Connelly *et al.* (1998) measured the vehicle's actual speed and distance with a laser speed and distance recording device. Primary school children said 'Yes, yes, …' repeatedly until the approaching vehicle reached a point at which they would no longer be prepared to cross in front of it, at which moment they said 'No'. This was the signal to measure the vehicle's speed and distance. Overall, children were setting similar distance thresholds regardless of the vehicle's approach speed. Moreover, judgements were inconsistent, particularly those of the 5- and 6-year-olds. This resulted in safe (i.e. taking the pre-determined crossing time into account) judgements for the lower speeds (< 55 kph), but also an increasing number of risky judgements for the higher speeds (> 56 kph) in particular for the 5- to 9-year-olds. At the highest speeds it were only the 11- to 12-year-olds who made safe decisions. Connelly also calculated the remaining distance and time between the front of the vehicle and the child at the moment the child would have arrived at the centre of the road, had they begun to walk just as they said 'No'. Both the remaining distance and time decreased with the vehicle's approach speed, underlining the finding that judgements were safest for the lowest speeds. Hence, primary school children appear generally overcautious, which is in agreement with the conclusion of Lee and co-workers. However, at higher vehicle speeds, judgements of whether a traffic gap is safe to cross become increasingly risky. Hence, the observation in most studies that the percentage in missed opportunities decreases with age might be caused by a shift from a distance to time strategy instead of setting narrower safety margins (cf. Demetre *et al.*, 1992).[3]

In sum, most authors agree that visual timing judgements of the crossability of traffic gaps change between 5 and 12 years of age. Remarkably, the judgements of the youngest children are the most cautious. It remains unclear, however, what induces the change in the children's ability to judge traffic gaps visually.

Crossing behaviour

With respect to crossing behaviour, a few developmental trends can be identified. The most frequent child pedestrian accident occurs when dashing out on the road, the percentage of which decreases with age (Van der Molen, 1981; Van Schagen and Rothengatter, 1997). Zeedyk *et al.* (2002) is the only experimental study that examined this issue by having children actually cross a road. They reported that, at a T-junction with a moving car, 75 per cent of the 5- and 6-year-olds were either running or skipping across the road, and that when crossing between parked cars half of the children demonstrated this behaviour.[4] Moreover, Limbourg and Gerber (1981) found that children between 3 and 7 years of age crossed the street diagonally instead of at a right angle (see also Ampofo-Boateng and Thomson, 1991). Likewise, the crossing times reported from the pretend road simulation studies tended to decrease with age. Also the inconsistency of the crossing times decreased with age (Lee *et al.*, 1984; Young and Lee, 1987). Some of the observed inconsistency may be due to children attempting to adapt their crossing speed to the time available to cross: the shorter the time, the faster the children tended to walk (Young and Lee, 1987). This ability to adapt walking while crossing warrants much research. In this respect, it is characteristic that only between 15 per cent and 40 per cent of the primary school children are reported to look while crossing the street (Rivara *et al.*, 1991; Zeedyk *et al.*, 2002). Finally, the pretend road simulation studies showed that the time between making a judgement and starting to cross a road systematically decreased with age. Likewise, the inconsistency of this starting delay decreased, indicating that with increasing age children hesitated less before crossing (Lee *et al.*, 1984).

To summarise, there is convincing evidence that the four component skills of road crossing improve during the primary school years. It appears that at 9 years of age children are increasingly aware that the visibility of oncoming traffic may be obstructed, and hence are able to select a safe site and route to cross. In contrast, although looking behaviour is suggested to improve from 7 and 8 years of age, even the 11-year-olds did not perform in the adult range. The ability to visually time crossing also undergoes changes between 5 and 12 years of age. Encouragingly, however, the youngest children appear more cautious. Although it is clear that the youngest children, in particular, often run, other developmental changes in crossing behaviour remain blurred. Because of obvious reasons, the developmental changes of the component skills are to a greater or lesser extent derived from simulation or laboratory studies instead of actual road-crossing behaviour. Hence, it is difficult to compare the developmental rates of the component skills. Nevertheless, it appears that looking behaviour is the most likely candidate as a rate limiter (cf. Thelen and Smith, 1994) for the development of road-crossing skill. As such, training or education programmes that are directed at improving children's looking behaviour (i.e. stopping at the line of vision, looking left–right–left, looking while crossing) might have the largest impact on their safety. Fortunately, there is a real possibility that children might be trained to adequate levels in looking behaviour, and also in selecting a safe site, visual timing, and crossing behaviour. Almost every single study reported that some of the younger children performed like adults. Although the majority of the studies did not report the children's traffic exposure, it seems reasonable to suggest that experience is an important contributor in the children's ability to cross a road safely. The next section, therefore, reviews the attempts that were undertaken to improve children's road-crossing skills.

4. Training programmes

The ultimate goal of training programmes and safety education is a decline in the number of children involved in traffic accidents. However, very large numbers of children would need to be trained before an impact on accident rates would be measurable (Rivara *et al.*, 1991). Therefore, researchers have chosen to evaluate the effects of training programmes on (the components of) road-crossing skill or knowledge of that skill. Firm conclusions about the effectiveness of a training programme can only be drawn from methodologically sound studies. These involve at least a comparison between an intervention and a control group and the verification of long-term effects of the intervention (cf. Duperrex *et al.*, 2002). Unfortunately, it is often considered undesirable to deny some children a training programme, and hence most studies have compared different forms of intervention. With this in mind, the effectiveness of training programmes that have attempted to improve children's ability to select a safe site and route, to look appropriately, to detect crossable gaps, and to actual cross the road, is evaluated.

Training to select a safe site

Most children under 9 years of age are poor at judging a safe place to cross the road (e.g. Ampofo-Boateng and Thomson, 1991). In a series of studies Thomson and Ampofo-Boateng (Ampofo-Boateng *et al.*, 1993; Thomson *et al.*, 1992, 1998), therefore, examined the effectiveness of roadside training in a real road environment and training using a tabletop scale model, or a combination of both. The 5-year-old children were either trained individually or in small groups by parents or highly qualified teachers. The six training sessions of half an hour were aimed at recognising dangerous sites and routes, and emphasised the importance of the visibility of vehicles. The training did not consist of drills, but attempted to improve the children's conceptual understanding. Roadside pre-tests, post-tests and follow up tests at about two and eight months after termination of the training were conducted. The children indicated the safe route by pointing and describing it, though they were never asked to actually walk across the road. It was found that both the roadside and the tabletop training led the children to select safer routes and sites (Ampofo-Boateng *et al.*, 1993; Thomson *et al.*, 1992, 1998). In one study (Ampofo-Boateng *et al.*, 1993), the trained children even performed like 11-year-old control participants. The latter training effect slightly deteriorated after a few months (Ampofo-Boateng *et al.*, 1993), which was not the case in the other studies (Thomson *et al.*, 1992, 1998). The authors concluded that in 5-year-olds, training substantially improves the ability to select safe sites and routes, and that these beneficial effects last at least as long as two months after the training has been terminated.

Notwithstanding these promising results, there is still the unexamined assumption in these studies that there is an automatic transfer from knowledge of perception (i.e. being able to point and describe the safest route) to roadside behaviour (i.e. actually walk across the road). Zeedyk *et al.* (2001) report two studies in which they attempted to address this point. The first study involved training 4- and 5-year-old children to identify safe and dangerous sites. A tabletop model, a board game and a set of illustrations were used. Knowledge was assessed after one week and after six months. Control children were only tested once. The small but significant increase in knowledge, which was brought about after a single 20-minute training session, was retained over six months. All interventions were equally effective. In the second study, Zeedyk *et al.* (2001) examined whether the same children were able to apply their knowledge to real traffic situations by inconspicuously filming the children's road-crossings that were made in the midst of completing a 'treasure trial'. The majority of children crossed the road at dangerous locations (e.g. between parked cars, or at a junction). No differences were found between the intervention and control group. That is, the greater knowledge of the trained group did not result in safer road-crossing behaviour.

To conclude, it has been shown that even 5-year-olds can acquire knowledge or can learn to identify what constitutes a safe site or route to walk across the road. Although these findings appear encouraging, it remains to be demonstrated that this leads to safer road-crossing behaviour. This lack of convincing intervention effects may be due to either the young age of the children (i.e. only 5-year-olds were trained), or perhaps more likely, to inherent limitations in the transfer of (perceptual) knowledge into action (cf. Goodale and Humphrey, 1998; see below section 5).

Training looking behaviour

In the previous section we argued that children's looking behaviour might be a rate limiting parameter in learning to cross a road safely. From the four component skills discussed here, children's ability to look satisfactorily seems to change at the slowest pace. Nevertheless, attempts to train children's looking behaviour are rather scarce. We found two such studies (Limbourg and Gerber, 1981; Rivara *et al.*, 1991). In both studies, children were conspicuously filmed while actually walking across the road before and after the training programme. The training programme of Limbourg and Gerber (1981) consisted of a film and a brochure that instructed parents to practice their 3- to 7-year-old children directly in real traffic situations. Parents were asked to analyse the own child's crossing behaviour and to demonstrate and explain correct behaviour. Correct behaviour comprised, among other things, stopping at the kerb and looking left and right. In their final experiment the authors reported dramatic improvements in both stopping at the kerb (10 per cent vs. 80 per cent) and looking left and right (20 per cent vs. 70 per cent).[5] They also reported, but did not further substantiate the claim, that the improvements were dependent on age and training frequency, and that looking behaviour deteriorated in a follow-up test after four months in all groups, but was still better in the experimental groups than in the control groups. Rivara *et al.* (1991) also used a school training programme that included role-playing, real traffic environments, and theoretical instructions (e.g. the children were taught to make eye contact with the driver). Important limitations of the study were that it did not involve a control group and that there was no verification of the long-term effects. No improvement in stopping at the kerb was found. However, the proportion of children who were looking left–right–left before crossing increased, but only after the parents were involved in the training. Finally there was a two- to threefold increase in the number of children who looked during crossing. In sum, these studies seem to indicate that children's looking behaviour can be trained. However, the findings need validation before we can draw firm conclusions.

Training visually judging 'crossable' traffic gaps

Young and Lee (1987) used the pretend road method to train children to visually judge whether or not traffic gaps are crossable. Five-year-olds were given nine to twelve sessions spread over six to twelve weeks of guided practice on the pretend road. The children received two types of feedback: i) they could see whether they reached the pretend kerb before the vehicle had passed the crossing line, and ii) the trainer reprimanded them if they behaved recklessly or urged them to watch more carefully if they were wasting large gaps. The 5-year-olds in this study performed very well on a single lane. They showed almost no tight fits (unlike their peers in Lee *et al.*'s 1984 study) throughout all the sessions. Moreover, the number of missed opportunities was less than the 7- and 9-year-olds (Lee *et al.*, 1984), and reached almost adult standard in two training sessions. On a two-way road, however, the children missed many more opportunities than the adults, and training only slightly reduced the number of missed opportunities. Demetre *et al.* (1993) aimed to extend these findings. The 5-year-old children received six training sessions on a two-way pretend road or on the two-step task (see section 3). The study included a 14-week and a long-term follow-up assessment (i.e. at six months). Both training programmes resulted in a reduction of the proportion of tight fits and missed opportunities committed by the children. These training effects did not appear very robust. After 14 weeks, reductions in tight fits were only found on the pretend road simulation, whereas reductions in missed opportunities were only present in the two-step task. The long-term follow-up failed to demonstrate any difference from the control group. In sum, although training on the pretend road revealed some promising short-term effects on visual timing skills, these improvements were not retained very long.

Training crossing behaviour

Limbourg and Gerber (1981) reported that after supervised practising in real traffic environments, there was an increase in the number of children who stopped at the kerb before crossing (but see Rivara *et al.*, 1991), which might indicate that fewer children would run across the road. The pretend road simulation training did not reveal systematic effects on crossing time (i.e. sometimes crossing time decreased, sometimes it increased, and sometimes it became more consistent) and the effects were not retained in the follow-up assessments. Likewise, the changes in time taken between making a judgement and starting to walk across (i.e. a decrease in starting delay and its inconsistency) the pretend road were no longer present four weeks after the termination of training (Demetre *et al.*, 1993; Young and Lee, 1987). Finally, Limbourg and Gerber (1981) found that an increasing number of children crossed at a right angle after their behavioural training programme.

5. The necessity to train the road-crossing action

It is now well established that action is inseparable from perception, and that perception is inseparable from action (e.g. Gibson, 1979). Moreover, perception in action is dissociated from perception in knowledge (Goodale and Humphrey, 1998). A major implication of this is that action can only be learned in the context in which it occurs, for example, crossing a road in a real traffic environment. Training on a real road has not been applied frequently because it can be dangerous for children. However, even mimicking the action as closely as possible either visually (e.g. learning to identify safe sites at the roadside) or motorically (e.g. practising on the pretend road) may not be sufficient for improvements in children's road-crossing behaviour to occur. At least that is the rather discouraging conclusion that emerges from the summary of the effectiveness of training programmes for children's component skills of road crossing. Even the pretend road studies did not succeed in bringing about long-term training effects. In fact, only Limbourg and Gerber (1981) reported an improvement in looking behaviour (i.e. stopping at the kerb, and looking left and right) of 3- to 7-year-old children in a follow-up assessment. Although the study appeared methodologically sound, the authors did not report any detail of the long-term training results. Notwithstanding this limitation, it is perhaps no coincidence that the training programme required the children to practise actual walking across the road (obviously, with supervision). There are also a few more studies that suggest that practising the act of road crossing is indispensable for a training programme to be successful. Unfortunately, these studies report a total score instead of separate scores for the component skills of road crossing. For example, Yeaton and Bailey (1978) found an increase of the overall road-crossing score that included waiting at the kerb, looking left and right, watching the vehicle distance, walking, and looking while crossing, even one year after termination of the training programme. Rothengatter (1984) had children practise road crossing in real traffic environments under parental supervision, and found that at the three-month follow-up assessment, 4- to 6-year-olds' road-crossing performance (as indicated by a sum score based on elements like stopping at the kerb, looking left and right, and speed and angle of crossing) was improved without concomitant improvements in traffic knowledge. In other words, there was no transfer between roadside behaviour and traffic knowledge. These findings underline the putative dissociation between perception in action and perception in knowledge, particularly with respect to road-crossing behaviour. Young children therefore require practice; safe road-crossing behaviour is learned by doing (cf. Rothengatter, 1984). In this context, the findings of Ampofo-Boateng, Thomson and co-workers with 5-year-olds who learned to perceptually distinguish dangerous sites and routes from safe ones should be interpreted with great care. The authors did not assess the children's ability during actual road crossing. Practice involving showing and explaining to children the real traffic environment does not automatically transfer to actual road-crossing behaviour (Zeedyk *et al.*, 2001).

In conclusion, the review suggests that training programmes in road-crossing behaviour may enhance safety if, and only if, children actually practise the behaviour itself. It is the degree of exposure to traffic that appears to be one of the most important determinants of safe road-crossing behaviour in young children. As several studies have shown, parents are capable of achieving improvements in their children's road-crossing behaviour (e.g. Limbourg and Gerber, 1981; Rivara *et al.*, 1991; Rothengatter, 1984). The disadvantage is that with parental training programmes it is difficult to assess relevant issues like the nature of the verbal instructions (e.g. explicit or implicit learning; see Masters *et al.*, 2002) and the type of feedback (e.g. knowledge of performance or results) or its frequency. Furthermore, it is perhaps fruitful to examine the additional effects of training by means of video or virtual reality (see chapter 3 by Plumert). However, we should be careful not to throw the baby out with the bath water. It is curious to find that most training efforts so far have been directed at 5-year-old children (e.g. Ampofo-Boateng *et al.*, 1992; Demetre *et al.*, 1993; Rothengatter, 1984; Thomson *et al.*, 1992, 1998; Young and Lee, 1987; Zeedyk *et al.*, 2001). We cannot be sure that the lack of transfer from increasing traffic knowledge to road-crossing behaviour in these young children is not due to the very young age of the participants. Perhaps in older children an increase in traffic knowledge transfers better to roadside behaviour. This is particularly important, because it is the older age group that is allowed to walk unaccompanied (see section 2). A study of Van Schagen and Rothengatter (1997) suggests that cognitive training of road-crossing skills might be beneficial in 6- and 7-year olds. They compared three groups of children who received a classroom cognitive instruction, a roadside behavioural training or a combination of both. Compared to the control group, all three interventions led to improved knowledge *and* road-crossing behaviour on an intersection. It is unknown, however, what aspects of road crossing were tested, and whether these effects were retained over longer periods.

Notes

1 However, there are some conflicting opinions. For instance, Rothengatter (1984) argues that quiet streets are particularly dangerous for younger children, and Grayson (1981) argues that crossing from the offside of a parked vehicle reduces the distance to be walked and that vehicle speed is lowest at junctions.

2 However, it is unclear whether or not in every single trial of these studies a vehicle was actually approaching.

3 Connelly *et al.* (1998), however, suggested that even adults primarily rely on distance.

4 Of course there is no causal relation between running and safe road-crossing behaviour. If a road is clear, it is safer to run across.
5 Table 5 (Limbourg and Gerber, 1981, p. 265) shows that also the two control groups performed better during the post-test, albeit to a lesser degree (i.e. stopping at the kerb 10 per cent vs. 30 per cent, and looking left and right 20 per cent vs. 35 per cent).

References

Ampofo-Boateng, K. and Thomson, J.A. (1991) Children's perception of safety and danger on the road. *British Journal of Psychology*, 82, 487–505.

Ampofo-Boateng, K., Thomson, J.A., Grieve, R., Pitcairn, T., Lee, D.N. and Demetre, J.D. (1993) A developmental and training study of children's ability to find safe routes to cross the road. *British Journal of Developmental Psychology*, 11, 31–45.

Chapman, A.J. and O'Reilly, D. (1999) Children's road safety. *The Psychologists*, 12, 390–2.

Connelly, M.L., Conaglen, H.M., Parsonson, B.S. and Isler, R.B. (1998) Child pedestrians' crossing gap thresholds. *Accident Analysis and Prevention*, 30, 443–53.

Cross R.T. and Mehegan, J. (1988) Young children's conception of speed: possible implications for pedestrian safety. *International Journal of Science Education*, 10, 253–65.

Demetre, J.D. and Gaffin, S. (1994) The salience of occluding vehicles to child pedestrians. *British Journal of Educational Psychology*, 64, 243–51.

Demetre, J.D., Lee, D.N., Grieve, R., Pitcairn, T.K., Ampofo-Boateng, K. and Thomson, J.A. (1993) Young children's learning on road-crossing simulations. *British Journal of Educational Psychology*, 63, 349–59.

Demetre, J.D., Lee, D.N., Pitcairn, T.K., Grieve, R., Thomson, J.A. and Ampofo-Boateng, K. (1992) Errors in young children's decisions about traffic gaps: experiments with roadside simulations. *British Journal of Psychology*, 83, 189–202.

Dhillon, P.K., Lightstone, A.S., Peek-Asa, C. and Kraus, J. (2001) Assessment of hospital and police ascertainment of automobile versus childhood pedestrian and bicyclist collisions. *Accident Analysis and Prevention*, 33, 529–37.

Duperrex, O., Bunn, F. and Roberts, I. (2002) Safety education of pedestrians for injury prevention: a systematic review of randomised controlled trials. *British Medical Journal*, 324, 1129–34.

Foot, H., Tolmie, A., Thomson, J. McLaren, B. and Whelan, K. (1999) Recognising the hazards. *The Psychologist*, 12, 400–2.

Gibson, J.J. (1979) *The Ecological Approach to Visual Perception*. Boston: Houghton Mifflin Company.

Goodale, M.A. and Humphrey, G.K. (1998) The objects of action and perception. *Cognition*, 67, 181–207.

Grayson, G.B. (1981) The identification of training objectives: what shall we tell the children? *Accident Analysis and Prevention*, 13, 169–73.

Hoffmann, E.R., Payne, A. and Prescott, S. (1980) Children's estimates of vehicle approach times. *Human Factors*, 22, 235–40.

Howarth, C.I., Routledge, D.A. and Repetto-Wright, R. (1974) An analysis of road accidents involving child pedestrians. *Ergonomics*, 17, 319–30.

Lee, D.N., Young, D.S. and McLaughlin, C.M. (1984) A roadside simulation of road crossing for children. *Ergonomics*, 27, 1271–81.

Limbourg, M. and Gerber, D. (1981) A parent training program for the road safety education of preschool children. *Accident Analysis and Prevention*, 13, 255–67.

Macpherson, A., Roberts, I. and Pless, I.B. (1998) Children's exposure to traffic and pedestrian injuries. *American Journal of Public Health*, 88, 1840–3.

Masters, R., Law, J. and Maxwell, J. (2002) Implicit and explicit learning in interceptive actions. In K. Davids, G. Savelsbergh, S.J. Bennett and J. van der Kamp (eds), *Interceptive Actions in Sport: Information and Movement* (pp. 126–43). London: Routledge.

Pitcairn, T.K. and Eldman, T. (2000) Individual differences in road crossing ability in young children and adults. *British Journal of Psychology*, 91, 391–410.

Plumert, J.M. and Schwebel, D.C. (1997) Social and temperamental influences on children's overestimation of their physical abilities: Links to accident proneness. *Journal of Experimental Child Psychology*, 67, 317–37.

Rao, R., Hawkins, M. and Guyer, B. (1997) Children's exposure to traffic and risk of pedestrian injury in an urban setting. *Bulletin of the New York Academy of Medicine*, 74, 65–80.

Rivara, F.P. (1990) Child pedestrian injuries in the United States. *American Journal of Diseases of Children*, 144, 692–6.

Rivara, F.P., Bergman, A.B. and Drake, C. (1989) Parental attitudes and practices toward children as pedestrians. *Pediatrics*, 84, 1017–21.

Rivara, F.P., Booth, C.L., Bergman, A.B., Rogers, L.W. and Weiss, J. (1991) Prevention of pedestrian injuries to children: effectiveness of a school training program. *Pediatrics*, 88, 770–5.

Road Accidents Great Britain (2000) London: Her Majesty's Stationery Office.

Roberts, I. (1993) Why have child pedestrian death rates fallen? *British Medical Journal*, 306, 1737–9.

Roberts, I., Carlin, J., Bennett, C., Bergstrom, E., Guyer, B., Nolan, T., Norton, B., Pless, I.B., Rao, R. and Stevenson, M. (1997) An international study of the exposure of children to traffic. *Injury Prevention*, 3, 89–93.

Rothengatter, T. (1984) A behavioural approach to improving traffic behaviour of young children. *Ergonomics*, 27, 147–60.

Routledge, D.A., Repetto-Wright, R. and Howarth, C.I. (1974) The exposure of young children to accident risk as pedestrians. *Ergonomics*, 17, 457–80.

Schwebel, D.C. and Plumert, J.M. (1999) Longitudinal and concurrent relations between temperament, ability estimation, and accident proneness. *Child Development*, 70, 700–12.

Stevenson, M.R. (1996). The validity of children's self-reported exposure to traffic. *Accident Analysis and Prevention*, 28, 599–605.

Thelen, E. and Smith, L.B. (1994) *A Dynamical Systems Approach to the Development of Action and Perception*. Cambridge, MA: MIT Press.

Thomson, J.A., Ampofo-Boateng, K., Lee, D.N., Grieve, R., Pitcairn, T.K. and Demetre, J.D. (1998) The effectiveness of parents in promoting the development of road crossing skills in young children. *British Journal of Educational Psychology*, 68, 475–91.

Thomson, J.A., Ampofo-Boateng, K., Pitcairn, T., Grieve, R., Lee, D.N. and Demetre, J.D. (1992) Behavioural group training of children to find safe routes to cross the road. *British Journal of Educational Psychology*, 62, 173–83.

Thomson, J.A., Tolmie, A., Foot, H.C., and Mclaren, B. (1996) *Child Development and the Aims of Road Safety Education: A Review and Analysis*. Report of the Department of Transport, London: Her Majesty's Stationery Office.

Towner, E.M.L., Jarvis, S.N., Walsh, S.S.M. and Aynsley-Green, A. (1994) Measuring exposure to injury risk in schoolchildren aged 11–14. *British Medical Journal*, 308, 449–52.

Van der Molen, H.H. (1981) Child pedestrian's exposure, accidents and behavior. *Accident Analysis and Prevention*, 13, 193–224.

Van der Molen, H.H., Rothengatter, J.A. and Vinjé, M.P. (1981) Blueprint of an analysis of the pedestrian's task. *Accident Analysis and Prevention*, 13, 175–91.

Van Schagen, I. and Rothengatter, T. (1997) Classroom instructions versus roadside training in traffic safety education. *Journal of Applied Developmental Psychology*, 18, 283–92.

Vinjé, M.P. (1981) Children as pedestrians: abilities and limitations. *Accident Analysis and Prevention*, 13, 225–40.

West, R., Train, H., Junger, M., West, A. and Pickering, A. (1999) Accidents and problem behaviour. *The Psychologist*, 12, 395–7.

Whitebread, D. and Neilson, K. (2000) The contribution of visual search strategies to the development of pedestrian skills by 4–11-year-old children. *British Journal of Educational Psychology*, 70, 539–57.

Yeaton, W.H., and Bailey, J.S. (1978) Teaching pedestrian safety skills to young children: an analysis and one-year follow up. *Journal of Applied Behavior Analysis*, 11, 315–29.

Young, D.S. and Lee, D.N. (1987) Training children in road crossing skills using a roadside simulation. *Accident Analysis and Prevention*, 19, 327–41.

Zeedyk, M.S., Wallace, L., Carcary, B., Jones, K. and Larter, K. (2001) Children and road safety: increasing knowledge does not improve behaviour. *British Journal of Educational Psychology*, 71, 573–94.

Zeedyk, M.S., Wallace, L. and Spry, L. (2002) Stop, look, listen, and think? What young children really do when crossing the road. *Accident Analysis and Prevention*, 34, 43–50.

5 Learning to draw and to write

Issues of variability and constraints

Karl S. Rosengren and
Gregory S. Braswell

1. Introduction

Drawing and writing are complex motor skills that emerge in the second year of life and exhibit significant changes over the next decade. In this chapter we examine drawing and writing skills together because these skills are constrained by similar influences, involve relatively sophisticated use of some sort of implement for leaving marks on a surface, and involve (at least in later periods of development) attempts to communicate information to other individuals. Additionally, writing typically emerges after drawing skills have become somewhat advanced. In this regard, early drawing skills can be viewed as precursors to later writing skills, and writing can be viewed as emerging out of these earlier drawing behaviours.

The main focus of the chapter is to explore how both of these skills change over the course of development. We first describe the changes in these skills using the traditional approach of describing how these skills change with age, then we present a theoretical framework (the TASC-based approach) for examining the changes in these skills over the time, and then we examine additional data from studies of drawing and writing that are consistent with this theoretical framework. We end with some recommendations for future research.

2. General trends in the acquisition of drawing and writing skills

The emergence of drawing and the changes that occur in drawing abilities over the course of development have long captured the attention of parents, teachers, and developmental researchers. One reason for the interest in children's drawings is that the drawings of young children appear quite different from those produced by older children and adults. A second reason for interest in children's drawings is that drawings made by children of the same age often show remarkable similarities. Due to these age-based similarities, some theorists have suggested that children's drawings can be used as a means of understanding how children of different ages think about the world (Case and Okamoto, 1996; DiLeo, 1973; Piaget and Inhelder, 1956). An additional reason for interest in children's drawings is that children with isolated and exceptional drawing skills (Selfe, 1977; Wiltshire, 1987) and isolated drawing deficits have been found (Stiles-Davis, 1988). Both of these findings suggest that the ability to draw may be to some extent influenced by the maturation of specific brain structures. This maturational perspective has dominated much of the past research on children's drawings.

Over the past 50 years vast quantities of children's drawings have been collected and used to create detailed developmental accounts of children's drawing (e.g. Cox, 1992; Eng, 1954; Goodnow, 1977; Kellogg, 1969; Willats, 1977; Gardner, 1980). These descriptive accounts of the emergence of drawing and writing suggest that children's first drawing attempts occur at about 18 months of age. These first drawings are usually described as 'scribbles', basically random marks across a page. Often these early scribbles are dominated by vertical lines and circular paths. Researchers disagree on whether children at this point are merely exploring the interaction between the implement and surface or actually trying to communicate specific ideas in these scribbles (Gardner, 1980). By age 3, many children produce copies of simple lines and circles. By age 4 children are usually able to combine vertical and horizontal lines to form a cross. At age 5, children can typically combine horizontal and oblique lines to form a triangle and by age 7, they can combine a series of oblique lines to form a diamond (Cox, 1992, p. 162).

Kellogg (1969) developed a different description of drawing development that went beyond the production of simple shapes. Her account described how children acquire certain 'concepts' of drawing that can be incorporated into more complex pictures as the child ages. For example, in her description children develop from the scribbling stage to the combine stage, where children acquire the ability to produce simple shapes. Next, in the aggregate stage, children begin to use simple shapes together to generate more complex figures, such as a face. Children then progress to the pictorial stage, where they attempt to draw objects in a more complex and realistic manner.

Although much of the drawing research has focused on the final product of children's drawings, researchers have also investigated *how* children draw (Gesell and Ames, 1946). Gesell and Ames investigated age differences in the directionality of strokes produced by children and adults when they were instructed to produce horizontal and vertical lines, circles, squares, triangles, and other geometric shapes. Similar to the research focusing on the final product, these researchers reported an age-based progression in stroke production. For example, Gesell and Ames found that young children first produce a cross as two parallel lines, then progress to constructing the cross from four lines all produced from a central position. In contrast, older children and adults typically produce a cross by first producing a vertical line drawn from the top to the bottom and then drawing a horizontal line from left to right through the centre of the vertical line.

Goodnow and Levine (1973) extended the work of Gesell and Ames (1946) and suggested that the development of drawing can be described in terms of the acquisition of a series of drawing principles that govern the production of both simple shapes and more complex figures. These production principles determine both where a figure might be initiated (e.g. topmost or leftmost part of the figure) and the order and direction of the strokes (e.g. draw all horizontal strokes left to right) needed to complete a figure. Like the product-centred accounts of children's drawing development, these early accounts were also highly descriptive, documenting an age-related acquisition of certain drawing principles without much attempt at understanding the origins of these principles. Researchers have extended this approach to describe the development of children's drawings of more complex figures (Golomb and Farmer, 1983; Goodnow, 1977; Van Sommers, 1984). One finding from this research is that young children tend to draw complex figures by starting with major components and progressing to the details.

It is during the later stages of early drawing development that children first begin to write letters and form words. Historically, in many Western cultures children first learned how to write when they entered the first or second grade of formal schooling (Sovik, 1993). This initial foray into writing often involved specific instruction regarding the 'correct' shape of letters and the 'correct' order and direction of strokes to produce those letters. Currently, it is not uncommon for young children to learn to write their names and the alphabet prior to entering formal schooling. The implication of children acquiring writing skills prior to the start of formal schooling is that the role of teachers may have changed from providing the 'initial' instruction in writing to 'correcting' children's early writing behaviours to conform to the preferred norm.

Regardless of how and when children first acquire early writing skills, children's early writing attempts are often characterized by an inability to control the proportions within a letter, an inability to control the size across letters, a seemingly arbitrary arrangement of letters on the paper, and the production of mirror images (Reimer *et al.*, 1975; Stennet *et al.*, 1972). With increasing age, accuracy (legibility) and speed of writing improve significantly (Sovik, 1993).

Acquisition of different grips

One area of research that cuts across both drawing and writing focuses on how children hold a drawing or writing implement. Most of this research has been descriptive in nature, examining the developmental progression from less 'mature' to more 'mature' grip configurations (Rosenbloom and Horton, 1971; Saida and Miyashita, 1979; Sasson *et al.*, 1986; Thomassen and Teulings, 1983; Ziviani, 1982, 1983). An assumption underlying this research is that the manner in which children hold a writing implement will impact on the quality of the drawing or writing product (Martlew, 1992; Ziviani and Elkins, 1986).

The descriptions of the acquisition of different grips suggest that children's earliest attempts to grip a writing implement often involve a palmar grasp, where the implement is held primarily between the palm and fingers. This is a powerful type of grasp that enables a child to produce firm, broad strokes. At the same time, this type of grasp makes the production of relatively fine movements difficult. If one tries, for example, to sign one's name as small as possible using this type of grip, one will find that the signature is likely to be less legible and larger than that produced with one's preferred grip.

As children age, they typically shift the writing implement away from the palm, and the thumb and the fingers begin to play a more dominant role in the grip. Typically by age 4 or 6, a tripod grasp emerges, which involves holding the implement firmly between the thumb and the first two fingers (Rosenbloom and Horton, 1971). At this stage of the development of grip configurations, the implement and the components of the hand are thought to be relatively fixed and unmoving. The final stage of grip development involves the acquisition of the 'preferred grip', the dynamic tripod. This grip is differentiated from a basic tripod grasp by small movements of the fingers and thumb. These small 'dynamic' movements are thought to enable the drawer to produce fine details with accuracy. By this maturational account, grip configurations are thought to reach maturity by about age 6 or 7 (Rosenbloom and Horton, 1971), an age where instruction in writing skills is often first introduced to children in formal school settings. Ziviani (1983) has shown, however, that children continue to modify and refine their grip configuration between the ages of 6 and 14.

3. Assumptions underlying past research

The majority of the past research on children's drawings seems to be driven by a number of underlying assumptions. The first assumption is that much of early drawing and writing ability is governed by the maturation of certain physiological structures (i.e. brain, arm, hand, and fingers) and develops in an endogenous manner, relatively unconstrained by factors external to the child. An additional assumption of past research, which is related to the emphasis on maturation, is the assumption that there is a relatively stable progression from the young child to the mature adult, with early products, grip configurations, production sequences, or representations, being replaced by more complex, sophisticated, and effective ones. Inherent in these accounts is a notion that at any given age both the products and processes of drawing are relatively stable and consistent both within a given child and across children of the same age. Indeed, much of the research in this area has been fuelled by what Lockman (2000) refers to as 'modal concerns', where researchers devote their energy to describing age norms for the emergence of a particular behaviour. These assumptions have also led to the use of children's drawings in various assessments that examine perceptual motor development (Bruinicks, 1978; Frankenburg *et al.*, 1990), cognitive development (Goodnough, 1926; Harris, 1963), and social-emotional development (Koppitz, 1968). All of these assessments are based on the notions that 'normal' children of a given age will produce highly similar products, grip configurations and production sequences, and that the drawing outcomes will be based on similar internal representations.

Perhaps due to the focus on the consistency and stability within children of a given age, there has been little emphasis on actually understanding the processes underlying change in children's drawing and writing. Recently, researchers in both motor and cognitive development have begun to recognise that variability within and across children is often more characteristic of development than is stability (Rosengren and Braswell, 2001; Siegler, 1994, 1996; Thelen and Smith,

1994). Indeed, Siegler and Thelen have both argued that variability plays a very important role in driving developmental change. Part of recognising that development is highly variable involves embracing the notion that development is a highly complex process involving both internal and external factors that constrain the developmental pathway. In the next section of this chapter we explore the concept of constraints and describe a particular theoretical account, the TASC-based approach (Rosengren and Savelsbergh, 2000) designed to investigate this complexity.

4. The TASC-based approach to perceptual–motor development

The TASC-based approach to perceptual motor development was developed by Rosengren and Savelsbergh (2000, 2001) in order to account for the high degree of variability that has been observed in development and in response to age-based accounts of development that implicitly place maturational factors in a central role in the developmental process. Rosengren and Savelsbergh (2000) argue that the primary focus of developmental researchers should not be on cataloguing age differences in children, but should be focused on the tasks that children are confronted with as they age. This emphasis on variation within specific tasks, rather than on age-based differences, is designed to shift the focus away from strictly maturational descriptions, to ones that incorporate how a variety of constraints impact on the emergence and development of specific behaviours.

Variability

Similar to other researchers in the domains of tool-use (Lockman, 2000), cognitive development (Siegler, 1996) and motor development (Thelen and Smith, 1994), Rosengren and Savelsbergh (2000) suggest that variability plays a very important role in development. Indeed, a central assumption of the TASC-based approach is that variability is an inherent characteristic of human behaviour. Variability is considered an evolutionary adaptation that enables an individual to explore the task space and to investigate the constraints that operate in a specific situation. From their perspective variability is highly adaptive, enabling the child to select from a variety of behaviours a behaviour (or in some situations a small set of behaviours) that leads to an optimal solution for a given task. Thus, the label 'TASC' is derived from an emphasis on *task*-related *adaptation* and *selection*, influenced by *constraints* both within and external to the child.

Learning and development

Rosengren and Savelsbergh (2000) have also made a distinction between developmental and non-developmental tasks. Developmental tasks are defined as those that are necessary for a child to solve in order for survival. By this definition, skills such as grasping objects and walking are viewed as solutions to the developmental tasks of obtaining food and moving to safety. Non-developmental tasks are associated with the acquisition of skills that are *not* necessary for survival. Drawing and writing skills have emerged to aid communication, but their overall survival value is less clear. Thus, these skills are viewed as solutions to non-developmental tasks. Rosengren and Savelsbergh (2000, 2001) argue that the term 'development' should perhaps be reserved to describe the emergence of behaviours related to solving developmental tasks, and the term 'learning' should be reserved for describing the emergence and change of behaviours related to solving non-developmental tasks. Thus, in their view, we should be talking about how drawing and writing skills are learned, not how they develop.

Constraints

A central aspect of the TASC-based approach is an emphasis on constraints. Drawing and writing skills are strongly influenced by a number of different types of constraints. Newell (1986) has described three broad types of constraints that influence motor skills and the manner in which they change over the course of development. These are environmental, organismic, and task constraints.

Environmental constraints

Environmental constraints refer to general characteristics of the world that in some way limit or shape behaviour. Gravity, general characteristics of surfaces, and the basic laws of physics (forces and their interaction) can be viewed as environmental constraints. With respect to drawing and writing, an important environmental constraint is the friction that arises from interaction between a drawing or writing implement and the surface. The actual friction produced in a particular situation, however, will depend on the force with which a child presses against the drawing or writing surface (an organismic constraint) and the specific characteristics of the implement and drawing surface (task constraints).

Organismic constraints

Organismic constraints refer to characteristics of the organism that serve to limit or shape behaviour. The physical structure of the child's hand and arm, biomechanical factors related to the structure of joints and muscles, general maturational factors, and the level of the child's perceptual and cognitive functioning all act as organismic constraints. Rosengren and Savelsbergh (2001) view the child's goal in relation to the task as one of the most important organismic contraints. The child's goal serves to organise the child's behaviour, providing a purpose and structure to what the child is trying to accomplish. In this sense, a child's drawing and writing behaviour is not purely the result of self-organisation, because the goal provides an overall organisational structure to the child's behaviour. With respect to drawing or writing, organismic constraints include such things as whether the child is right or left handed, how much experience they have had with drawing and writing, his or her overall level of motivation to achieve some goal, the force that he or she is imparting on the surface with the implement, and the goal the child has for this given task.

Task constraints

Task constraints refer to properties of the specific task or problem that the child or adult is confronting. With respect to drawing and writing, task constraints include such things as the characteristics of the drawing implement (size, shape, and colour of the implement, hardness of the writing tip, etc.) and drawing surface (orientation with respect to gravity, hardness, shape, and colour of the drawing or writing surface, etc.). Additional task constraints may include specific instructions given to the child, and the presence of a peer, parent, or teacher during the drawing or writing episode.

Impact of constraints

As a child or adult engages in the drawing or writing process these different types of constraints interact to limit the range of possible behaviours that a child or adult can produce. These constraints also serve to create particular movement opportunities for the child. In a given situation, the three types of constraints always interact to determine a set of possible outcomes that can be produced, given the particular configuration of constraints and their interaction. For example, the type of implement (a crayon or piece of chalk) and the type of surface (a piece of paper or sidewalk) interact with the child's physical abilities and lead the child to adopt a particular grip configuration. Changing the implement changes the frictional characteristics of the tasks, and potentially enables the child to adopt a different grip configuration that might enable her to produce a different range of possible outcomes. For example, if a child wants to draw a picture on the sidewalk with a piece of chalk, the interaction between the chalk and the sidewalk leads to high levels of friction which necessitate that the child adopt a more powerful grip to hold the chalk. At the same time, adopting a powerful grip makes it more difficult for the child to produce more fine details in her drawing. In this instance, the grip configuration and the nature of the implement interact and may influence the child to make her drawing larger than initially desired, and to choose certain types of images to make (ones lacking small, fine detail) over others.

Methodological considerations

From a TASC-based approach, researchers should place less emphasis on determining age-based norms and more emphasis on investigating issues related to variability in behaviour. Much of the research methods we currently have in developmental science are based on the assumption that behaviours are relatively stable and the analytic techniques generally focus on analysing mean differences (Rosengren and Braswell, 2001). Focusing on variability, rather than stability, may entail collecting different types of data that enable researchers to focus on variation rather than stability, and developing new analytic techniques for investigating aspects of variability (Rosengren and Braswell, 2001; Van Geert and Van Dyk, 2002). An initial step in the TASC-based approach is to document variability in the behaviour as a child engages in trying to solve a particular problem or task.

5. Variability in the acquisition of drawing and writing skills

Although much of the past research on the acquisition of drawing and writing skills has focused on stable products and patterns produced by children at specific ages, a number of researchers have acknowledged that the drawing and writing process is actually more heterogeneous than is typically reported.

A basic assumption of the TASC-based approach is that variation in drawing and writing performance will occur as a function of changing constraints. Organismic constraints will change as the child gains better control over their hands and arms as a function of both maturation and experience. Organismic constraints will also change as the child's goals change from exploring the impact of making marks on a piece of paper or wall to communicating ideas on some surface. Task constraints will change as the specific tasks the child is confronted with change. These changes may involve variations in the instructions a child is given in a particular drawing session, or variations in the frictional coefficients as a child attempts to draw with a different drawing implement. Constraints always interact, so changing one constraint impacts on the entire system, yielding significantly different outcomes.

Variability in grip configuration

A number of researchers have reported variation in grip configurations in children of the same age. In a series of studies of the writing behaviour of 5- to 7-year-old children, Blote and her colleagues (Blote and Van der Heijden, 1988; Blote *et al.*, 1987) found that roughly 40 per cent of the children used a grip other than the dynamic tripod. Examining the acquisition of grip configurations cross-culturally, Saida and Miyashiti (1979) report that Japanese children acquired the dynamic tripod grip much earlier than British children described by Rosenbloom and Horton (1971). Saida and Miyashita (1979) suggest that cultural differences in grip acquisition may be due to differential experiences, specifically the use of chopsticks in Japan.

Blote *et al.* (1987) also reported some variability in the grip configurations of individual children. For example, they found that many of the 6-year-old children began drawing with a tripod grip, but shifted to a power grip, such as the palmar grip, over the course of the drawing session. Likewise Greer and Lockman (1998) have reported considerable variability in grip configurations and pen positioning within individual 3-year-old children. By 5 years of age the variability in these children's grip configurations and pen positioning was reduced substantially. Greer and Lockman (1998) suggest that the variability observed in early writing behaviour stems from children exploring what the pen and writing surface afford, and a decrease in variability occurs as children discover particular behaviours that maximise stability and efficiency of the motor skill.

Organismic constraints

The biomechanics of the fingers, hand and arm provide a set of organismic constraints on the drawing process. Stroke directionality appears to be particularly susceptible to biomechanical constraints (Van Sommers, 1984). Children and adults tend to produce vertical lines from top to bottom, perhaps because finger and hand flexion, which involve moving the writing implement downward or inward toward the body, is more efficient than extension (Thomassen *et al.*, 1992; Van Sommers, 1984).

The strongest evidence for biomechanically-driven stroke directionality comes from data on horizontal line production. When producing horizontal lines, right-handed individuals prefer to draw from left to right, whereas left-handed individuals prefer to draw in the opposite direction (Van Sommers, 1984). In both instances horizontal line production tends to proceed from the body's midline outward. This effect has been demonstrated for adults (Van Sommers, 1984) as well as children of various ages (Gesell and Ames, 1946; Scheirs, 1990). Also, this effect is not limited to the production of solitary lines or simple geometric figures. In a study by Glenn *et al.* (1995), right-handed children often produced components of a human figure from left to right, and left-handed children often produced the same components from right to left. Thus mirror production occurs in the production of both simple horizontal strokes and the sequencing of parts in more complex figures. Although Van Sommers (1984) noted few age-related differences in directionality preferences, others (e.g. Braswell and Rosengren, 2000; Goodnow and Levine, 1973) have found that older right-handed drawers exhibited stronger directionality preferences than younger drawers. This result suggests that biomechanics appear to play an increasingly important role in determining stroke directionality with age as individuals become more experienced, efficient drawers.

Another type of organismic constraint that influences the manner in which children draw and write are various cognitive principles. These principles may also be thought of as constraints that operate on the process of drawing. Many researchers have proposed that the production of entire figures as well as individual strokes are constrained by abstract principles. For instance, Phillips and colleagues have posited that planning the sequence and placement of strokes to produce an image is largely driven by procedural representations (Phillips *et al.*, 1978; Phillips *et al.*, 1985). That is, children and adults follow a set sequence to produce a triangle, stick figure, Necker cube, and so on. While individuals may rely on procedural representations for constructing well-practised forms, this may not always be the case. Again, a focus on modal concerns may have led researchers to overlook substantial variability in the production sequences used in drawing. Indeed, a number of researchers have found considerable intrapersonal variability in the production of drawing shapes and complex figures, and this finding reveals the limits of this notion of set procedures (Braswell and Rosengren, 2000; Van Sommers, 1983).

Instead of procedural representations, others have proposed that more general abstract principles guide the process of drawing. For example, Goodnow and Levine (1973) proposed a series of general principles for starting figures (start principles) and for stroke directionality (progression principles). The four start principles include starting with the leftmost point, starting at the uppermost point, starting a vertical line from top to bottom, or if drawing a figure with a left oblique starting with the left oblique from top to bottom. If there is a conflict between starting at the topmost point versus the leftmost point, the former predominates.

The three progression principles entail drawing horizontal lines from left to right, vertical lines from top to bottom, and threading. Threading is used to describe the situation where an individual completes a figure or part of a figure without lifting the implement from the surface. For example, in drawing a triangle, one can draw three separate and distinct lines, lifting the implement off of the surface between the drawing of each stroke or one can draw the triangle in a more continuous manner by not lifting the implement off the surface and threading.

In Goodnow and Levine's (1973) study, adherence to the start position principles increased across age groups. Use of threading, however, increased then decreased over the various child and adult age groups, whereas the other two progression rules followed an opposite pattern (because threading overrides them). As discussed above, stroke directionality, aside from threading, may be driven primarily by biomechanics. However, start position may be guided more by cognitive constraints, given that handedness has little effect on the propensity to start figures from the top and/or left (Van Sommers, 1984).

Many of these cognitive constraints are shaped by cultural influences, particularly by literacy and education. For example, it has been suggested that counter-clockwise circle production by older children and adults in Western cultures is primarily based on educational experience (Thomassen and Teulings, 1979). Cross-cultural comparisons have also demonstrated that differences in writing systems are often related to differences in stroke production.

Interestingly, even though the text as a whole proceeds in opposite directions across the Hebrew and Roman writing systems, few differences in stroke directionality have been noted between Hebrew and Roman alphabets (Goodnow *et al.*, 1973). This is probably because both systems primarily rely on left-to-right strokes within letters. However, one might expect to find differences for a writing system such as Arabic, in which words *and* individual characters are written from right to left. Lieblich *et al.* (1975) examined differences in stroke production between Jewish and Arab Israeli children in kindergarten through eighth grade. While copying vertical lines both Jewish and Arab children typically proceeded from top to bottom. However, an interesting difference was discovered in how these two groups produced horizontal lines. The Jewish children of all ages mainly drew from left to right. Drawing from right to left became more prevalent across age groups for the Arab children, as they became more experienced with their handwriting system.

Differences in stroke directionality have also been found between Roman letters and Chinese characters. Wong and Kao (1991) asked children in Hong Kong to draw Goodnow and Levine's (1973) geometric stimuli. Overall, Goodnow and Levine's drawing principles were more prevalent among the Chinese sample than the original sample collected in the United States, except for starting with a vertical line. The Chinese children also adhered to starting at the top and the starting at the leftmost point at a younger age than children in the United States. Given these various differences in production principles across cultures, the significance of having experience with particular writing systems is clear.

Task constraints

As described previously, task constraints include the characteristics of the drawing or writing implement, the characteristics of the surface being drawn on, the orientation of the drawing surface, and any instructions given to the child. Changing task parameters and instructions exerts a significant impact on drawing and writing, and is quite well documented (Arrowsmith *et al.*, 1994; Barrett *et al.*, 1985; Burton, 1980; Chen, 1985; Davis, 1983, 1984; Golomb, 1973; Kossyln *et al.*, 1977; Lewis *et al.*, 1993; Light, 1985; Sitton and Light, 1992; Taylor and Bacharach, 1982). In this section we explore more closely the impact of changing task constraints on the child's drawing behaviour. We begin with a brief description of some of our own work on children's grip configurations then discuss the impact of changing instructional demands.

We have conducted two studies designed to examine the effect of changing task constraints on young children's grip configurations (Rosengren *et al.*, 1998). One of the main goals of the study was to examine whether children's grip configurations were actually as stable as previous research has suggested. In the first study, 3-year-old children were presented with a wide range of different drawing implements (ten different ones), ranging from a very thin pencil (that broke if too much force was applied) to a very thick piece of chalk. A number of 8½-by-11-inch sheets of printer paper were provided to the children. The instructions given to the children were simply to produce a drawing or series of drawings, but to try and use all of the different implements over the course of the drawing. The children's drawing behaviour was videotaped, and two independent coders coded the children's overall grip configurations, changes in the grip configurations, and changes children made within the particular grip configurations. The grip configurations coded included a palmar grasp, a digital grasp, a modified tripod grasp, a tripod grasp, and a dynamic tripod grasp. The changes in grip configurations that were recorded included movement of the thumb or fingers within a particular grip configuration and changes in flexion and extension of specific fingers.

The overall result from this study was that children made a lot of changes in both their overall grip configuration and within particular grip configurations. All of the children changed their grip configuration at least once over the course of the ten-minute drawing session, with children averaging about 12 changes in their overall grip configuration. Changes were also quite common within particular grip configurations. Children averaged 47 different within-grip changes. This is a considerable degree of variability.

In a second study, the implement characteristics were kept the same (in this case a set of markers was used), but we varied the task instructions. In this study, children were asked to perform a number of different tasks, including drawing horizontal lines as fast as possible, drawing vertical lines as fast as possible, copying a series of simple shapes (a cross, triangle, square, and circle), and free drawing. It was assumed that the free drawing task might lead the children to produce drawings with some fine details and thus elicit more use of the dynamic tripod. Children's grip configurations were not as variable in this study, though variation rather than stability was still the norm. Two-thirds of the children (12/18) exhibited one or more changes in their grip configurations over the course of this study and all of the children exhibited changes within particular grip configurations.

The results of both of these studies suggest that for 3-year-olds, grip configurations clearly vary as a function of the implement and task. Rather than primarily exhibiting immature grip configurations, children seem to be exploring the dynamics of the task situation. This exploration involves trying out a variety of different grip configurations. Fewer grip changes were seen in adults, but even adults exhibited some variation in their grip configurations.

A central assumption of much of the work on children's drawing and writing is that the manner in which a child holds his or her drawing or writing implement relates to the quality of the final product (Martlew, 1992). We explicitly examined this issue by investigating whether the quality of children's shape-copying varied by grip configuration or by variability in grip configuration. Two independent coders rated the quality of the children's copied shapes using a 4-point scale (0 = unrecognisable scribble, 1 = clearly a shape, but not clear that the drawing was of the target shape, 2 = clearly the target shape, but one dimension of the shape varied by at least 50 per cent from the target, and 3 = an accurate copy of the target shape). The results were then averaged across the shapes and children were categorised as producing either high- or low-quality drawings. We then examined whether grip configuration or variability in grip configuration were related to drawing quality. We found no overall effect of grip configuration, but we did find a significant effect of grip variability. Children who varied their grip configurations a lot tended to produce poorer-quality copies than children who did not vary their grip very much.

Task constraints also influence both stroke directionality and the starting point of figures. For example, in a study of children's shape copying, Braswell and Rosengren (2000) found that modal start position (top, bottom, left, right) and directionality of strokes (left to right, right to left) varied considerably as a function of the shape the children were copying. The majority of the 4- to 5-year-olds in this study began crosses and triangles at the top of the shape, but started circles at the bottom of the shape.

Task effects on the drawing product

Much of the research investigating task effects on children's drawings suggests that children of a particular age do not produce uniform products across specific tasks, and that the products are quite sensitive to task demands. For example, children who typically draw tadpoles to represent the human form may produce more complete pictures when given partially drawn figures or models (Golomb, 1973). Even children who are able to produce conventional human figures will alter their images when the task is varied. In one study, Sitton and Light (1992) asked 4- to 6-year-olds to draw a man, a woman, a boy, and a girl both individually and in contrasting pairs (man/woman, boy/girl). The researchers examined whether children included different defining features (e.g. gender- and age-typed hair and clothing) in their drawings. The older participants, but not the younger ones, specified more characteristics that identified the figures when they were asked to draw the contrasting pairs than when asked to draw only individuals.

Similar task effects have been demonstrated for the depiction of mugs, which are often drawn in canonical orientation even when the handle of the mug is not visible to the drawer (Davis, 1983, 1984; Lewis *et al.*, 1994; Taylor and Bacharach, 1982). For example, Davis (1983) demonstrated that 5- and 6-year-olds are able to draw a mug with its handle turned away, as they see it, when it is placed in contrast with a mug placed in its canonical orientation. Also, the nature of the stimulus itself exerts a strong effect regardless of the instructions given. Young children will often produce more accurate pictures when copying two-dimensional stimuli instead of three-dimensional stimuli (Chen, 1985).

Instructions (task constraints) often interact with the age of the child (an organismic constraint). For example, young children (4-year-olds) often will not alter their drawing behaviour across different instructions. Yet slightly older children will adapt their drawing behaviour to fit the instructions. It is likely that younger children may not have enough appropriate options within their graphic repertoire, may not fully attend to the instructions, or that the measures used in the past investigations are not sensitive enough to capture any variability across instructions (Barrett *et al.*, 1985). Once children acquire a sufficient range of drawing skills, they produce different drawings as a function of changing task demands (Davis, 1983). In general, it appears that communicative contexts exert strong effects on the end product of drawing, yet these effects interact with organismic constraints, such as the age and ability of the child.

Researchers have also found that changing instructions may influence the process of drawing as well as the product. In particular, the sequence and direction of specific strokes in the production of an image may vary as a function of the task. For example, right-handers typically produce horizontal lines from left to right. However, when drawing arrows, the direction of the arrow often dictates the directionality of the horizontal stroke (Van Sommers, 1984). If the arrow points to the left, many right-handers will draw the horizontal stroke from right to left.

The effects of changing task instructions have been cleverly shown with respect to drawing ambiguous figures. For example, the order of strokes has been found to vary depending upon whether the same ambiguous figure is described as a man with a telescope or as a cocktail with a cherry (Van Sommers, 1984; Vinter, 1999).

The order of stroke production in which larger graphic units are produced also appears to be context-dependent (Van Sommers, 1984). For example, the order in which two letters are drawn may be influenced by the instructions given to the drawer (e.g. draw A in front of B versus A behind B).

Overall, the research suggests that children and adults are quite sensitive to changing task constraints. In this way, drawing may be equated with other complex systems that show sensitivity to changing initial conditions. The fact that the drawing outcome is found to vary significantly with changing task constraints makes a purely maturational account of drawing untenable.

Interaction of constraints

The importance of one type of constraint compared to another may vary across drawing episodes and even within a particular drawing episode. For example, cognitive constraints appear to largely determine the starting point of a figure, whereas organismic constraints drive the directionality of subsequent strokes. Furthermore, one type of constraint may override the other at times. For example, horizontal line directionality appears to be mainly dependent on biomechanical constraints, yet it is often influenced by cognitive constraints. Four examples illustrate this point. First, the right-handed Arab children in Lieblich *et al.*'s (1975) study increasingly produced horizontal strokes contrary to biomechanical preferences as they became more experienced with using the Arabic alphabet. Second, directionality of circle production has been shown to depend on whether the drawer makes rapid strokes or slow, deliberate strokes (Thomassen and Teulings, 1979). Third, the meaning of a graphic symbol often plays a role in how it is reproduced. Right-handed adults, who typically draw horizontal lines from left to right, will often draw the horizontal component of a left-pointing arrow in the direction of the arrow, that is, from right to left (Van Sommers, 1984). Fourth, planning considerations often override biomechanical preferences. This often occurs during anchoring. Anchoring involves drawing new strokes outward from previously drawn lines. This technique is thought to be used to ensure accuracy (Thomassen, 1992; Van Sommers, 1984), although there are many potential instances when it may conflict with biomechanical constraints. Such instances were explored in a study by Braswell and Rosengren (2000). Four- to 7-year-olds and adults copied a picture of a house with a sun and a picture of a smiling face with hair. The authors examined the use of anchoring to produce hairs at the top of the face picture and the rays around the sun in the other picture. Interestingly, the degree to which both hairs and sunrays were anchored declined across age. In fact, many older participants often anchored the rays around the bottom of the sun and drew rays inward around the top of the sun. These participants therefore demonstrated more of a preference for top-down stroke production. One possible explanation for this pattern is that younger children may rely more upon anchoring, because of its accuracy benefits, than older drawers who have more manual control.

Based on the literature reviewed, multiple sources of evidence demonstrate that cognitive and biomechanical constraints interact in various, complex, ways. Some planning considerations, such as anchoring, may sometimes conflict with (if the previous stroke is below or to the right of the new stroke) and sometimes match (if the previous stroke is above or to the left of the new stroke) biomechanical constraints. Also, the meaning assigned to an image may override or match directionality preferences based on anatomical structure (e.g. drawing arrows that face right or left). The parameters of the drawing task (e.g. pitting speed vs. accuracy) and the cultural milieu (especially in terms of writing systems) in which one becomes an experienced drawer provide other contexts in which these various constraints interact. Together, these and other factors help shape the interplay between constraints on drawing behaviour.

6. Recommendations for future research

If we adopt the TASC-based approach to the acquisition of drawing and writing skills, a number of directions for future research are apparent. First, we must continue to explore variation in the drawing and writing behaviour of young children. A central goal of this exploration will be to determine when variability and stability are the norm and when they are indicative of behavioural problems. Clearly, more longitudinal studies of children's drawing and writing behaviour need to be conducted in order to investigate changes in variability over time. In conjunction with these studies, we need to develop more sophisticated techniques for examining variability and changes in variability over time (Rosengren and Braswell, 2001).

Second, we need to focus more on identifying the constraints that are operating as a child performs a particular task. We also need to explore how these constraints influence behaviour. In addition, we need to explore how these constraints change over time and how these changes influence the behaviour of a child engaged in a particular task. For example, it might be the case that in the early stages of writing acquisition, letter reversals commonly seen in young children arise primarily from biomechanical constraints that govern the directionality of strokes. One implication of this is that right-handed children might produce different types of letter reversals than left-handed children. As far as we know this issue has not been investigated. With increasing age, cognitive constraints may override these biomechanical constraints. This process may not occur in children who continue to produce letter reversals. By identifying the constraints that are relevant in a particular task and by examining how these change over time, we may be able to develop better intervention techniques for children who exhibit delays in the acquisition of some behaviours.

Third, we need to examine in much greater detail how various constraints interact to lead to a particular behaviour. Constraints do not work in isolation; they interact with each other to produce a particular range of behaviours that satisfy the current goal of the child. With respect to grip configurations, finger strength (an organismic constraint) may interact with frictional components of the implement and surface (an environmental constraint) to determine whether a child adopts a particular grip configuration. In our view, behaviours should always be viewed as emerging from the interaction of constraints as a child approaches a particular task with a specific goal in mind.

Children's drawings are inherently interesting. Unfortunately, much of the focus of past research has been on cataloguing the modal aspects of children's drawing and writing behaviour. This 'modal concern' (Lockman, 2000) has been based on the assumption that much of drawing and writing behaviour is governed by maturational processes. Yet, much of the research on drawing and writing behaviour indicates a considerable degree of variability, not just between children of different ages, but also between children of the same age, and even in individual children over repeated drawings. Future research in this area must strive to understand the causes of this variability and the role of variability in the acquisition of drawing and writing skills.

References

Arrowsmith, C.J., Cox, M.V. and Eames, K. (1994) Eliciting partial occlusions in the drawings of 4- and 5-year-olds. *British Journal of Developmental Psychology*, 12, 577–84.

Barrett, M.D., Beaumont, A.V. and Jennett, M.S. (1985) Some children do sometimes do what they have been told to do: task demands and verbal instructions in children's drawing. In N.H. Freeman and M.V. Cox (eds), *Visual Order: The Nature and Development of Pictorial Representation* (pp. 176–87). Cambridge: Cambridge University Press.

Blote, A.W. and Van der Heijden, P.G.M. (1988) A follow-up study on writing posture and writing movement in young children. *Journal of Human Movement Studies*, 14, 57–74.

Blote, A.W., Zielstra, E.M. and Zoetewey, M.W. (1987) Writing posture and writing movement in kindergarten. *Journal of Human Movement Studies*, 13, 323–41.

Braswell, G.S. and Rosengren, K.S. (2000) Decreasing variability in the development of graphic production. *International Journal of Behavioural Development*, 24, 153–66.

Bruininks, R.H. (1978) *Bruininks–Oseretsky Test of Motor Proficiency*. Circle Pines, MN: American Guidance Service.

Burton, J. (1980) Representing experience from imagination and observation. *School Arts*, 80, 26–30.

Case, R. and Okamoto, Y. (1996) The role of central conceptual structures in the development of children's thought. *Monographs of the Society for Research in Child Development* (Serial No. 246).

Chen, M.J. (1985) Young children's representational drawings of solid objects: a comparison of drawing and copying. In N.H. Freeman and M.V. Cox (eds), *Visual Order: The Nature and Development of Pictorial Representation* (pp. 157–75). Cambridge: Cambridge University Press.

Cox, M. (1992) *Children's Drawings*. New York: Penguin.

Davis, A.M. (1983) Contextual sensitivity in young children's drawings. *Journal of Experimental Child Psychology*, 35, 478–86.

Davis, A.M. (1984) Noncanonical orientation without occlusion: children's drawings of transparent objects. *Journal of Experimental Child Psychology*, 37, 451–62.

DiLeo, J.H. (1973) *Children's Drawings as Diagnostic Aids*. New York: Brunner/Bazel.

Eng, H. (1954) *The Psychology of Children's Drawings*, second edition. London: Routledge and Kegan Paul Ltd.

Frankenburg, W.K., Dodds, J. and Archer, P. (1990) *Denver II Technical Manual*. Denver, CO: Denver Developmental Materials.

Gardner, H. (1980) *Artful Scribbles*. New York: Basic Books.

Gesell, A. and Ames, L.B. (1946) The development of directionality in drawing. *Journal of Genetic Psychology*, 68, 445–61.

Glenn, S.M., Bradshaw, K. and Sharp, M. (1995) Handedness and the direction and sequencing in children's drawings of people. *Educational Psychology*, 15, 11–21.

Golomb, C. (1973) Children's representation of the human figure: The effects of models, media and instructions. *Genetic Psychology Monographs*, 87, 197–251.

Golomb, C. and Farmer, D. (1983) Children's graphic planning strategies and early principles of spatial organization in drawing. *Studies in Art Education*, 24, 87–100.

Goodenough, F.L. (1926) *The Measurement of Intelligence by Drawings*. New York: World Books.

Goodnow, J. (1977) *Children's Drawing*. London: Fontana/Open Books.

Goodnow, J.J., Friedman, S.L., Bernbaum, M. and Lehman, E.B. (1973) Direction and sequence in copying: the effect of learning to write in English and Hebrew. *Journal of Cross-Cultural Psychology*, 4, 263–82.

Goodnow, J.J. and Levine, R.A. (1973) 'The grammar of action': sequence and syntax in children's copying. *Cognitive Psychology*, 4, 82–98.

Greer, T. and Lockman, J.J. (1998) Using writing instruments: invariances in young children and adults. *Child Development*, 69, 888–902.

Harris, D.B. (1963) *Children's Drawings as Measures of Intellectual Maturity*. New York: Harcourt, Brace and World.

Kellogg, R. (1969) *Analyzing Children's Art*. Palo Alto, CA: Mayfield.

Koppitz, E. (1968) *Psychological Evaluation of Children's Human Figure Drawings*. London: Grune and Stratton.

Kosslyn, S.M., Heldmeyer, K.H. and Locklear, E.P. (1977) Children's drawings as data about internal representations. *Journal of Experimental Child Psychology*, 23, 191–211.

Lewis, C., Russell, C. and Berridge, D. (1993) When is a mug not a mug? Effects of content, naming, and instructions on children's drawings. *Journal of Experimental Child Psychology*, 56, 291–302.

Lieblich, A., Ninio, A. and Kugelmass, S. (1975) Developmental trends in directionality of drawing in Jewish and Arab Israeli children. *Journal of Cross-Cultural Psychology*, 6, 504–11.

Light, P. (1985) The development of view-specific representation considered from a socio-cognitive standpoint. In N.H. Freeman and M.V. Cox (eds), *Visual Order: The Nature and Development of Pictorial Representation* (pp. 214–30). Cambridge: Cambridge University Press.

Lockman, J.J. (2000) A perception–action perspective on tool use development. *Child Development*, 71, 137–44.

Martlew, M. (1992) Pen grips: their relationship to letter/word formation and literacy knowledge in children starting school. *Journal of Human Movement Studies*, 23, 165–85.

Newell, K. M. (1986) Constraints on the development of coordination. In M. Wade and H.T.A. Whiting (eds), *Motor Development in Children: Aspects of Coordination and Control* (pp. 341–60). Dordrecht: Martinus Nijhof.

Phillips, W.A., Hobbs, S.B. and Pratt, F.R. (1978) Intellectual realism in children's drawings of cubes. *Cognition*, 6, 15–33.

Phillips, W.A., Inall, M. and Lauder, E. (1985) On the discovery, storage and use of graphic descriptions. In N.H. Freeman and M.V. Cox (eds), *Visual Order: The Nature and Development of Pictorial Representation* (pp. 122–34) Cambridge: Cambridge University Press.

Piaget, J. and Inhelder, B. (1956) *The Child's Conception of Space*. London: Routledge and Kegan Paul.

Reimer, D.C., Eaves, L.C., Richards, R. and Crichton, J. (1975) Name printing as a test of developmental maturity. *Developmental Medicine and Child Neurology*, 17, 486–92.

Rosenbloom, L. and Horton, M.E. (1971) The maturation of fine prehension in young children. *Developmental Medicine and Child Neurology*, 13, 3–8.

Rosengren, K.S. and Braswell, G.S. (2001) Variability in children's reasoning. In H. W. Reese and R. Kail (eds), *Advances in Child Development and Behaviour*, Vol 28, San Diego: Academic Press.

Rosengren, K.S., DeGuzman, D., Pierroutsakos, S. and Braswell, G.S. (1998) Task constraints on children's grip configurations during drawing. Unpublished manuscript.

Rosengren, K.S. and Savelsbergh, G.J.P. (2000) A TASC based approach to perceptual motor development. Paper presented at the Motor Development Research Consortium, Bowling Green, Ohio.

Rosengren, K.S. and Savelsbergh, G.J.P. (2001) The TASC based approach to learning and development. Paper presented at Development, Learning and Practice: What is the Difference? Alsager, United Kingdom.

Saida, Y. and Miyashita, M. (1979) Development of fine motor skill in children: manipulation of a pencil in young children ages 2 to 6 years old. *Journal of Human Movement Studies*, 5, 104–13.

Sasson, R., Nimmo-Smith, I. and Wing, A.M. (1986) An analysis of children's penholds. In H.S.R. Kao, G.P. van Galen and R. Hoosian (eds), *Graphonomics: Contemporary Research in Handwriting* (pp. 93–106). Amsterdam: North-Holland.

Scheirs, J.G.M. (1990) Relationships between the direction of movements and handedness in children. *Neuropsychologia*, 28, 742–8.

Selfe, L. (1977) *Nadia: A Case of Extraordinary Drawing Ability in an Autistic Child*. London: Academic Press.

Siegler, R.S. (1994) Cognitive variability: a key to understanding cognitive development. *Current Directions in Psychological Science*, 1, 1–5.

Siegler, R.S. (1996) *Emerging Minds: The Process of Change in Children's Thinking*. Oxford: Oxford University Press.

Sitton, R. and Light, P. (1992) Drawing to differentiate: flexibility in young children's human figure drawings. *British Journal of Developmental Psychology*, 10, 25–33.

Sovik, N. (1993) Development of children's writing performance: some educational implications. In A.F. Kalverboer, B. Hopkins and R. Geuze (eds), *Motor Development in Early and Later Childhood: Longitudinal Approaches* (pp. 229–46) Cambridge: Cambridge University Press.

Stennet, R.G., Smythe, P.C. and Hardy, M. (1972) Developmental trends in letter printing skills. *Perceptual and Motor Skills*, 34, 182–6.

Stiles-Davis, J. (1988) Spatial dysfunctions in young children with right cerebral hemisphere injury. In J. Stiles-Davis, M. Kritchevsky and U. Bellugi (eds), *Spatial Cognition: Brain Bases and Development* (pp. 251–72) Hillsdale, NJ: Erlbaum.

Taylor, M. and Bacharach, V.R. (1982) Constraints on the visual accuracy of drawings produced by young children. *Journal of Experimental Child Psychology*, 34, 211–329.

Thelen, E. and Smith, L.B. (1994) *A Dynamic Systems Approach to the Development of Cognition and Action*. Cambridge: MIT Press.

Thomassen, A.J.W.M. (1992) Interaction of cognitive and biomechanical factors in the organization of graphic movements. In G.S. Stelmach and J. Requin (eds), *Tutorials in Motor Behavior: II* (pp 249–61). Amsterdam: North-Holland-Elsevier.

Thomassen, A.J.W. and Teulings, J.L.H.M. (1979) The development of directional preference in writing movements. *Visible Language*, 13, 299–313.

Thomassen, A.J.W. and Teulings, H.L.H.M. (1983) The development of handwriting. In M. Martlew (ed.), *The Psychology of Written Language*. New York: John Wiley.

Thomassen, A.J.W., Meulenbroek, R.G.J. and Hoofs, M.P.E. (1992) Economy and anticipation in graphic stroke sequences. *Human Movement Science*, 11, 71–82.

Van Geert, P. and Van Dijk, M. (2002) Focus on variability: new tools to study intraindividual variability in developmental data. *Infant Behavior and Development*, 25, 340–74

Van Sommers, P. (1983) The conservatism of children's drawing strategies: at what level does stability persist? In D. Rogers and J.A. Sloboda (eds), *The Acquisition of Symbolic Skills* (pp. 65–70). New York: Plenum Press.

Van Sommers, P. (1984) *Drawing and Cognition: Descriptive and Experimental Studies of Graphic Production Processes*. Cambridge: Cambridge University Press.

Vinter, A. (1999) How meaning modifies drawing behaviour in children. *Child Development*, 70, 33–49.

Willats, J. (1977) How children learn to draw realistic pictures. *Quarterly Journal of Experimental Psychology*, 29, 367–82.

Wiltshire, S. (1987) *Drawings*. London: J. M. Dent.

Wong, T.H. and Kao, H.S.R. (1991) The development of drawing principles in Chinese. In J. Wann, A.M. Wing and N. Søvik (eds), *Development of Graphic Skills* (pp. 93–112). New York: Harcourt Brace Jovanovich.

Ziviani, J. (1982) Children's prehension while writing: a pilot investigation. *British Journal of Occupational Therapy*, 45, 306–7.

Ziviani, J. (1983) Qualitative changes in dynamic tripod grip between seven and 14 years of age. *Developmental Medicine and Child Neurology*, 25, 535–9.

Ziviani, J. and Elkins, J. (1986) Effect of pencil grip on handwriting speed and legibility, *Educational Review*, 38, 247–57.

6 Constraints in children's learning to use spoons

Dominique van Roon, John van der Kamp and Bert Steenbergen

1. Introduction

In 1943 Gesell and Ilg charted the chronological milestones of self-feeding with a spoon. Recapitulating, 'at 15 months the infant may grasp a spoon and insert it into the dish. Filling however is poor, and if the infant brings the spoon to the mouth she is apt to turn the spoon upside down before it enters the mouth. Three months later, the infant is capable of filling the spoon, but still has difficulty inserting the spoon into the mouth and frequently turns the spoon in the mouth. The infant spills a considerable amount of food. Around her second birthday, the child inserts the spoon in the mouth without turning and there is still moderate spilling. At the age of 3 girls show little spilling and may have a supinate grasp of the spoon' (Gesell and Ilg, 1943, p. 242).

Although Gesell and Ilg gave an intuitive and perhaps appealing picture of the changes that occur when young children learn to feed themselves with a spoon, it is far from complete. For instance, infants need to discover that a spoon affords scooping food from the bowl during meals, and not banging on the table. They must also learn to understand that the spoon must be grasped at the handle and not at the bowl, and they need to select a suitable grip pattern from a large variety of possible grips. Moreover, as Gesell and Ilg emphasised, infants must come to terms with spilling food. They must learn to fill the spoon, transport it smoothly into the mouth, the opening of which must be precisely co-ordinated with movements of the hand and head, and they must empty the spoon in the mouth without turning the spoon. Furthermore, because self-feeding, and thus spoon use, is a culturally embedded practice, children must learn to adopt the social demands at mealtimes. Finally, these requirements often result in quite different ways of handling in disabled children, and may even necessitate specially designed spoons to make the act of self-feeding with a spoon possible.

Achieving insight into the process of learning to use a spoon at mealtimes requires an explanation of all these issues. Given the rich variety of issues, a general framework on the development and learning of action is indispensable before a coherent explanation of the process of learning to use a spoon can be sought. Newell (1986, 1989) has offered such a general framework, in which he argues that development and learning emerge from the changes in constraints imposed on action. According to him, the regularity in the development of action is determined in large part by these (changing) constraints imposed on action. Constraints do not serve as a single-factor explanation for development, nor do they prescribe actions. Rather, they exclude some actions. Constraints limit the possible number of movement solutions or action patterns. Development is driven by changes in the constraints on action that, particularly in the first few years of life, may change dramatically. Newell distinguishes three categories of constraints that interact to induce a (new) action pattern for any activity for a particular organism: organismic, environmental and task constraints. The organismic constraints reside in the organism. Typical organismic constraints are body weight, height, shape, functional synaptic connections, and the status of the child's central nervous system. As we will illustrate below, it is especially in children with movement disorders that the role of these constraints in the development of tool use becomes salient. The environmental constraints, in contrast, appear to have only a minor influence in the development of tool use, except of course for the role of gravity when spilling food. Environmental constraints are external to the organism and relatively time-independent. They reflect the general ambient conditions like gravity and the optic array. However, it is important to realise that in Newell's (1986, 1989) description environmental and task constraints are only distinct according to the experimental or specific conditions on action. Formulated simply, environmental constraints are not manipulated in an experiment, while task constraints are. Finally, Newell (1986, 1989) mentions three types of task constraints: 1) the goal of the task, 2) implements or machines specifying or constraining action patterns (physical constraints like cars, bicycles, but also, of course, tools for grasping or transporting objects such as spoons) and 3) rules specifying or constraining the action patterns. Examples are the non-physical rules that can be found in sports or the cultural habits during mealtimes. These different categories of task constraints will appear to be important in learning to use a spoon for self-feeding.

In the remainder of this chapter we will identify the constraints on learning to use a spoon for self-feeding in children. To this aim, Newell's categorisation of constraints serves as a guide. First, the role of the different types of task constraints (i.e. goal, implements, and rules) on the early learning of using the spoon for self-feeding is discussed. Subsequently, the role of organismic constraints is dealt with through an examination of spoon-handling in children with spastic tetraparesis. The chapter concludes with some remarks on the (ergonomic) design of spoons, which follow from an understanding of how children's learning to use spoons for self-feeding is constrained.

2. Task constraints I: the goal of the task

At mealtimes, the goal of feeding is to convey food efficiently from the dish to the mouth, while at the same time meeting certain cultural expectations. To accomplish this goal, it is essential that the orientation of the spoon be such that the concave side of the bowl faces upward (Steenbergen *et al.*, 1997). To convey food from dish to mouth, this orientation should be established and maintained when picking up the spoon, inserting it into the food, loading the spoon, transporting the loaded spoon from dish to mouth, emptying the spoon into the mouth, and removing the spoon from the mouth (cf. Connolly and Dalgleish, 1989, 1993). These components of the feeding action mutually constrain each other. Approximately until the end of the first year, the parent feeds the child, but control of feeding is gradually transferred to the infant as the skill of using a spoon and, eventually, cultural habits are learned. As a first step, around the end of the first year, children are frequently given a spoon at mealtimes. There have been reports of infants playing with the spoon, i.e. repeatedly putting it into the mouth, banging it on the table, dipping the spoon into the dish, dropping it on the ground, transferring it from hand to hand and so on (Connolly and Dalgleish, 1989; Gesell and Ilg, 1943; Valsiner, 1997). Presumably, these exploratory actions drive the discovery of what the spoon affords or, stated differently, the selection of actions that are appropriate to the goal. Obviously, during mealtimes the spoon serves for self-feeding, not for banging or dropping. Unfortunately, this very first phase of learning the goal of self-feeding with a spoon has only received scant attention.

McCarty, Clifton, and Collard (1999) presented 9-, 14-, and 19-month-old children with a spoon loaded with food, and also with items that had no clear goal (e.g. a toy attached to a handle), with the handle alternately oriented to the left and right. The 9-month-olds put the bowl of the spoon into their mouth more often than the toy and grasped the spoons and toys differently (i.e. the spoon evoked more radial grips, see figure 6.1). In a second study, in which loaded spoons were included besides tools like hammers and hairbrushes, McCarty, Clifton and Collard (2001) again observed that 9-month-olds brought the spoon to the mouth in about two-thirds of the trials, but did not perform appropriate actions with the other tools. According to McCarty *et al.* (1999, 2001), these findings show that even for the 9-month-olds the spoons afforded the goal of obtaining food, whereas the other items had a variety of apparently non-functional uses, such as visual examination, mouthing and haptic exploration. Interestingly, when the bowl of the spoon was oriented toward the preferred hand, the majority of the 9-month-olds was observed to grasp the bowl of the spoon with their preferred hand and/or place the handle into the mouth. Most 14-month-olds picked up the spoon by the handle with their preferred hand and placed the bowl into the mouth. When necessary, they made a correction of the grip configuration during transport. The 19-month-old children planned the grip in advance and used the hand at the handle-side, so that corrections were superfluous (McCarty *et al.*, 1999, 2001). Based on these observations McCarty *et al.* (1999, 2001) proposed a model for the development of planning. Learning to use spoons for self-feeding is described as a shift in the moment at which children evaluate a sequence of actions. At first, the evaluation occurs after the whole self-feeding action is completed (feedback strategy), followed by an evaluation in the middle of the action sequence (partially planned), and eventually the action is evaluated in advance (fully planned).[1] However, the model leaves largely unanswered how the affordance of self-feeding with a spoon is discovered in the first place. How does an infant learn the action properties of the spoon properties and how does the child learn to differentiate the spoon from

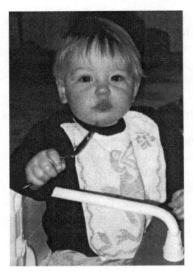

Figure 6.1 A 13-month-old girl using a transverse palmar radial grip

other tools or objects (such as a knife or fork) and so on? It remains to be seen whether development of planning will also be identified as a constraint in this early phase of learning to use spoons.

In sum, there is some evidence that children differentiate between the goal of the spoon and other items at 9 months of age. Appropriate and efficient use of the spoon for self-feeding, nonetheless, does not emerge before the end of the first year. Connolly and Dalgleish (1989, 1993) provided the most detailed description of the changes that occur in the use of spoons during feeding in children aged 1 to 2 years. During this period, children show a shift from movements of the shoulder to movements of the wrist joint when filling the spoon and an increased use of elbow and shoulder flexion during transport of the spoon to the mouth. In addition, movement trajectories become more fluent and the number of errors is reduced. These changes are paralleled by changes in grip configurations. Early in the second year, children use a large variety of grip configurations, sometimes adding up to eight. Since only relatively few patterns allow for efficient loading, transporting and emptying the spoon into the mouth, it is only after a few months that the inefficient grips (e.g. ulnar grips that make it extremely difficult to remove food from the spoon) drop out of the initial repertoire. Another tendency that was observed is an increasing use of more flexible configurations that permit intrinsic movements of the spoon (Connolly and Dalgleish, 1989, 1993; see also Achard and Von Hofsten, 2002). The majority of the 1- to 2-year olds held the spoon in the palm of the hand with the digits tightly flexed around the spoon into a fist (figure 6.1). Recently, McCarty *et al.* (1999) and Achard and Von Hofsten (2002) have confirmed the prevalence of transverse palmar radial grips in the second year of life. At the end of the second year, however, there is a growing tendency to grasp the spoon with the ulnar fingers curled around the spoon and the forefinger

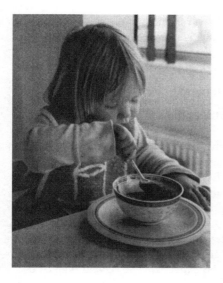

Figure 6.2 A 23-month-old girl using a transverse digital radial grip

extended or flexed back on the handle (Connolly and Dalgleish, 1989; figure 6.2). This configuration becomes dominant in children aged between 2 and 4 years (Steenbergen *et al.*, 1997). The (clenched) transverse digital radial grip makes intrinsic movements of the spoon, and thus a more precise control of the spoon, possible. Furthermore, it is observed that children predominantly position the hand at the end of the handle, although early in the second year the hand is sometimes placed closer to the bowl (Achard and Von Hofsten, 2002; Connolly and Dalgleish, 1989, 1993; Steenbergen *et al.*, 1997). These adaptations during the second year and thereafter result in greater precision and flexibility. One behavioural consequence is reduced spillage and, hence, an optimisation of accomplishing the goal of using a spoon for self-feeding. These observations may reflect an initial freezing and subsequent unfreezing of the available degrees of freedom, and support the concept of proximo-distal organisation of co-ordination in learning to use spoons for self-feeding (cf. Bernstein, 1967; Connolly and Dalgleish, 1989; Steenbergen *et al.*, 1997; Van der Kamp and Steenbergen, 1999).

The next section deals with the degrees of freedom problem in somewhat more detail, but first it needs to be emphasised that 2-year-old spoon users do not manipulate the spoon in the same way as adults do. It is probably not before 4 years of age that the adult grip (see figure 6.4), which may or may not be the supinate grip referred to by Gesell and Ilg (1943), becomes predominant. According to Connolly and Dalgleish (1989, p. 899), the advantage of this configuration is not the precision of movements as such, but rather the variety of movements that are available. It leads to 'convenience and economy of action' (p. 899), suggesting that the emergence of the adult grip reflects a further optimisation of accomplishing the goal of conveying food from the dish into the mouth. However, it is proposed in the fourth section that it may be a non-physical rule that is the primary constraint inducing the adult grip configuration. First, however, another type of task constraint identified by Newell, physical implements that constrain the action patterns, will be dealt with.

3. Task constraints II: physical implements

In the previous section we suggested that the optimisation of accomplishing the goal of conveying food from the dish into the mouth with a spoon may be understood in terms of mastering the control of the redundant degrees of freedom. That is, the gradual change from transverse palmar radial to (clenched) transverse digital radial grips during the second year may reflect a shifting balance between, on the one hand, the necessity to reduce the number of independent variables to be controlled and, on the other hand, the requirement that degrees of freedom remain that can actively be controlled in response to changing task demands. One way to test this claim is by manipulation of task constraints to make the accomplishment of the goal of self-feeding with a spoon more difficult. In that case, an increasing number of transverse palmar grips might be expected. The second type of task constraint, viz. physical implements that constrain or specify the action pattern, may be an important constraint on actualising such a manipulation.

Steenbergen *et al.* (1997; see also Van der Kamp *et al.*, 1993) manipulated the geometrical relation between the bowl and the handle of the spoon. In normal spoons the axis of the handle continues into the bowl. To use a spoon as a tool for loading and transporting food, this particular relation between the bowl and handle is not mandatory. As long as the individual is able to orient the bowl in such a way that the concave side faces upwards so that it affords holding the substance, the spoon can be used for self-feeding. Steenbergen and co-workers presented 2- to 4-year-old children with six spoons (figure 6.3), one of which was the conventional spoon, the other five were bent at the intersection of the bowl and the handle. The children were asked to load the spoon with dry uncooked rice and transport it from one basket to the other. In all instances the children brought the scoop into

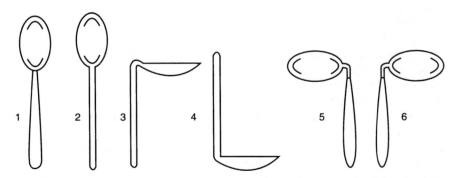

Figure 6.3 The spoons used by Steenbergen *et al.* (Adapted from Steenbergen *et al.*, 1997)

the rice with the concave side facing up. That is, all children perceived the (bent) spoons to afford loading and transporting the rice, although they were not always successful in accomplishing this goal. In particular in the case of spoon three only half of the scooping attempts resulted in transporting rice. The conventional spoon was predominantly grasped with a transverse digital radial grip (figure 6.2) at the end of the handle – a grip configuration that first becomes apparent at the end of the second year (Connolly and Dalgleish, 1989). However, the children varied their grip configuration in such a way that the functional act of scooping was preserved. The handling mode was contingent upon the relative occurrence of successful and unsuccessful transport attempts. The control problems posed by spoon three resulted in a prevalence of transverse *palmar* radial grips (figure 6.1) positioned close to the bowl. This grip pattern is similar to that observed in 1-year-olds during their first successful attempts of self-feeding with a spoon. Steenbergen *et al.* (1997) argued that this highly rigid handling mode, in which compensatory movements of the individual fingers are excluded, may point to the principle of freezing degrees of freedom as a solution to the control problem.

At mealtimes it is not solely the spoon but also implements like the dish, plate or bowl that function as task constraints upon the act of self-feeding. Recently Achard and Von Hofsten (2002) have explored the ability of 12- to 17-month-old children to feed themselves with a spoon when the food had to be retrieved through a slit in a lid placed over the plate. The lid constrained both the access to the semi-liquid food as well as the retrieval. Without the lid the most frequently shown grip configuration was the transverse palmar radial grip, of which the relative occurrence decreased with age. That is, at about 17 months half of the grips employed by the children were (clenched) transverse digital grips. The spoon was held by the end or middle part of the handle. However, the introduction of the lid with the slit affected the way the children grasped the spoon, the adaptations observed being dependent on age. In the 12-month-olds the lid induced more non-functional and ulnar grips and a concomitant decrease in the more flexible transverse digital grips. In contrast, the eldest children were holding the spoon in similar ways in the no-lid and lid-present conditions. In the lid-present conditions the children held the spoon more often at the middle of the handle, and sometimes even at or close to the bowl. In this condition there was a slight, but significant decrease in the number of attempts in which the bowl of the spoon was oriented with the concave side up. Again, the adaptations in grip configuration can be interpreted as a shifting balance between the need to maintain control over the act of self-feeding with a spoon and the requirements of precision and flexibility. As in the experiment of Steenbergen *et al.* (1997), the increasing demands on control resulted in a decrease in flexible grips that permitted intrinsic or compensatory movements of the fingers (i.e. a transverse digital radial grip positioned at the end of the handle of the spoon). Whereas more experienced children were more inclined to change to rigid handling modes (i.e. a transverse palmar radial grip positioned nearer to the bowl; Steenbergen *et al.*, 1997), inexperienced young children more often tended to use inappropriate grips (e.g. ulnar and interdigital grips sometimes positioned at the bowl; Achard and Von Hofsten, 2002).

In sum, these studies provide some evidence that the changes in learning to use a spoon for self-feeding, together with other changes (see section 2) in children aged from 1 to possibly 4 years, reflect an initial freezing and a subsequent unfreezing of the available degrees of freedom. The intrinsic or compensatory finger movements that become manifest during this learning process allow for a more efficient accomplishment of the goal of conveying food from the dish into the mouth. This gain in flexibility and efficiency is accompanied by a reduced spillage of food. Apart from perhaps the urge not to spill any food, these changes are primarily induced by the changing interaction of constraints related to the goal of the task and the (configuration of the) implements. Only after these constraints are dealt with to a certain degree, might task constraints defined by cultural habits become more important in learning to use a spoon during meals (although we do not want to suggest that this is a strictly sequential process).

4. Task constraints III: non-physical rules

Surprisingly little is known about the development of the adult grip. In the adult grip the spoon is held between the pulp surfaces of the opposed thumb and index finger, which may or may not be curled around the handle, and lying around the lateral surface of the third digit (Connolly and Dalgleish, 1989, p. 899; figure 6.4). The adult grip is barely observed before 4 years of age (Connolly and Dalgleish, 1989; Steenbergen *et al.*, 1997), but it was found to be the predominant grip configuration in adults (Van der Kamp and Steenbergen, 1999). We were not able, however, to trace any reliable observation about children's first consistent use of the adult grip at mealtimes (cf. chapter 5 by Rosengren and Braswell). In comparison to the transverse palmar and digital radial grips, in the adult grip or its clenched version, with the fingers tightly flexed, the orientation of the spoon in the hand is radically different. Why do the transverse palmar and digital radial

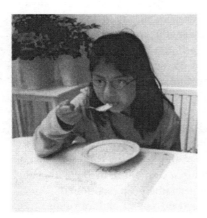

Figure 6.4 An 8-year-old girl using an adult grip

grips give way to adult grip configurations? This question is even more pertinent because the fist-type grip configurations are quite successful for conveying food from the dish into mouth without spillage, certainly around the age of 4. Connolly and Dalgleish (1989) speculate about its convenience and economy for action. Rather, we would like to argue here that it is predominantly the non-physical task-constraints on self-feeding, viz. cultural habits and etiquette, that induce the change from a fist-type to an adult-type grip configuration. In the absence of developmental data, we will illustrate this argument through a cultural-historical analysis (Valsiner, 1997), assuming that the context of children's mealtimes has changed in clearly specifiable ways in human history. An analysis of the transformation of cultural practices during mealtimes in the broadest sense (including, for instance, the changes in the specific tools, feeding utensils, special chairs for children, and so on) that has taken place during the past centuries may perhaps lead us to the cultural habits that nowadays constrain children's learning to use a spoon at mealtimes.

In his classic work *The Civilizing Process: The Development of Manners* Norbert Elias (1978) described the cultural history of practices during mealtimes in the European cultures from the sixteenth to the nineteenth century as an increasing differentiation of the individual participant's food and food-use utensils from communal usage (see also Muchembled, 1988). That is, the European cultural traditions of eating have been transformed from sharing a communal dish from which food was taken by hand, towards a highly differentiated social organisation of mealtimes where each participant has a varied set of food-handling tools (plates, bowls, glasses, forks, spoons, knives etc.) for his or her private use (cf. Valsiner, 1997). The transformations in mealtime practices were a reflection of increasing thresholds of embarrassment and a sense of shame. Body image became more and more negatively valued.[2] To put it bluntly, over the ages the body and bodily fluids like sweat, spittle, urine and so on became 'dirty things'. They evoked an intensifying sense of disgust that resulted in a compulsion towards self-control. Taboos arose, for instance, on bodily contact with one's table-companions. This resulted in the transformation of the mealtime practice, in which both new implements (e.g. single chairs with a clear distance from the neighbour as a replacement for benches on which people had sat closely together) and rules of good manners were introduced. One of these rules prescribed how the spoon ought to be grasped. The spoon had to be held with 'three fingers rather than the whole fist, as peasants do it' (Teutenberg, 1998, p. 157; Forbes, 1969; Schürmann, 1998).[3] There is some agreement among authors that this 'three-finger grip' rule became fashionable during the late seventeenth and eighteenth century (Forbes, 1969; Schürmann, 1998), but probably at different rates in different social groups (Muchembled, 1988). Although it is hazardous to conclude definitely that this 'three-finger-grip' is the adult grip and not the transverse digital radial grip, present-day etiquette still prescribes a 'three-finger grip' where the spoon should be held just like a pen (Groskamp-ten Have, 1983), undoubtedly the adult grip (cf. Connolly and Elliott, 1984; chapter 5). In short, we suggest that the change from fist-type grip configuration to adult-type grip configuration, which nowadays is an important milestone in children's learning to use a spoon, first took place in the seventeenth and eighteenth centuries. However, there is more to the story. Interestingly, the desired grip configuration also affected the design of the spoon. That is, it 'required the flat handles still in use today in the late seventeenth century because at that time it became customary to hold them with three fingers rather than with the whole fist' (Schürmann, 1998, p. 175; see also Forbes, 1969). As a consequence, the customary medieval spoons (often denoted as fist spoons!) with the short, thick round handle disappeared (figure 6.5). Why the 'three-finger grip' rule was so significant that it even affected the shape of the spoon remains unanswered. Cultural historians prefer social status as a basis for the transformation of table manners. Nevertheless, although it might be speculated that in times when most people were illiterate, handling a spoon like a pen might serve to dissociate one from lower social ranks, the taboo on bodily contact appears to be the more likely explanation. The adult grip permits the spoon to be manipulated by rotation of wrist and forearm, the gain being a larger variety of movements available (Connolly and Dalgleish, 1989). Most importantly, in contrast to the transverse radial grips, the adult grips enable the loading, transport and emptying of the spoon to be performed without outward movement of the elbow. Hence, the adult grip configuration makes it easier to comply with the taboo on bodily contact at mealtimes. It seems that nowadays this functional significance of the adult grip configuration is forgotten, as is the origin of many other cultural habits.

The contemporary mealtime practice in Europe-rooted societies is an outcome of the cultural histories of these societies. One of the rules that has emerged from this development is the habit of using an adult grip configuration when eating with a spoon. Children entering the mealtime practice have to learn to come to terms with this non-physical task constraint. Exactly when and how they do this remains unknown. Children are likely to observe and imitate how others (e.g. parents and siblings) behave at mealtimes and perhaps parents 'correct' their children's grip configuration.

5. Organismic constraints

So far we have discussed what appears to be an overwhelming influence of task constraints on children's learning to use a spoon for self-feeding. This is not to say that environmental and organismic constraints are unimportant: task constraints do not act in isolation! Especially in children with motor disorders, the interaction

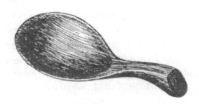

Figure 6.5 A sixteenth-century wooden fist spoon (Adapted from Forbes, 1969)

between task and organismic constraints on learning to use spoons becomes clearly manifest. In particular, here we will focus on spoon use in children with cerebral palsy. 'Cerebral palsy (CP) is an inclusive term used to describe a number of chronic non-progressive disorders of motor function, which occur in young children as a result of disease of the brain' (Ingram, 1966, p. 337). It can be caused by, for instance, an oxygen shortage at or around birth, intra-uterine infection, prematurity or a brain tumour at a very young age. In approximately 60 per cent of the children with cerebral palsy the brain damage results in spasticity (Sugden and Keogh, 1990). Spasticity in turn is a motor disorder characterised by a velocity-dependent increase in tonic stretch reflexes that results in an inappropriate and excessive activation of skeletal muscles (see chapter 10 by Steenbergen, Utley, Sugden and Thiemann, and chapter 11 by Ledebt). A recent series of reaching and grasping studies by Steenbergen and co-workers has shown that in children with spastic hemiparesis (one impaired body-side) the distal musculature is more affected than the proximal musculature. These children perform movements more slowly and less fluently, they have difficulties generating the right amount of force when grasping an object, and the functional range of motion of the elbow joint at the impaired body-side is reduced. To be able to perform the task succesfully they increase the involvement of the trunk (Steenbergen *et al.*, 1996; Steenbergen, 2000; Steenbergen *et al.*, 2000; Van Thiel and Steenbergen, 2001; see also Cirstea and Levin, 2000). This movement (re)organisation may be characterised as a reduction of the degrees of freedom in order to comply with the task demands.

Depending on the severity of the impairment, children with spasticity encounter various problems with activities of daily life, including self-feeding (cf. Reilly and Skuse, 1992). Obviously, in children with spastic tetraparesis, in which both sides of the body are affected, these problems are even more pronounced. The degree to which these problems present themselves reflects the specific interaction between the organismic constraint (i.e. severity of the disorder) and the various task constraints (i.e. goal, implement and non-physical rules). In the remainder of this section, only the interaction of the organismic contraint with the goal and implement task contraints will be dealt with.

Severely affected individuals have difficulties accomplishing the goal of conveying food from the dish into the mouth with a conventional spoon or cannot realise that goal without much spilling. Sometimes, these individuals are not able to feed themselves. There are only a few reports that tested specially designed 'spoons' to help individuals with severe spasticity to eat independently (e.g. Shaw and Wright, 1982; Wyckoff and Mitani, 1982; Yuen, 1993). The effectiveness of these adapted task implements varies. Shaw and Wright (1982), for instance, tested a so-called two-handle spoon in individuals with cerebral palsy. The two-handle spoon can be grasped with both hands, thereby reducing uncontrolled movements. By using this spoon, two patients were able to accomplish the task independently for the first time. One of the subjects did so 'while fixating to stabilize movements' (p. 46), which might point to freezing part of the redundant degrees of freedom of the system. The two-handle spoon improved some aspects of eating in nine other individuals, but in the remaining seven independent eating was not improved.

In moderately affected spastic individuals difficulties involve the optimisation of self-feeding with a spoon. With optimisation we mean that, as in learning to use spoons in children, a balance is sought between, on the one hand, controllability (managing the redundant degrees of freedom) and, on the other hand, flexibility (being able to feed without spilling). It is important for this balance that the gain in flexibility, which would result in a reduced spillage of food, should not go at the expense of decreased controllability. To explore this issue, we tested a group of adolescents who were diagnosed as suffering from spastic tetraparesis with a group of healthy young adults on a spoon-use task. The task was to transport a spoon filled with four pieces of popcorn to the mouth and empty it. Our first aim was to describe the differences in eating styles, and our second to compare the effectiveness of two ergonomic spoons (figure 6.6) to that of a conventional one.

Remarkably, only a few pieces of popcorn were spilled (less than 10 per cent), but on average the individuals with tetraparesis tended to spill a little more (table 6.1). The movement (re)organisation, however, differed substantially among both groups. As Table 6.1 shows, the spastic participants moved more slowly and less fluently as compared to the adults without cerebral palsy. The larger movement duration was due to a lengthening of both the acceleration phase and the deceleration phase. The movement of the wrist was always upwards and towards the mouth. With respect to the involvement of the head during the eating task, three different 'strategies' could be discerned (table 6.2). In approximately half of the trials a 'head forwards and downwards' strategy was used. Here, the head and the hand with the spoon were moving towards each other. In these trials, the involvement of the head could be expressed as a percentage: the head covered a larger part of the total distance in the tetraparetic group (m = 24 per cent, sd = 7 per cent) in comparison to the control group (m = 13 per cent, sd = 6 per cent; $F(1,10) = 6.89$, $p < 0.05$). In the remaining trials a 'head forwards and upwards' or a 'head backwards and upwards' strategy was used.[4] Together, these findings show a slowing down of the movement and a larger proximal involvement. These results are in line with earlier findings on spoon use in adults without cerebral palsy (Van der Kamp and Steenbergen, 1999). In this study, participants were to eat kale and water with a spoon. A slowing down of the complete movement was observed for water as compared to kale and this was accompanied by an increased amount of trunk involvement. These findings were interpreted as a 'freezing' of degrees of freedom in order to cope with the increase in task complexity (i.e. higher accuracy demands). In the present study the amount of spilled popcorn was virtually equal among the tetraparetic and the healthy participants. This may indicate that the tetraparetic participants reorganised their movements in an efficient way, as adults without cerebral palsy do when a liquid substance has to be transported.

The second purpose of this study was to explore the effectiveness of the two ergonomic spoons (figure 6.6). Adaptations in ergonomic spoons for individuals with CP are primarily based on expert notions of occupational therapists and physiotherapists, but their effect on movement co-ordination has never been systematically investigated. It seems that the two ergonomic spoons used in this experiment were designed mainly to increase the stability of the movement system

Table 6.1 Means (and standard deviations between subjects) of the wrist kinematics

	Spoon 1	Spoon 2	Spoon 3	Group effect
% spilled popcorn				
Tetraparetic group	4.3 (5.5)	8.9 (11.0)	6.8 (10.9)	n.s.
Control group	0.0 (0.0)	0.4 (1.0)	1.3 (3.1)	
Movement time (ms)				
Tetraparetic group	1,786 (610)	1,753 (753)	1,669 (604)	$F_{(1,11)} = 6.02$, $p < 0.05$
Control group	1,019 (154)	1,099 (259)	1,088 (270)	
Mean velocity (mm/s)				
Tetraparetic group	160 (29)	184 (63)	181 (60)	$F_{(1,1)} = 9.69$, $p < 0.01$
Control group	268 (62)	282 (75)	290 (86)	
Max. velocity (mm/s)				
Tetraparetic group	323 (68)	354 (98)	361 (107)	$F_{(1,1)} = 5.32$, $p < 0.05$
Control group	459 (112)	481 (141)	512 (156)	
Acceleration time (ms)				
Tetraparetic group	851 (359)	748 (285)	645 (191)	$F_{(1,11)} = 7.23$, $p < 0.05$
Control group	449 (68)	472 (104)	497 (135)	
% to peak velocity				
Tetraparetic group	47.1 (12.4)	44.3 (7.4)	39.7 (8.4)	n.s.
Control group	44.0 (4.8)	43.5 (4.1)	45.7 (4.5)	
Zero-crossings (number/s)				
Tetraparetic group	7.4 (2.0)	7.1 (2.1)	7.0 (1.8)	$F_{(1,11)} = 28.82$, $p < 0.001$
Control group	1.7 (0.6)	2.9 (1.7)	2.9 (1.7)	

Table 6.2 Head movement strategies

		Forwards(−)/backwards(+)		Upwards(−)/downwards(+)	
	% of trials	Mean (SD)	Range	Mean (SD)	Range
Tetraparetic group					
Forwards and downwards	47.6	−69 (50)	−245 … −2	+31 (30)	1 … 136
Forwards and upwards	22.7	−17 (19)	−94 … 0	−16 (18)	−73 … −1
Backwards and upwards	29.7	+34 (36)	0 … 162	−53 (39)	−149 … −7
Control group					
Forwards and downwards	53.1	−38 (25)	−99 … −2	+24 (20)	0 … 74
Forwards and upwards	23.1	−9 (7)	−24 … 0	−8 (6)	−28 … 0
Backwards and upwards	23.8	+12 (9)	0 … 37	−26 (13)	−52 … −5

Note: Means, SD and ranges are in mm.

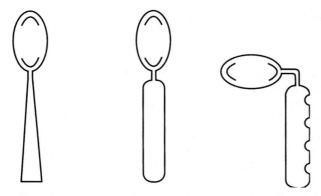

Figure 6.6 A conventional (1) and two ergonomic spoons with a thick handle (2) and a thick and bent handle (3)

(i.e. to increase controllability). The thicker stem elicits transverse radial palmar grips and a consequence of the bend is that wrist rotation is less necessary. Probably, using these spoons will not increase the flexibility of the system, but it is possible that the increased stability enlarges the potential to deal with perturbations (and hence spillage will be reduced).

The three spoons appeared equally effective; that is, the differences in the amount of spilled popcorn were negligible (table 6.1). Moreover, the kinematics were similar for the spoons in both the tetraparetic and the adults without cerebral palsy. Even the two spastic participants who normally ate with the spoon with the bent handle showed this same pattern. This might challenge the use of these particular ergonomic spoons. Still, for individuals who are more severely disabled or when eating liquid food (larger accuracy demands) the use of these ergonomic spoons may appear to be more advantageous.

6. Ergonomic design

There is high practical value in this work, especially in the field of ergonomic design. Van Dieën and Kingma (chapter 2) consider ergonomics as the optimisation through design of the interaction between the human and the man-made environment. Optimisation through design can be reformulated as a change in the interaction of constraints imposed on action by changing the task implement constraints (cf. Newell, 1986). Hence, adaptations to the spoon (i.e. the task implement constraint) should be directed at facilitating 1) learning to convey food from the dish into the mouth and/or learning to reduce food spillage, and 2) learning to comply with cultural habits such as the right-handed adult grip. Knowing the action capabilities of the (non)-disabled child is contributory to the effectiveness of these adaptations in design. To conclude the present chapter, we point to some ergonomic issues.

Optimisation of accomplishing the goal of the task

Probably the first study directed at restoring the ability to eat independently with a spoon in disabled individuals was reported in 1948 by Bernstein and Salzgever (in Gurfinkel and Cordo, 1998, pp. 10–12). According to Gurfinkel and Cordo (1998) Bernstein even had his own laboratory at the Moscow Institute of Prosthetic Appliances. Based on three-dimensional movement recordings of an individual with an intact arm, who ate with a spoon, Bernstein designed an arm prosthesis in which pronation and supination movements of the artificial wrist were combined with elbow flexion and extension. This prosthesis would enable an amputee to eat with a spoon. Notice that Bernstein's efforts were primarily directed at the organismic constraint and not at the design of the spoon. To recapitulate section 5, attempts to devise a spoon that facilitated independent eating led to mixed success (Shaw and Wright, 1982; Wyckoff and Mitani, 1982; Yuen, 1993). Given the large variety of forms and severities of disorders in individuals who cannot eat independently, it seems inevitable that designing efforts should be aimed at the single individual. Still, ergonomic spoons with thick or bent handles (figure 6.6) are most commonly used. To find out whether or not the use of these spoons actually results in a reduction of food spillage or more efficient movement co-ordination, more research is required.

Moreover, these ergonomic spoons, in particular the ones with a thick handle, may or may not impede the use of an adult grip configuration in motorically disabled individuals. It is obvious, however, that the reduction in spillage is a much more important challenge than compliance with cultural expectations.

Compliance with non-physical rules

As we argued in section 4, the design of the conventional spoon in west-European-rooted cultures reflects the social conventions about its use. Its flat handle, for instance, was introduced to induce an adult grip configuration (figures 6.4 and 6.5). However, the large variety of contemporary spoons that are available for infants and toddlers may, through their form, even better reflect the cultural expectations that children become socialised eaters within their society. As an example, infants' and toddlers' spoons are sometimes constructed to promote the use of one hand over the other. The bent handle of these spoons (cf. figure 6.3, spoon 5) makes it easier to use the right hand while self-feeding and at the same time makes left-hand use of the spoon increasingly difficult (cf. Valsiner, 1997). Although infants and toddlers may learn to comply with cultural expectations, one may wonder whether the bent handle does not interfere with learning to use a spoon for self-feeding: McCarty et al. (1999) showed that only after 19 months of age children picked up the spoon with their non-preferred hand, when the handle of the spoon was oriented towards the non-preferred body side. Moreover, Steenbergen et al. (1997) found that in 2- to 4-year-old children the spoon in which the handle was bent to the right (cf. figure 6.3, spoon 6) induced more grasps close to the bowl. Both findings suggest developmental tendencies that may interfere with the specific cultural constraints of the 'right-handed' spoon.

Acknowledgements

The present chapter was written while the authors were supported by grants awarded by the Netherlands Organization for Scientific Research (NWO).

Notes

1 Earlier, Connolly and Dalgleish (1989) had proposed a similar model that emphasised the correct sequencing of actions and the inclusion of feedback loops in children's learning to use a spoon. However, an alternative interpretation might be that these changes reflect a changing interaction between ventral and dorsal visual systems (Creem and Proffitt, 2001; Milner and Goodale, 1995; Van der Kamp and Savelsbergh, 2000).
2 It is probably no coincidence that it was around the same time that Descartes proposed his dichotomy of body and mind.
3 Table manners were (and are) partly spread through books on good manners. Unfortunately, the authors do not provide the original sources from which the 'three-finger grip' rule is obtained. However, it is highly probable that it may be found in eighteenth-century books on good manners.
4 In these trials the percentage of head involvement could not be reliably assessed.

References

Achard, B. and Von Hofsten, C. (2002) Development of the infant's ability to retrieve food through a slit. *Infant and Child Development*, 11, 43–56.

Bernstein, N. (1967) *The Co-ordination and Regulation of Movements*. Oxford: Pergamon Press.

Connolly, K. and Dalgleish, M. (1989) The emergence of a tool-using skill. *Developmental Psychology*, 25, 894–912.

Connolly, K and Dalgleish, M. (1993) Individual patterns of tool use by infants. In A.F. Kalverboer, B. Hopkins and R. Geuze (eds), *Motor Development in Early and Later Childhood* (pp. 174–204). Cambridge: Cambridge University Press.

Connolly, K. and Elliott, J. (1972) The evolution and ontogeny of hand function. In N. Blurton Jones (ed.), *Ethological Studies of Child Behaviour* (pp. 329–84). London: Cambridge University Press.

Cirstea, M.C. and Levin, M.F. (2000) Compensatory strategies for reaching in stroke. *Brain*, 123, 940–53.

Creem, S.H. and Proffitt, D.R. (2001) Grasping objects by their handles: a necessary interaction between cognition and action. *Journal of Experimental Psychology: Human Perception and Performance*, 27, 218–28.

Elias, N. (1978) *The Civilizing Process: The Development of Manners*. Oxford: Basil Blackwell.

Forbes, W.A. (1969) *Antiek bestek: korte ontwikkelingsgeschiedenis van mes, lepel en vork (Ancient cutlery: a short history of the evolution of the knife, spoon and fork)*. Bussum, the Netherlands: Van Dishoeck.

Gesell, A. and Ilg, F.L. (1943) *Infant and Child in the Culture Today. The Guidance of Development in Home and Nursery School*. New York: Harper and Brothers Publishers.

Groskamp-ten Have, A. (1983) *Hoe hoort het eigenlijk? (How should we behave?)*. Amsterdam: Becht.

Gurfinkel, V.S. and Cordo, P.J. (1998) The scientific legacy of Nikolai Bernstein. In M.L. Latash (ed.), *Progress in Motor Control, Vol. 1: Bernstein's Traditions in Movements Studies* (pp. 1–19). Champaign, IL: Human Kinetics.

Ingram, T.T.S. (1966) The neurology of cerebral palsy. *Archives of Disease in Childhood*, 41, 337–57.

McCarty, M.E., Clifton, R.K. and Collard, R.R. (1999) Problem solving in infancy: the emergence of an action plan. *Developmental Psychology*, 35, 1091–101.

McCarty, M.E., Clifton, R.K. and Collard, R.R. (2001) The beginnings of tool use by infants and toddlers. *Infancy*, 2, 233–56.

Milner, A.D. and Goodale, M.A. (1995) *The Visual Brain in Action*. Oxford: Oxford University Press.

Muchembled, R. (1988) *L'invention de l'homme moderne: sensibilités, moeurs et comportements collectifs sous l'Ancien Régime*. Paris: Fayard.

Newell, K.M. (1986) Constraints on the development of coordination. In M.G. Wade and H.T.A. Whiting (eds), *Motor Development in Children: Aspects of Coordination and Control* (pp. 341–60). Dordrecht, The Netherlands: Martinus Nijhoff.

Newell, K.M. (1989) On task and theory specificity. *Journal of Motor Behavior*, 21, 92–6.

Reilly, S. and Skuse, D. (1992) Characteristics and management of feeding problems of young children with cerebral palsy. *Developmental Medicine and Child Neurology*, 34, 379–88.

Schürmann, T. (1998) Cutlery at the fine table: innovations and use in the nineteenth century. In M.R. Schrürer and A. Fenton (eds), *Food and Material Culture*. Proceedings of the fourth symposium of the international commission for research into European food history (pp. 171–83). East Lothian: Tuckwell Press Ltd.

Shaw, G. and Wright, C. (1982) A two-handle spoon: an aid for independent eating. *American Journal of Occupational Therapy*, 36, 45–6.

Steenbergen, B. (2000) The planning and co-ordination of prehension movements in spastic hemiparesis. PhD thesis, University of Nijmegen, the Netherlands.

Steenbergen, B., Hulstijn, W., De Vries, A. and Berger, M. (1996) Bimanual movement coordination in spastic hemiparesis. *Experimental Brain Research*, 110, 91–8.

Steenbergen, B., Van der Kamp, J., Smitsman, A.W. and Carson, R.G. (1997) Spoon handling in two- to four-year-old children. *Ecological Psychology*, 9, 113–29.

Steenbergen, B., Van Thiel, E., Hulstijn, W. and Meulenbroek, R.G.J. (2000) The coordination of reaching and grasping in spastic hemiparesis. *Human Movement Science*, 19, 75–105.

Sugden, D.A. and Keogh, J.F. (1990) *Problems in Motor Skill Development*. Columbia, SC: University of South Carolina Press.

Teuteberg, H.J. (1998) The German bourgeois at the dining table: structural changes of meal manners, 1880–1930. In M.R. Schrürer and A. Fenton (eds), *Food and Material Culture*. Proceedings of the fourth symposium of the international commission for research into European food history (pp. 133–70). East Lothian: Tuckwell Press Ltd.

Valsiner, J. (1997) *Culture and the Development of Children's Action: A Cultural-Historical Theory of Developmental Psychology*, 2nd edn. New York: John Wiley and Sons.

Van der Kamp, J. and Savelsbergh, G. (2000) Action and perception in infancy. *Infant Behavior and Development*, 23, 237–51.

Van der Kamp, J. and Steenbergen, B. (1999) The kinematics of eating: bringing the food to the mouth or the mouth to the food? *Experimental Brain Research*, 129, 68–76.

Van der Kamp, J., Steenbergen, B. and Smitsman, A.W. (1993) Preliminaries for a natural physical approach to tool-use in children. In S.S. Valenti and J.B. Pittenger (eds), *Studies in Perception and Action II* (pp. 329–32). Hilsdale, NJ: Lawrence Erlbaum Associates, Inc.

Van Thiel, E. and Steenbergen, B. (2001) Shoulder and hand displacements during hitting, reaching, and grasping movements in hemiparetic cerebral palsy. *Motor Control*, 5, 166–82.

Wyckoff, E. and Mitani, M. (1982) The spoon plate: a self-feeding device. *American Journal of Occupational Therapy*, 36, 333–5.

Yuen, H.K. (1993) Self-feeding system for an adult with head injury and severe ataxia. *American Journal of Occupational Therapy*, 47, 444–51.

Part II
Health sciences

7 Reflexes reflected

Past and present of theory and practice

Motohide Miyahara and Koop Reynders

1. Introduction

Neurological conditions that disturb co-ordinated movements include involuntary movements, such as abnormal reflexes, synkinesia, dyskinetic movements, and ataxia. Abnormal reflexes are of particular interest because the theoretical views on them have been changing considerably during the last century, and yet they are still used as a basis for assessment and intervention. The classic anatomical definition of reflex is 'an unvoluntary and relatively stereotype response to a specific sensory stimulus' (Gordon and Ghez, 1991, p. 565). As such, if reflexes are innately programmed and involuntary, then some previously so-called reflexes, such as the stepping reflex and postural reflex, can be no longer considered reflexive. At the same time, the assessment and intervention focus on reflexes has also been undergoing rapid change. To understand present-day practices, it would be useful to see them in the light of a historical perspective. In this chapter the reflex theory, the dynamic systems theory, and the neuronal group selection theory will be reviewed looking at the particular 'reflex' that each theory focuses on. In the discussion that follows, a strategy to advance health science will be noted from a philosophy of science framework.

2. Tonic reflexes: the reflex theory and practice

Tonic neck reflexes and tonic labyrinthine righting reflexes have been seen as obligatory, unchanging and primitive reflexes because they were initially recognised in those animals more primitive than monkeys. For example, while falling, a cat first erects the head by labyrinthine righting reflex, then rights up the rest of the body by cervical righting reflex before landing on the ground. Magnus (1924) suggested that these reflexes had been lost in the process of attaining upright walking because human arm function differs from the forelimb function among four-legged animals in balancing, reaching and grasping. When a dog drinks water at ground level, for example, the head and front legs need to be flexed, whereas the hind legs are extended. The symmetric tonic neck reflex thus serves four-legged animals functionally, and therefore should remain permanently.

This is not the case in humans. As typical infants grow up, primitive reflexes are usually integrated into functional behaviours and go unnoticed. Otherwise, they disrupt later motor development. In the presence of the asymmetric tonic neck reflex, for instance, the arm is extended to the side to which the infant is looking, thus preventing the infant from rolling or reaching toward an object in close proximity. The persistence of tonic reflexes has been, therefore, considered as a primary cause of delay in achieving motor milestones among young children and as a reason for difficulty in performing co-ordinated movements among children with movement disorders.

Clinically, prolonged emergence or re-emergence of primitive reflexes have been regarded as abnormal and pathological when they persist after certain periods during early childhood or reappear after brain damage. The hierarchical centres in the central nervous system (i.e. spinal and/or brain stem, midbrain, cortical) were assigned to each reflex based on experiments using decerebrate animals (Magnus, 1924) and classified into the ontogenetic stages of locomotor development (i.e. apedal, quadrupedal, bipedal) in children (Fiorentino, 1963). It was assumed that the cortex gradually started to take both facilitatory and inhibitory roles over the reflexes as young children matured (McGraw, 1945). When abnormal primitive reflexes were recognised in children with cerebral palsy, for instance, physio-therapists used to focus on the inhibition of the postural reflexes and the facilitation of voluntary movements (e.g. Bobath and Bobath, 1957; Rood, 1954).

So-called abnormal reflexes seemed not so abnormal to some researchers, however. For example, Fukuda (1984) identified tonic neck reflexes in athletes who were exerting their maximum muscle power as baseball players pitched and caught a ball, soccer players performed heading, and judoists and sumo wrestlers threw their opponents. Although those athletes were engaged in voluntary movements, the involuntary tonic reflexes occurred without their awareness, serving as an integral part of goal-directed motor behaviours. In that context, the tonic neck reflexes, though they had emerged in adults, were neither abnormal nor pathological.

The notion of obligatory and reproducible reflexes has also been challenged. Touwen (1976) found a wide variability in the presence and absence of infant reflexes among typically developing infants. According to Stein and Capaday (1988) and Rothwell (1994), proprioceptive reflexes are particularly changeable, variable, and influencible. Henderson (1986) questioned the validity of calling the reflexes abnormal, and considered it inappropriate to include the reflexes in screening procedures. Nevertheless, evaluation of tonic reflexes is still practised in clinical settings among paediatricians (e.g. Liptak, 1998), neurologists (e.g. Adams and Victor, 1993), physiotherapists (e.g. Watter, 1996), occupational therapists (Porr and Rainville, 1999), and also by coaches in disability sport settings (Mushett *et al.*, 1995).

Although practitioners may still examine reflexes, their use of terms and their views on the role of reflexes have changed considerably. Terms such as reflexive movements, and postural patterns, reactions, or responses, seem to be preferred by contemporary clinicians. The centre of each reflex is no longer considered localised. For instance, an obligatory and sustained tonic neck reflex is now regarded as a sign of pyramidal or extrapyramidal motor abnormality at any age (Adams and Victor, 1993). It is reasonable that Touwen (1984) questioned the use of adjective, 'primitive' for the reflexes.

Therapeutic emphasis on the inhibition of tonic reflexes has also changed. Bobath (1969) accepted the finding that the inhibitory positions would inhibit voluntary movements as well as involuntary reflexes in children with spasticity. She recommended inhibiting crucial reflexes only, and stressed the role of therapists in guiding voluntary movements. To date, this trend has been inherited. For example, Watter (1996) de-emphasises the inhibition of unwanted reflexive responses for children with minor co-ordination dysfunction because the inhibition would decrease the children's total function. Instead, the facilitation of positive support is encouraged with weight-shift reaction. The altered perspective is most symbolically represented by B. Bobath's rejection of the term, 'posture reflex mechanism' in favour of 'posture *control* mechanism' (Mayston, 1997).

3. Stepping movements: the dynamic systems theory and practice

Neonates exhibit rhythmical stepping movements if held in an upright position with the feet touching the floor. This response used to be called stepping reflex, and was believed to be observable only during a period from birth till about five months of age. After this reflexive period, no stepping seemed to occur by virtue of cortical inhibition until deliberate stepping emerged (McGraw, 1945). Thus, the stepping reflex was considered analogous to tonic reflexes; observable only at early life, inhibited if infants mature normally, and unrelated to later voluntary movements which appear after an inhibitory or stable period.

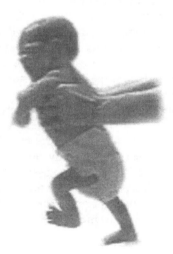

Figure 7.1 The stepping reflex

This classic view of stepping reflex was challenged by Zelazo *et al.* (1972) who reported that their infants had not gone through the inhibitory phase when the infants had practised stepping daily. In fact, the infants continued to step ceaselessly until they walked independently, earlier than usual. Zelazo (1983) interpreted the later sustained stepping in terms of Skinnerian conditioning, and stated that stepping 'progressed from a reflexive to an instrumental response' (p. 107). To explain the maintained stepping movements, Thelen (1983) devoted her attention to the role of physical weight and muscle strength. She hypothesised that infants in the stable period could step if they had sufficient strength or less body mass on their legs. The hypothesis was tested and supported by the demonstration of seemingly disappeared stepping when infants were submerged in the water (Thelen *et al.*, 1984) or held over on a treadmill (Thelen, 1986). It was concluded that the stepping had not disappeared but transformed itself into mature walking as a result of the self-organisation of dynamic systems, including muscle strength, balance, postural control, physical mass, and proportion (Thelen and Cooke, 1987). Newborn stepping was therefore related to later walking, and the old reflexive hypothesis on early stepping was refuted.

How can the dynamic systems theory be applied to practice? As far as stepping reaction is concerned, continuous stepping practice seems to promote earlier walking. For infants with Down syndrome who are known to start walking late, between 13 and 48 months of age, stepping training might help overcome otherwise late walking. The constraints on walking that are unique to infants with Down syndrome consist of short limbs, muscular hypotonia, laxity at the joints, and resultant body instability. Visual impairment and overweight may be additional constraining factors. Ulrich *et al.* (1992) manipulated the body weight and stability of infants with Down syndrome by supporting them on a motorised treadmill, and successfully elicited stepping movements. Ulrich *et al.* (2001) further trained a group of infants with Down syndrome on a treadmill, and demonstrated that the trained infants started to walk earlier by 101 days than did control infants with Down syndrome. It is hoped that treadmill training will become a supplement of standard medical treatment for infants with Down syndrome. Were treadmill training to be used as a supplementary treatment, the exercise should be placed in a meaningful context for children as the dynamic systems theory emphasises both contextual and task factors in their treatment.

In discussing the application of the dynamic systems theory to the practice of physiotherapy, Kamm *et al.* (1990) proposed to assess all subsystems involved, to focus on the system in its transition, and to control specific parameters such as the central nervous system, muscle strength, motivation, and context. With regard to the central nervous system, early intervention used to be encouraged for infants with motor disorders under the assumption that the system is still plastic and has a potential to self-organise functional patterns. The neuronal group selection theory fully integrates the dynamic systems theory and the principle of neuromuscular plasticity.

Primary variability

Activity of epigenetically determined, grossly specified primary neural repertoires

Neural system explores by means of self-generated activity, and consequently by
self-generated afferent information, all motor possibilities available within
neurobiological and anthropometric constraints set by evolution

Abundant variation in motor behaviour

Occurring during foetal life and infancy

Selection

Experiential selection of effective motor patterns and their associated
neuronal groups

Transient minor reduction in variation of motor behaviour

Abundant variation in motor behaviour

Occurring during infancy at function-specific ages

Secondary or adaptive variability

Creation of secondary neural repertoires with a large collection of parallel
channels due to exposure to a multitude of experiences

Mature situation
Task constraints: ability to adapt each movement exactly and efficiently to task-
specific conditions
No task constraints: multiple motor solutions or strategies for a single motor task

Onset: function-specific from mid-infancy onwards
Starting to bloom at 2–3 years; mature in adolescence

Figure 7.2 Motor development in light of Edelman's Neuronal Group Selection Theory
(Source: Hadders-Algra, 2000a. Copyright MacKeith Press)

4. Postural adjustments: the neuronal group selection theory and practice

Clinical evidence has demonstrated that the nervous system has the capability of self-organisation and plastic adaptation to the environment throughout the life span, even after brain damage (Kidd *et al.*, 1992). Edelman (1987) applied the mechanism of synaptic plasticity to the brain network model, and proposed the neuronal group selection theory. To explain co-ordinated movement, the theory assumes a global mapping which allows for perception–action coupling, or input–output correlations in Edelman's term. Global mapping consists of re-entrant connections in the complex sensory–motor circuits encompassing both cortical and subcortical regions. The circuits are variant in nature, and form *selected neuronal groups*, or 'interconnected neurons that tend to share functional properties and to discharge in a temporally correlated fashion' (Sporns and Edelman, 1993, p. 967). Edelman (1993) claims that variation and selection within the neuronal groups contribute to the solution of Bernstein's problem of inverse kinematics (further details see Sporns and Edelman, 1993).

Can the neuronal group selection theory be applied to describe, predict, and control the development and disorders of movement co-ordination? The theory has been considered useful not only in explaining variation in normal motor development (Hadders-Algra, 2000a), but also in understanding and treating developmental motor disorders (Hadders-Algra, 2000b). Hadders-Algra (2000a) applied the neuronal group selection theory to neuromotor development, and depicted three developmental phases: 1) the primary variability phase during the fetal and infant periods, 2) the selection phase during infancy and at function-specific age, and 3) the secondary or adaptive variability phase from mid-infancy onwards with a culmination at 2 to 3 years of age. Although primary variability is subject to neurobiological and anthropometric constraints, goal-directed motor behaviours are explored right from the beginning. Large cortical networks with unspecific synaptic connections are rearranged into smaller networks with specific connections during the developmental learning process. These function-specific selections of neural groups are made for postural adjustment, locomotion, speech, etc. The secondary or adaptive variability permits an efficient and precise motor solution by tuning into either specific task constraints or task-specific strategies. Phase-specific deficits in neuronal networks manifest themselves as deficiencies in postural adjustments among infants with different types of cerebral palsies (Hadders-Algra, 2000b; Hadders-Algra *et al.*, 1999), minor neurological dysfunction (Hadders-Algra, 2000b) and periventricular leucomalacia (Hadders-Algra, 2000b; Hadders-Algra *et al.*, 1999). In each study, Hadders-Algra and her colleagues prescribed phase- and deficit-specific intervention strategies for the improvement of postural adjustments. The efficacy of specific intervention, however, needs further clinical verification.

5. Discussion

Regarding competing views on the development of science, Popper (1963) argues that scientific knowledge grows as old theories are falsified and replaced by new theories that are more powerful in explanatory depth and predictive power over a wider range of phenomena. In contrast, Kuhn (1962) maintains that scientific theories, or paradigms, shift from an old one to an incompatible new one when an anomaly is perceived in the old paradigm and the new paradigm is generated to adjust to the anomaly. Paradigms are defined as 'universally recognised scientific achievements that for a time provide model problems and solutions to a community of practitioners' (Kuhn, 1962, p. viii). Did the theoretical transitions of reflex phenomena occur in the objectively progressive manner that Popper imposes on the growth of scientific knowledge, or in the non-cumulative manner Kuhn recognises from the historic pattern of scientific revolutions?

As far as tonic reflexes are concerned, modifications were made only in regard to auxiliary hypotheses, such as the interpretation of their manifestation and disappearance, the notion of localised centres, and the phylogenetic comparison. The basic mechanical assumption from a sensory receptor through neural tracts to a motor effector remains unchallenged. Indeed, dynamic systems theorists such as Kamm *et al.* (1990) accepted the notion of primitive reflexes, of which tonic reflexes are part, as a stable solution. Moreover, Hadders-Algra (2000a, 2000b) maintained that a synthesis of the reflex theory and the dynamic systems theory was achieved by the neuronal group selection theory. Thus, both the dynamic systems theory and the neuronal group selection theory seem to embrace the reflex theory. These theoretical developments may well, on the one hand, be regarded as a growth of scientific knowledge rather than as paradigm shifts.

On the other hand, neither the dynamic systems theory nor the neuronal group selection theory meets all three requirements that Popper (1963) assigned to new objective theories. According to these requirements new theories should 1) be simple, powerful, and unifying ideas, 2) be independently testable, explain, and predict at least as much empirical content as their predecessor, and 3) be better testable, and explain and predict a wider range of phenomena than old theories. Many would agree that both the dynamic systems theory and the neuronal group selection theory satisfy the first requirement. However, it is questionable if these two new theories meet the second and third requirements.

For instance, the 'reflex' that each theory focused on was not the same. Of course, the refutation of one 'reflex' phenomenon is not sufficient to undermine the entire reflex theory. However, to say the least, the new theories have not yet tested, explained, and predicted the whole empirical content that the reflex theory covered. Popper's alternative to an objective, logical, and ontological theory is a subjective, psychological, and epistemological theory. If the dynamic systems theory and the neuronal group selection theory do not yet fulfil the requirements to be categorised as objective ontological theories, then they can be considered either as subjective epistemological theories, or as new paradigms. Because the two new theories are still under development, it is probably premature to determine which of Popper's categories they fall into. Instead, let us explore the third possibility of new paradigms.

Provided that the dynamic systems theory and the neuronal group selection theory are new paradigms, the fact that they use different 'reflex' phenomena to refute the old reflex theory is no longer an issue. Kuhn (1962) used a mathematical term, incommensurability, to indicate the difficulty in comparing different theories point by point. The reason why the three theories dealt with different 'reflexes' might be, if not on an ad hoc basis, attributed to incommensurability of paradigm shifts. Kuhn (1962) states that 'paradigms gain their status because they are more successful than their competitors in solving *a few problems* that the group of practitioners has come to recognise as acute'. In doing so, a new paradigm does not necessarily preserve the gains of an old paradigm, as paradigms do not evolve in a cumulative manner. So far, the 'reflex' in the spotlight of each theory seems to have solved some problems that health practitioners faced. What is important for health scientists and practitioners is to retain the benefits of old theories because they may still serve for problem-solving in practice. As a solution beyond the dichotomy between Popper's objectivism and Kuhn's relativism, R.J. Bernstein (1983) proposed to focus on practical tasks and practical rationality. What is needed is for those who engage in health science and who work on movement co-ordination in children to concentrate on practical tasks and practical rationality in order for further theoretical sophistication and clinical advancement.

References

Adams, R.D. and Victor, M. (1993) *Principles of Neurology*, 5th edn. New York: McGraw Hill.

Bernstein, R.J. (1983) *Beyond Objectivism and Relativism: Science, Hermeneutics, and Praxis*. Philadelphia: University of Pennsylvania Press.

Bobath, B. (1969) The treatment of neuromuscular disorders by improving patterns of co-ordination. *Physiotherapy*, 55, 18–22.

Bobath, K. and Bobath, B. (1957) Control of motor function in the treatment of cerebral palsy. *Physiotherapy*, 43, 295–303.

Edelman, G.M. (1987) *Neural Darwinism: The Theory and Neuronal Group Selection*. New York: Basic Books.

Edelman, G.M. (1993) Neural Darwinism: Selection and re-entrant signaling in higher brain function. *Neuron*, 10, 115–25.

Fiorentino, M.R. (1963) *Reflex Testing Methods for Evaluating CNS Development*. Springfield: IL: Thomas.

Fukuda, T. (1984) *Statokinetic Reflexes in Equilibrium and Movement*. Tokyo: University of Tokyo Press.

Gordon, J, and Ghez, C. (1991) Muscle receptors and spinal reflexes: the stretch reflex. In E.R. Kandel, I.H. Schwartz and T.M. Jessel (eds), *Principles of Neural Science*. London: Prentice Hall International.

Hadders-Algra, M. (2000a) The neuronal group selection theory: a framework to explain variation in normal motor development. *Developmental Medicine and Child Neurology*, 42, 566–72.

Hadders-Algra, M. (2000b) The neuronal group selection theory: promising principles for understanding and treating developmental motor disorders. *Developmental Medicine and Child Neurology*, 42, 707–15.

Hadders-Algra, M., Brogren, E., Katz-Salamon, M. and Forssberg, H. (1999) Periventricular leucomalacia and preterm birth have different detrimental effects on postural adjustments. *Brain*, 122, 727–40.

Hadders-Algra, M., Van der Fits, I.B., Stremmelaar, E.F. and Touwen, B.C. (1999) Development of postural adjustments during reaching in infants with CP. *Developmental Medicine and Child Neurology*, 41, 766–76.

Henderson, S. (1986) Problems of motor development: some theoretical issues. *Advances in Special Education*, 5, 147–86.

Kamm, K., Thelen, E. and Jensen, J.L. (1990) A dynamical systems approach to motor development. *Phyiscal Therapy*, 70, 763–72.

Kidds, G., Lawes, N. and Musa, I. (1992) *Understanding Neuromuscular Plasticity: A Basis for Clinical Rehabilitation*. London: Edward Arnold.

Kuhn, T. S. (1962) *The Structure of Scientific Revolutions*. Chicago: University of Chicago Press.

Liptak, G. S. (1998) The child who has severe neurologic impairment. *Pediatric Clinics of North America*, 45, 123–68.

Magnus, R. (1924) *Körperstellung*. Berlin: Verlag von Julius Springer.

Mayston, M.J. (1997) *Course Notes: Normal Postural Control Mechanism*. London: The Bobath Centre.

McGraw, M.B. (1945) *The Neuromuscular Maturation of the Human Infant*. New York: Columbia University Press.

Mushett, C.A., Wyeth, D.O. and Richter, K.J. (1995) Cerebral palsy. In B. Goldberg (ed.), *Sports and Exercise for Children with Chronic Health Conditions*. Champaign, IL: Human Kinetics.

Popper, K.R. (1963) *Conjectures and Refutations: The Growth of Scientific Knowledge*. London: Routledge and Kegan Paul.

Porr, S.M. and Rainville, E.B. (1999) *Pediatric Therapy: A Systems Approach*. Philadelphia: F.A. Davis

Rood, M. (1954) Neurophysiological reactions as a basis for physiotherapy. *Physical Therapy Review*, 34, 9–23.

Rothwell, J. (1994) *Control of Human Voluntary Movement*, 2nd edn. London: Chapman Hall.

Sporns, O. and Edelman, G.M. (1993) Solving Bernstein's problem: a proposal for the development of coordinated movement by selection. *Child Development*, 64, 960–81.

Stein, R. and Capady, C. (1988) The modulation of human reflexes during functional motor tasks. *Trends in Neuroscience*, 11, 328–32.

Thelen, E. (1983) Learning to walk is still an 'old' problem: a reply to Zelazo (1983). *Journal of Motor Behavior*, 15, 139–61.

Thelen, E. (1986) Treadmill-elicited stepping in seven-month-old infants. *Child Development*, 57, 1498–506.

Thelen, E. and Cooke, D.W. (1987) Relationship between newborn stepping and later walking: a new interpretation. *Developmental Medicine and Child Neurology*, 29, 380–93.

Thelen, E., Fisher, D.M. and Ridley-Johnson, R. (1984) The relationship between physical growth and a newborn reflex. *Infant Behavior and Development*, 7, 479–93.

Touwen, B.C. (1976) *Neurological Development in Infancy. Clinics in Developmental Medicine*, No. 58. London: S.I.M.P.

Touwen, B. (1984) Primitive reflexes: conceptional or sematic problem? In H.F. Prechtl (ed.), *Continuity of Neural Functions from Prenatal to Postnatal Life* (pp. 115–23). Philadelphia: J. B. Lippincott.

Ulrich, B.D., Ulrich, D.A. and Collier, D.H. (1992) Alternating stepping patterns: Hidden abilities of 11-month-old infants with Down syndrome. *Developmental Medicine and Child Neurology*, 34, 233–9.

Ulrich, D.A., Ulrich, B.D., Angulo-Kinzler, R. and Yun, J.K. (2001) Treadmill training in infants with Down syndrome: evidence-based developmental outcomes. *Pediatrics*, 108, 84–91.

Watter, P. (1996) Physiotherapy and the growing child. In Y.B. Burns and J. MacDonald (eds), *Physiotherapy and the Growing Child* (pp. 415–32). London: W. B. Saunders.

Zelazo, P.R. (1983) The development of walking: new findings and old assumptions. *Journal of Motor Behavior*, 15, 99–137.

Zelazo, P.R., Zelazo, N.A. and Kolb, S. (1972) 'Walking' in the newborn. *Science*, 176, 314–15.

8 Children's co-ordination and developmental movement difficulty

Helen E. Parker and Dawne Larkin

1. Introduction

During typical development, experience and maturation interact to influence the development of musculoskeletal and neuromotor systems, which enable children's motor skills to improve with increasing age. It is conventional to see the development of movement skill co-ordination as age-related but not age-determined. This aspect is highlighted in the typical variation for learning motor skills and the individual differences in motor performance of any group of same-aged children. However, there are some children who exhibit difficulty co-ordinating their movement and for whom learning fine and gross motor skills is very hard. For some, such children are seen to have a delay in motor development; however, as this chapter will clarify, it is our view that the developmental pathway of these children is different compared to their typically developing peers. The interaction between the child, the environment, and culturally demanding motor tasks contributes to the difference in developmental outcome.

This chapter presents a review of literature including examples from our research into the problems experienced by children with co-ordination difficulties. We present information on the differences in motor abilities, the effects associated with other constraints affecting skill development, and differences in functional skill performances. The last section is directed towards the practical application of this knowledge to intervention and discusses the importance of early intervention in shaping the child's own developmental pathway, and the different intervention models, including our task-based model, that have been used in the physical education and therapy domains.

2. What is developmental movement disorder?

Up to 20 per cent of young children find performing and learning motor skills very difficult. Their motor skills are impaired to the degree that they cannot successfully participate in sports and games with their peers. Their movement problems include a variety of difficulties such as continual misjudgement of distance and time (e.g. bumping into objects and people, tripping over, failing to catch balls), inability to co-ordinate complex movements necessary to participate in age-appropriate sports and games (e.g. running, kicking, catching, and throwing), and difficulties in manipulative skills, such as in writing, copying, drawing, and dressing. The key issue in movement dysfunction is that children are unable to perform the required actions of daily living in a culturally acceptable way. Arnheim and Sinclair (1979) said that these children 'have motor learning difficulties and display asynchronous and inefficient motor behaviour when attempting to carry out movement tasks that they would commonly be expected to accomplish under reasonable circumstances' (p. 256).

There are many terms in the literature to describe the motor difficulties of children. Terminology is usually linked to the perspective of the professional – the educational, the medical, or the therapeutic (for reviews see Cermak *et al.*, 2002; Miyahara and Register, 2000; Peters *et al.*, 2001). The terms include motor learning difficulty, poor co-ordination, clumsiness, dyspraxia, minimal brain disorder/dysfunction, sensory integrative disorder, perceptual–motor disorder, and more recently, developmental co-ordination disorder (DCD; American Psychiatric Association, 1987; 1994) and specific developmental disorder of motor function (SDDMF; World Health Organization, 1992). Clinical diagnostic criteria identifying DCD and SDDMF specify a marked impairment in the development of motor co-ordination. The DCD diagnostic criteria include significant interference with academic achievement and/or performance of activities of daily living, but exclude a diagnosable medical condition such as cerebral palsy, hemiplegia, or muscular dystrophy (American Psychiatric Association, 1994). As physical educators, however, it is our view that understanding movement disorder and how to alleviate the problem is important, whether or not the disorder adversely impacts on the academic performance of the child. From the perspective of the physical educator, movement difficulties interfere with motor development and consequently impact on the child's development of social relationships and a healthy, active lifestyle.

The estimated prevalence of motor disorder varies from 6 per cent to as high as 22 per cent (Gubbay, 1975; Kadesjo and Gillberg, 1999; Keogh, 1968; Larkin and Rose, 1999) for children aged from 5 to 11 years. The ratio of males to females who are identified with developmental movement disorder varies. Our clinical figures have changed over the past years. In 1986, there was one girl to every nine boys in our developmental movement skills programme. But by 1990, this ratio had changed from 1:5 to, most recently, in 2001 1:3. However, surveys of motor skills in the wider population of children, as distinct from the clinical referrals, reveal that gender distribution is more equal. For example, Larkin and Rose (1999) in a sample of 846 children found that 50 per cent of children identified as having movement problems by a standardised screening tool were girls. Gubbay reported a similar distribution (1975). By contrast, in a Swedish population study, Kadesjo and Gillberg (1999) report that the ratio of males to females ranges from 4:1 to 7:1. It is unclear what contributes to these differences across cultures. In part it may reflect the different assessment tools used in these population studies. In the Australian samples there is a clear difference between the clinical referral bias toward boys and the incidence of motor impairment in population surveys. Perhaps there is still a greater social pressure on boys to excel at sport in comparison to girls and therefore boys with relatively poor co-ordination are more noticeable to parents and professionals than girls with similar movement difficulties (Revie and Larkin, 1993a).

What are the long-term effects of motor co-ordination problems in children? Some teachers, clinicians, and medical practitioners still assume that motor impairment is due to motor delay and that children with motor problems will grow out of their motor difficulties. However, recent research has shown that motor problems can have long-term effects. Losse and colleagues (1991) reported that children identified as clumsy at 6 years of age continued to have motor difficulties as well as social, emotional, and educational problems at 16 years. Other studies (Cantell *et al.*, 1994; Rasmussen and Gillberg, 2000) have supported the view that there can be long-term effects in children with developmental co-ordination disorder (for a review see Cantell and Kooistra, 2002). It seems that movement co-ordination problems can result in a life-long disability, and that problems encountered in childhood may persist well into adulthood (Fitzpatrick, 2000; Kirby and Drew, 1999). Consequently it is important for the physical educator and coach to address the problem as early as possible and develop positive strategies to reduce long-term effects.

The early identification and subsequent intervention of motor co-ordination difficulties such as DCD or dyspraxia can impact positively on the developmental pathway. The developing musculoskeletal, neuromuscular and cardio-respiratory systems are responsive to the demands placed on them by physical activity. The child who has co-ordination difficulties needs specialised attention at an early age to reduce the movement problems and ensure more optimal development of these systems. Early intervention also avoids the attendant psychosocial stigma that can arise from looking awkward in movement skills and failing to cope with physical play activities. Being able to participate in the physical activity of their peer group helps the child to socialise in their play environment. Later in this chapter we will give an overview of task-specific intervention methods that aim to facilitate all-round motor development.

Motor difficulties can impact negatively on the psychosocial aspects of young people's lives. A follow-up survey of 86 teenagers who had attended a motor skill development programme as primary school children, found that their physical self-perceptions were still relatively negative compared to those of normally co-ordinated peers (Larkin and Parker, 1997). Among other low physical self-perceptions, adolescents with poor co-ordination perceived themselves to have lower levels of physical activity, endurance, and sports competence. As adolescents they participated in significantly fewer physical activities out of school time and had more sedentary hobbies, such as watching TV, computing, reading, and listening to music. Interestingly, both normally and poorly co-ordinated teenagers were similar in their perceptions of the benefits of physical activity, although the poorly co-ordinated group reported significantly higher barriers to physical activity than their normally co-ordinated peers (Larkin and Parker, 1999). With respect to the influence of attitudes of parents and adolescents to the benefits of physical activity, there was a significant correlation between parents' perception of barriers and those of adolescents. If parents reported high barriers then the normally co-ordinated adolescents were also more likely to report higher barriers too. However, for the adolescents with poor co-ordination a positive response to the benefits of physical activity was linked with perceptions of fewer barriers to physical activity. This finding suggests that if skills and knowledge of physical activity are provided through an early intervention programme then access to physical activity may be improved for this group.

In a survey of 380 8- to 12-year-old children who were classified as either poorly, moderately, or well co-ordinated, Rose *et al.* (1994) measured the perceived social support from parents, teachers, classmates and best friends using Harter's Social Support Scale (Harter, 1985). This tool uses a 4-point scale, based on the degree of agreement the child has with particular statements about support. For example, statements such as, 'Some kids don't get asked to play games with classmates very often but other kids often get asked to play in games with their classmates' were read to the children who nominated which statement was most like them and whether it was 'really true' or 'sort of true'. The children with movement difficulties recorded lowest perceived social support scores, with significantly lower ratings for classmates and best friend support. Overall the psychosocial profile of the children with co-ordination difficulties was poorer than their co-ordinated peers. They had lower self-perceptions in the scholastic domain as well as the athletic domain (Rose *et al.*, 1997), low motivation for challenging activities (Rose *et al.*, 1998) and the girls with poor co-ordination also had the highest performance anxiety (Rose *et al.*, 1999). It appeared from these data and other studies that children with poor co-ordination experience more psycho-social problems, greater loneliness and isolation, and greater exclusion and ridicule in the playground (Schoemaker and Kalverboer 1994; Smyth and Anderson, 2000).

Identification

Identification of children with motor difficulties often takes longer than it should and causes a certain amount of anxiety for the parents and the child (Dyspraxia Foundation, 1998). There are a number of factors that contribute to the difficulties with identification. We will briefly address two important issues for movement specialists: a) how well different tests identify motor dysfunction, and b) the importance of professional development for accurate identification by testers.

Burton and Miller (1998) report that there are approximately 45 different assessment batteries readily available for assessing movement skills. Of these, several prominent tools are used to identify children with movement problems. These include the Bruininks–Oseretsky Test of Motor Proficiency (BOTMP; Bruininks, 1978), the Basic Motor Ability Test – revised (Arnheim and Sinclair, 1979), the McCarron Assessment of Neuromuscular Development (McCarron, 1982), the Test of Gross Motor Development – 2nd edition (Ulrich, 2000), the Test of Motor Impairment (TOMI-H; Stott *et al.*, 1984), and its most recent revision the Movement Assessment Battery for Children (MABC; Henderson and Sugden,

1992). Each of these test batteries includes items which sample different areas of motor performance such as balance control, fine motor skills, gross motor skills, and speed and agility. It is important for the physical educator to be aware of the strengths and weaknesses of these popular tests (for review see Burton and Miller, 1998).

One of the issues that constantly worries practitioners as well as movement scientists is the lack of agreement between tests when they are used to identify children with movement problems. Few studies have explored the identification accuracy of these well-cited assessment tests. Quite different detection rates emerge from these studies and different children are selected by different tests. For example, Riggen *et al.* (1990) evaluated the concurrent validity between the TOMI-H and the BOTMP short form for measuring motor deficit in 41 children. The impaired–nonimpaired classification for each test was based on the 15th percentile performance standard and the overall proportion of agreement of these classifications was a relatively high 0.88 (88 per cent decision consistency). However, closer scrutiny revealed that the BOTMP identified only four motor impaired cases, whereas the TOMI-H identified nine of the 41 children, which represents a low 44 per cent agreement and points to poor decision consistency between the tests.

In a similar study, Maeland (1992) examined the concurrent validity between the Test of Motor Proficiency (TMP; Gubbay, 1975) and the Test of Motor Impairment (TOMI-H; Stott *et al.*, 1984) for identifying motor impairment in a group of 223 children. Of children deemed clumsy by the TOMI-H 15th percentile standard cut score, TMP identified 53 per cent, and the overall proportion of agreement was 0.51. Even the agreement rate for identifying children without impairment was only 50 per cent. Maeland (1992) found that the concurrent validity between the tests was inadequate.

Recently, we (Tan *et al.*, 2001) conducted a comparison between the BOTMP short form and the MAND using the 15th percent cut standard. Based on intitial testing with the MABC, 26 children were identified with motor impairment and 26 children, who were age- and gender-matched, were identified as controls without motor impairment. From the subgroup of 26 children with motor impairment, only 8 children were identified by the BOTMP short form, whereas a total of 23 children were identified by the MAND. The overall decision agreement between the BOTMP short form and the MAND was only 8 of 23 cases, a low 0.35 agreement level.

Based on the initial classification of the MABC, we found that the MAND was nearly three times more sensitive than the BOTMP short form for identifying children with motor impairment (81 per cent compared to 31 per cent). Our results provide support for the findings reported by Kaplan and colleagues (Kaplan *et al.*, 1998). They reported that only 26 per cent of children identified below the cutoff for impairment on the MABC were identified below the impairment cutoff on the BOTMP short form for a sample of children with learning and attention problems. Using the 15th percentile cut score to make motor impairment decisions with the BOTMP short form seems very conservative. Despite its wide use for identifying children with movement problems, the number of children missed by the BOTMP short form is a concern

It is clear from the above studies that tests differ with regard to their discrimination accuracy. Certainly it is important to recognise the deficiencies any test has. We need more research to develop objective, reliable and valid tests, ones that include items that can be objectively scored, that provide reliable information, that have up-to-date norms and are culturally appropriate to the children being tested. Chow *et al.* (2001) in Hong Kong, Miyahara *et al.* (1998) in Japan, and Rosblad and Gard (1998) in Sweden showed discrepancies in the use of the MABC in their respective countries. These studies caution us that we should not assume that a test item that discriminates motor proficiency well in one culture will apply to other cultures.

Each of the above tests requires a degree of expertise to administer and is typically the domain of clinicians, human movement specialists and therapists. Teachers are generally not trained to use them nor are these tests appropriate to guide physical education instruction. Without training in movement observation and analysis, it is difficult for professionals to identify children with co-ordination difficulties. This is clearly the case from our data (Revie and Larkin, 1993a), which showed that primary school teachers often mis-identified children, such that girls who were identified had very severe co-ordination difficulties while boys who were identified by teachers ranged from the bottom 5th percentile up to the 70th percentile on Arnheim and Sinclair's (1979) test of motor proficiency. It is clear that we need better training of professionals in movement observation and analysis if we are to improve the accuracy of identification of children with co-ordination difficulties.

A heterogeneous group

It is widely accepted that children with motor difficulties are a heterogeneous group (Cratty, 1994; Dewey and Kaplan, 1994; Hoare, 1994; Miyahara, 1994; Morris and Whiting, 1971; Wann *et al.*, 1998; Wright and Sugden 1996). A number of co-ordination subgroups have emerged from cluster analysis of children's performances on a range of sensory, perceptual and motor tasks (Hoare, 1994; Macnab *et al.*, 2001). For example, Hoare (1994) described five subgroups within a pool of 80 children identified as having motor difficulties. Scores were obtained from a number of tests that measure kinaesthetic acuity, visual perception, visual–motor integration, manual dexterity, static and dynamic balance, and gross motor co-ordination. Twenty-eight per cent of the children with poor co-ordination scored below average on gross motor co-ordination and kinaesthetic acuity. A second cluster comprised 25 per cent of children who scored above the mean average for visual perception and visual motor tasks but performed on average (for a group with DCD) for each of the other tasks. A smaller cluster of 19 per cent of children comprised those who experienced difficulty in visual motor tasks and visual perception as well as static balance. Another cluster, 17.5 per cent of the sample, performed above average in kinaesthetic acuity and running, and close to average on the other tasks by comparison with the other children with poor co-ordination. The smallest cluster, 10 per cent, exhibited difficulties in manual dexterity, static balance and gross motor co-ordination.

Using different tasks, Wright and Sugden (1996) identified four subgroups within their developmental co-ordination disorder sample. From the 69 Singaporean children aged between 6 and 9, using the MABC checklist, they found that the largest cluster (61 per cent) were those children who displayed difficulties when time was under their own control and the environment was stable. The second cluster (14 per cent) performed better when left to their own timing in a stable environment and exhibited difficulties when asked to adapt to external forces. The third cluster consisted of 17 per cent of the children who performed best in tasks that used their hands quickly from a stable position but performed poorly when the environment changed. The last cluster had the smallest number (7 per cent). These exhibited greatest difficulty manipulating their hands at speed and also performed poorly on the dynamic balance tasks.

From these studies it is interesting to note the difficulties seen in the subgroups are not common to all children with motor co-ordination difficulties. Some tasks are performed relatively well by comparison to others. Miyahara (1994) concluded that motor timing and co-ordination problems are subgroup-specific. So where children's performances lack fluency and co-ordination the assumption is that they have poor timing. However, this may not be the case. At one extreme there would be some children who have relatively rigid and overly stable motor systems that may be insensitive to environmental information and will display highly inaccurate timing adaptations to externally set tempos. At the other extreme, children may be quite sensitive to such information and show high variability in self-paced tempos. It might be expected that most children with motor co-ordination difficulties might fall between these two extremes and the amount of variability in their performance would depend on the nature of the task, the tempos they are trying to match and the environmental circumstances.

It is important that we recognise that subtypes exist within the population of children with motor difficulties. Accurate assessment and accurate interpretation of measures are important if we are to target intervention to the individual's needs.

Motor impairment is often observed in children with other diagnosed disorders. For example, children with learning and attention problems often have motor co-ordination problems too (Beyer, 1999; Harvey and Reid, 1997; Kadesjo and Gillberg, 2001). Although it can be concluded that some children with Attention Deficit Hyperactivity Disorder (ADHD) have motor control problems, it remains to be seen whether subtypes in attention disorders have distinctly different motor profiles from each other. In the current DSM-IV diagnostic classification (APA, 1994), the ADHD is described as including three types – the hyperactive/impulsive subtype, the inattentive subtype and a combined subtype. Our recent research (Hummelshoj, 1999; Larkin *et al.*, 2000) with a sample of 32 boys aged between 6 and 11 years showed that the inattentive subgroup had significantly lower motor proficiency, based on the neuro-developmental index of the McCarron (1982) test, than the combined subgroup or age-matched controls. In looking at the gross motor average scores within the test, the inattentive group had the worst performance, followed by the combined group and then the control group. Only the inattentive group had significantly poorer fine motor scores compared to either of the other two groups. A discriminant analysis based on the fine and gross motor scores of the children correctly classified 93 per cent of children into their respective groups; that is, into the inattentive group, the combined disorder group and the control group. Overall the results showed that the groups with ADHD differed from the control group and the inattentive group had the most impaired motor profile.

3. Differences in motor control of children with co-ordination difficulties

This section will be looking at the neuromuscular responses of children with co-ordination difficulties; specifically reaction time (RT) and EMG patterning. Williams (2002) has completed a comprehensive review of the difficulties and differences exhibited by these children.

Reaction time

This measure is of interest because it is viewed as an indicator of the degree of integrity of the neuromuscular pathways and the ability of the system to respond to environmental information/stimuli rapidly. With respect to reaction time to visual and kinaesthetic stimuli, Smyth and Glencross (1986) showed that, in a simple and two-choice reaction time key-press response 5-year-old children with co-ordination difficulties responded more slowly to the kinaesthetic but not visual stimuli. However, Henderson *et al.* (1992) found that children aged 8 to 11 years had significantly slower visual RTs (367 ms) than age matched controls (326 ms). Williams and Burke (1998, cited in Williams, 2002) studied the RTs for unimanual and bimanual reaching tasks in children with and without DCD. Data showed there was little difference in the RT in initiating one- compared to two-handed movements between the groups; however, children with DCD took significantly longer to initiate a bimanual response than a unimanual response. For both symmetrical and asymmetrical (each hand moving simultaneously to targets at different distances) tasks children with DCD had significantly slower RTs (315 ms and 312 ms) than control children (269 ms and 274 ms). They interpreted the difference in the bimanual RTs to indicate a difference in motor planning processes in the children with DCD because each limb is treated as a separate entity rather than as a co-ordinated whole (or co-ordinative structure). Huh *et al.* (1998) also analysed the variability with which children with DCD initiated single and bimanual reaching movements and found that the DCD children were significantly more variable in RT than their normally co-ordinated peers. In our lab, Raynor (1998) used a visual reaction time task and showed that children with co-ordination difficulties had both slower motor times and slower reaction times than age-matched peers. Overall, children with DCD tend to have longer RTs as well as more variable RTs.

Timing and rhythm

A co-ordinated action is well timed, fluent and smoothly performed, and rhythm requires precise timing. However, children with motor difficulties show inefficient, poorly timed movements and seem to lack natural rhythm. Over the past decade research has been trying to determine whether these timing problems are related to poor internal timing control (self-pacing) or to deficient perception of external beat information (external pacing).

For example, studies of timing control under external pacing conditions in 6- to 11-year-old children with co-ordination problems highlight poor timing consistency when they are required to maintain a predetermined pace or to synchronise their tapping with an auditory metronome (Geuze and Kalverboer, 1987, 1993, 1994; Greene and Williams, 1993; Williams *et al.*, 1992). In Williams and colleagues' (1992) study, most children with DCD showed time lags in matching the tempo and drifted between early, anticipatory and too late responses. This contrasted with the accurate synchronicity showed by control children. The studies by Williams *et al.* (1992) and Lundy-Ekman *et al.* (1991) attributed the poor timing to a faulty central timer mechanism. However, Lundy-Ekman *et al.* (1991) also indicated that poor force control may be a problem for some. Although it is difficult to clearly separate timing from force in movement control, these results concur with the characteristic heterogeneity in those with movement co-ordination difficulties.

A recent study by Volman and Geuze (1998) looked at dynamical systems explanations of stability and entrainment in tapping variability. Children aged 7 to 12 years tapped at self-paced and paced modes using single and bi-finger patterns. As the visual metronome increased its frequency (in 0.8 Hz steps), children with DCD were less able to keep pace and switched from anti-phase, alternate tapping to in-phase tapping at a lower critical frequency than the non-DCD group. Children with DCD also required more time to re-establish timing stability after such a switch in co-ordination pattern, and this stability of pattern was maintained across a narrower range of frequencies. This appeared to point to a potential lack of flexibility in the system and highlighted how vulnerable a child with DCD is to a changing sensory environment. As others had previously reported, Volman and Geuze identified different timing subgroups. One group was characterised by very poor bimanual co-ordination patterns but stable single hand co-ordination, a second group had the reverse characteristics and a third group had both poor bimanual and poor single hand co-ordination.

The question that is less clear is: do children with DCD also have difficulties with timing when they are allowed to choose their tapping tempo? We addressed this question in our research into self-paced timing control in children with movement co-ordination dysfunction. The studies looked at the rhythmic consistency in 6- to 11-year-olds in tasks that included self-paced one-hand and two-hand tapping (both in-phase and anti-phase co-ordination), foot tapping and rhythmic jumping (Parker *et al.*, 1997; Parker *et al.*, in preparation). Sometimes children changed their tapping pace according to an instruction to go faster or slower (Chng, 1996) and sometimes children synchronised tapping speed with a metronome (Hennessey, 1998). So that we could determine the degree of stability of tapping the tempo, tapping trials were of 30s duration. The children's motor co-ordination level was objectively scored using the MAND test (McCarron, 1982), with children being classified as having DCD if their scores fell one standard deviation or lower than the age norms.

Linked to what we already knew about the existence of different subtypes of DCD, Parker *et al.* (1997) found timing control differences specific to particular tasks between three groups – children with gross motor problems, those having combined fine and gross motor difficulties, and those who were normally co-ordinated. The preferred speed of performance was not different between the groups; however, the variability of timing in tapping was different. The fine and gross motor impaired group had more problems than the others with hand tapping, but the variability of foot tapping and repetitive jumping was similar among the three groups. We concluded that it was premature to assume that timing difficulties were necessarily the same for all children with DCD or expressed the same in all tasks.

Another study (Parker *et al.*, in preparation) also examined timing stability in self-paced tapping, this time with one or two hands. The consistency of tapping improved with age, as Williams *et al.* (1999) and Greene and Williams (1993) had also reported for externally paced tapping, however timing consistency was significantly lower overall in the children with DCD. The 10-year-old children with DCD performed like normally co-ordinated 6-year-olds, whereas in the normally co-ordinated group timing consistency had plateaued around 8 to 10 years. When the children with DCD tapped with two hands in an alternate manner, the coupling between the hands improved the timing stability of each hand, particularly for the least rhythmic one. In contrast, both hands became more variable when tapping in-phase than when tapping singly. Volman and Geuze (1998) also identified a subgroup of children with DCD who had poor single- compared to two-hand timing control. Thus, even when able to choose the tempo of hand tapping, children with DCD find the co-ordination demands of in-phase, symmetrical tapping more demanding with respect to timing consistency than an alternate tapping pattern.

As an extension of this work, Chng (1996) conducted a study to examine whether children could change pace and still maintain rhythmic stability in single-hand tapping. In each pace change, trial participants began tapping at their own self-chosen tempo for the first 10s and then changed to the 'twice as fast' or 'half as slow' tempos on command. They attempted to sustain that new tempo for the rest of the 30s trial. As before, we found an age-related improvement in tapping variability for all children, with children with DCD having higher variability of timing than their normally co-ordinated peers. With respect to changing speed, normally co-ordinated children were more accurate in scaling their speed to twice or half pace compared to the DCD children and were also able to produce a consistent baseline tempo. In older children with DCD, slow pace trials resulted in a drift to faster tapping at baseline. So although these children were able to change pace as instructed, they were unable to maintain a stable, self-selected tempo and changed pace within only a limited range of tempos. The 6-year-olds with DCD had the most limited range of volitional tapping rates of all.

The most recent study in this series by Hennessey (1998) focused on the particular responses within 5- to 11-year-old children in the DCD population to external pacing tasks. We were interested in whether there were children who were temporally rigid and insensitive to the metronome tempos and who therefore might display highly inaccurate timing adaptation to external tempos, especially tempos different to their intrinsic, preferred tempo. Alternatively, were there children who were overly sensitive to external pacing, such that they found it difficult to stabilise a preferred tempo and instead showed high variability and instability in self-paced tapping? Children performed single-hand tapping at their comfortable, self-chosen pace for a whole 30 seconds (baseline pacing consistency). Subsequent trials involved 10s self-paced tapping followed by 20s paced by an auditory metronome at 60, 90, 120, 180, 240, and 300 beats per minute presented in a fixed ascending order.

This study again confirmed that the self-pacing stability of children with DCD was lower compared to the normally co-ordinated controls. In beat-matching trials, children with DCD were less accurate in adjusting from self-chosen to the imposed pace, regardless of which hand was used. Tapping accuracy for all children, however, was higher when the imposed metronome tempo was most similar to that preferred under self-pacing and the accuracy decreased for tempos both slower and faster than this 'local minima'. All children had difficulty synchronising at tempos higher than 120 bpm. The tapping variability of the older DCD group was like the younger, normally co-ordinated children. Overall, synchronisation inaccuracy and variability was higher for the children with DCD, and especially for the younger DCD group. The young DCD group tended to tap faster and with greater variability than the other children, with each hand, and did not appear to be entrained to the metronome tempo unless it matched their preferred tempo.

In summary, studies have highlighted the greater timing difficulties in rhythmic tapping that children with DCD have when performing either self-paced or metronome-paced tasks compared to normally co-ordinated children. These timing features characterise a group who appear very much 'limited-paced' and who are relatively insensitive to environmental pacing information, but who also have poor internal timing control. Therefore these children may be especially vulnerable to failure in tasks that require consistent, repetitive actions (serial, closed tasks) whereas some may have added difficulty with tasks involving complex timing of movement to information from the external environment (open tasks).

4. Interacting constraints on skill co-ordination

Physical fitness

Generally, children with poor motor co-ordination are less physically active than normally co-ordinated children (Bouffard *et al.*, 1996). Evidence is also mounting from our work that these children are less physically fit. Poor fitness can constrain the ability of the child to perform optimally so compounding their difficulty in learning new motor skills. Data from Larkin and Hoare (1991), O'Beirne *et al.* (1994) and Hands *et al.* (2000) indicate the degree of difficulty these children have. Generally, the children score below the 25th or 30th percentile level of age-matched standards from the Australian Schools Fitness standards (Pyke, 1986). This level represents the minimal standard for physical health in children. Measuring *aerobic capacity* is difficult for children with motor co-ordination problems, as running for extended periods, for example, the 1.6 km run which is the standard endurance test, is hard for them. We have found better success with the Manitoba 800m run from the Manitoba Physical Fitness Performance Test (Manitoba Department of Education, 1980). Recently, we have trialled the multi-stage shuttle fitness test in which children run 20m laps to a set cadence which increases in pace. We obtained encouraging results, especially if the child has an exercise buddy running with them encouraging them to stick at it. The endurance score is the number of completed laps. Nevertheless, whichever protocol is used, these children perform poorly, generally below the 25th percentile level. Preliminary studies on monitoring these children's heart rates show that they are peaking very rapidly and staying very high. The physical effort of performing motor skills is very high and these children are working physically very hard, which is contrary to popular perceptions that these children are lazy and not trying hard enough.

In measuring *anaerobic capacity*, usually a 50m sprint is used, which is relatively simple to administer. For the poorly co-ordinated group percentile ranks for sprint time range from below the 5th to 65th percentile, however, 70 per cent of these children scored at or below the 10th percentile for running speed. O'Beirne and colleagues (1994) measured anaerobic capacity using the Wingate 30s bicycle test and found that children with poor co-ordination reached similar heart rates to their age-matched co-ordinated peers but had significantly lower power.

A similar pattern of low scores for children with poor co-ordination is seen for *muscular strength* and *endurance*. There are a number of tests that we have used with these children – grip strength, the number of sit ups in 60s, curl ups, modified push ups and standing broad jump. As a group children identified with co-ordination difficulties perform well below the 50th percentile on Australian and Canadian population norms (for a review see Hands and Larkin, 2002). One of the difficulties with the measurement of muscular strength and endurance is that co-ordination is important for test performance and co-ordination difficulties can interfere with the accurate measurement of fitness. However, research with simple tasks requiring less co-ordination adds to the evidence that children with co-ordination problems have low levels of strength and power. Using a simple isometric knee extension and knee flexion task, Raynor (2001) found significantly lower peak torques in children with DCD. The children with DCD also had lower peak torques and power output on an isokinetic extension-flexion task.

For further constraints on motor performance, one needs to look at the *somatotype* of these children. Although there are children with co-ordination difficulties who are very slender, the results of a number of studies show that groups with DCD are more endomorphic with relatively high fat levels and increased body weight (Larkin *et al.*, 1989; Raynor, 1989). Being relatively heavy adds to the difficulty in performing weight-bearing tasks and tasks that require body projection such as running, hopping, jumping and absorption skills of landing. The physical effort of generating sufficient propulsion to get off the ground, to absorb the landing forces, and to control balance on landing is a challenging task for these children. For children with both motor impairment and low levels of physical activity, increased endomorphy is a severe constraint on the learning and control of motor skills.

The overall picture of poor basic fitness in children with co-ordination difficulties raises an important issue for physical education teachers and others involved in remedial or compensatory motor skill programmes. With poor fitness, children who already have difficulty controlling movement and performing motor skills have fewer 'physical resources' on which to draw. With less physical activity, these fitness capacities are not developed and the motor skills themselves become much harder to learn and perform. Less physical activity involvement, lower than optimal fitness capacity and poorer co-ordination abilities combine to create a downward spiral of negative effect resulting in even poorer skills.

Assessment of physical fitness capacities is very important when working with children whose motor co-ordination is poor. However, it is also important to recognise that there is an interaction between these – low fitness constrains the ability to perform, and a low skill level creates poor fitness through low environmental challenge to the developing neuromuscular system. An intervention programme with poorly co-ordinated children should combine both skills teaching and physical fitness activities, and individualising the programme to the specific deficiencies and strengths and needs of the child.

Balance and postural control

One of the common features of the child with movement co-ordination difficulties is poor balance and postural control. It is possible that this poor control is a pervasive underlying constraint on the performance of other gross motor skills in which central/core stability is important to the limb manipulations (e.g. overarm throwing, kicking a ball). Extensive testing of children with co-ordination difficulties indicates that many of these children score poorly on measures of static and dynamic balance. Armitage (1993) found that children with DCD (n = 40) maintained static balance for a shorter time. Although the mean maximal one-foot static balance time increased with age in the DCD groups (11.4s in the 5- to 6-year-old and 18.5s in the 8- to 9-year-old DCD groups), both groups had shorter balance times than both the younger and older controls (21.3s and 29.2s respectively). The DCD group also had increased sway by comparison to co-ordinated controls (Armitage, 1993). On a more dynamic task using a bipedal stance and exploring the stability limits of the task space, Przysucha and Taylor (2000) reported that children with DCD were limited in their exploration by contrast to the control group.

Wann *et al.* (1998) compared the sensitivity to environmental information in adults and children with and without DCD. When children with DCD aged 8 to 9 years were asked to stand in a simple upright position with their eyes open, they showed both significantly more sway (7.37 cm) than control children (3.5 cm) as well as nursery school children (4.89 cm) or adults (4.86 cm). When the eyes were closed the sway increased in children with DCD in contrast to the other groups, whose sway did not change significantly. Children were placed in a moving room where the surround was moved (i.e. oscillated at approximately 0.17 Hz) and displaced 40, 80 and 120 per cent of the base of support of the individual. The sway was synchronised with the sway of the room to some degree for all individuals, with 76 per cent of exposures for children with DCD, 72 per cent for control children, 80 per cent for nursery school children, but only 35 per cent exposures for adults. Regardless of age and developmental level, the dominant frequency of postural sway was approximately that of the movement of the room, indicating the coupling of visual information as part of postural control. In terms of peak frequency of sway, children with DCD seem to be more like the 4- to 5-year-old children. Young children are more affected by perturbations of optic flow, showing responses that are directly coupled with the visual motion. Wann *et al.* speculated that the stronger reliance on vision in children with DCD may indicate either a slower developing capacity to process proprioceptive information or a slower developing capacity to effectively integrate proprioceptive and visual information.

In terms of postural control, there is a lot of evidence about the establishment of postural synergies in response to unexpected balance perturbations such as tripping and slipping. In the ages from around 7 to 10, postural synergies, in terms of speed and consistency of muscle response, become refined, although children as young as 15 months show similar synergies. These postural synergies relate to the pattern of activation of the muscles in the legs and trunk. Williams and Woollacott (1997) examined postural responses in children with DCD aged 6–7 and 9–10 years of age. They stood on a force platform with their eyes open and their feet shoulder-width apart, and the platform was unexpectedly shifted in either a forward or backward direction creating posterior and anterior sway, respectively. The speed with which the postural synergy was activated (that is, the latency and the pattern of the sequence) was investigated. They found that onset latencies in the postural muscles to counteract anterior sway in children with DCD were particularly variable compared with age-matched control children. However, the variability of onset for backward sway was not different between DCD and control children. Importantly, the variability in response to forward sway was present in both the younger and older children with DCD. In typically developing children, the emerging postural synergy that is expected in response to both forward or backward sway is a distal-to-proximal patterning leg muscle activation. In these children the pattern was present on every perturbation trial. However, on 28 per cent of trials for young children with DCD, the activation of upper leg muscles preceded activation of the stretched ankle muscles. For older children with DCD this proximal–distal pattern was present on 17 per cent of trials. And only two-thirds of younger children with DCD and one-third of older children with DCD showed the normal proximal–distal pattern of activation on at least 40 per cent of balance perturbation trials. The aberrant postural muscle patterning seemed to be, typically, thigh muscles followed by ankle then trunk and then neck muscles. The trunk control of children with DCD during many tasks such as landing after jumping is particularly poor (Larkin and Hoare, 1991). These patterns of muscle activation point to different, less efficient organisation of postural responses in children with DCD.

5. Differences in performance of functional skills

Running and walking technique

Efficient locomotion is one of the important fundamental actions in motor development. However, children with movement impairment show particularly inefficient patterns. They often trip over obstacles in their path, ascend steps in a hesitant way, fall off-balance when trying to walk along lines, and so on. Playground games such as tag, hopscotch and rope skipping are really difficult for these children. Hoare and Larkin (1988), in a kinematic analysis of locomotor techniques in children with DCD, showed that there was a general lack of ability to propel the body forward and upward in jumping and hopping tasks. For jumping, the children failed to exhibit fully extended limbs at takeoff. The child with DCD finds it difficult to transfer weight smoothly from one leg to another in running. This results in movement that looks jerky and does not flow. In walking, for example, Larkin and Hoare (1991) have listed the following common problems: poor head control with head position down rather than erect, upper arms being held sideways with elbows bent in high guard position, failure to swing arms in opposition with leg action, jerky transition from limb to limb, excessive hip flexion, pronounced asymmetry in gait, wide base of support, short steps, heavy foot strike with flat foot, and walking on toes rather than heel–toe, or excessive toe-in or toe-out gait.

Hopping technique

Hopping is one of the challenging skills that typically developing children begin to perform on one leg around 3 to 4 years of age. For children with movement difficulties, this task is very hard because it requires sophisticated postural control and good muscle strength to support the body weight on one limb while producing enough force to propel the body off the ground and then control the landing. The hop can be repetitive, in-place or over distance. Hop for distance is one of the tasks in the Gross Motor Screening Test of Larkin and Revie (1994) because it is such a good predictor of children with DCD (Hoare, 1991). Armitage and Larkin (1993) reported on the asymmetry in performance in hop for distance of young (5–6 years) and older (8–9 years) poorly co-ordinated children compared to age-matched normally co-ordinated peers. They found a significant main effect for co-ordination but not for age. The percentage difference between the performance of the limbs for the poorly co-ordinated group was 29 per cent on average, compared to 13.9 per cent difference for the normally co-ordinated children. Performance asymmetry between the right and left limbs is expected in normal development. Denckla (1974) reported that developmentally younger children have a tendency to greater limb asymmetry in hopping. Not only does the hop develop later in these children but also the asymmetry is more pronounced.

In Larkin and Hoare (1991), a listing of common problems in hopping exhibited by children with movement difficulties includes: unsteady head upsetting balance, excessive trunk lean leading to unstable hopping, trunk stability problems, arms not being used to aid upward drive but held out for balance, extraneous arm movements that disturb balance, inadequate flexion in the ankle joint especially during unweighting, failure to extend the joints of the lower limb during propulsion, flexing at the hip, knee and ankle rather than full extension at lift off, non-support leg being lifted forward or out to the side and not swinging to assist the hop, heavy landings, the support foot turning in, causing circling in hopping, hopping flat-footed rather than using the forefoot, lack of rebound between hops, a short flight time, inconsistency in height and rhythm of hops, and exaggerated difference in the performance of the two limbs.

Jumping and landing

Jumping requires the child to develop enough muscular force through reciprocal contraction to project the body to flight as well as, importantly, absorbing forces on landing. If the child cannot absorb forces, enormous pressure is placed on the joint structures, which could predicate the finding that landing 'hurts' and they are less likely to jump high. Poorly co-ordinated children need to be directly taught to land by giving at the ankle, knee and hip, and taught the efficient use of the arms to slow the body. They need to learn how to control the trunk and head so as not to topple the body forwards. Larkin and Hoare (1991) identify common persistent problems in symmetrical jumping such as a lack of flexion in the knee during unweighting or preparation, and the arms not swinging backwards so that they are ready to assist with propulsion. Arms often hang limply at the side or actively working against the jump. There is often excessive joint flexion during the unweighting, especially at the hip, which is usually attributed to the trunk taking an excessive lean forwards before there is a hip extension, which drives the trunk vertically as if the child is trying to lift themselves off the ground rather than to push against the ground. There is poor control of the head during flight, and insufficient flexion of the knee during flight to bring the feet out in front of the body.

There can be asymmetric action of the arms and asymmetric propulsion of the lower limbs with one leg leading the other at takeoff. There is inadequate extension of the lower limbs during the propulsion phase, and heavy landing with limited flexion of the ankle, knee, and hip to absorb the momentum. Often the landing is unstable and the child falls forwards or backwards.

Throwing and catching

Being able to control objects such as balls is fundamental to children's play. In Larkin and Revie's (1994) screening test a bounce and catch test item is included. Within the Movement Assessment Battery for Children, one of the areas tested is in ball projection and reception skills. Over-arm throwing is also included in the Test of Gross Motor Development (Ulrich, 2000).

Overarm throwing is a basic fundamental pattern that is used in many sports that children learn later on and so acquisition of this pattern is quite important. Children with movement difficulties really show inefficient overarm throwing patterns. There are many detailed descriptions of the pattern of an efficient overarm throw. In its basic form, it requires the child to be in an asymmetric side on position with the tennis ball held in the hand to wind up and transfer weight on to the back foot, with a vigorous step forward as the throwing hand moves down and back, bending at the elbow to bring the ball behind the head. The drive forward initiated by the step forward is continued with a strong rotation of the trunk beginning with the hips rotating forward followed by the shoulders, a segmented rotation in Roberton and Halverson's descriptions. As the shoulders are brought square, the upper arm leads the throw with the ball in the hand lagging behind the leading elbow. Finally, a vigorous extension of the arm at the elbow, to ball release and then the follow-through of the throwing arm down and across the body.

In children with movement difficulties, there are many problems that are characteristic. These are, according to Larkin and Hoare (1991): head control is poor, eyes not focused on the target, there is limited preparatory action, often with an 'over-shoulder' wind up rather than a down-and-back wind up, base for support is too wide or too narrow, there is no transference of weight, and the trunk moves more in a flexion action rather than a rotation action. The arm itself does not segment to successively add segments into the force of the throw; often the forearm leads the shoulder and the elbow. The ball release is often poorly timed and you see the finger and hand control is poor at ball release. The follow-through is lacking or uncontrolled and is not along the flight of the ball. The non-throwing arm is not used to assist the throw and it rarely points at the target to assist in getting the shoulders side-on or the body side-on to the target. There are many extraneous movements of the non-throwing arm. Children with movement impairment often show isolated action of elbow movement, and the rest of the body does not contribute to the flow of the action.

Catching is also a difficult basic skill for children with movement problems. It requires the ability to control the object with the hands with fine, well-timed grasping and appropriate flexion of the elbows to absorb the force of the oncoming ball. Catching also requires visual tracking of the object to predict where to place the hands, how to position the hands and when to grasp the ball. With good observational skills, the teacher can use catching to identify difficulties with tracking and hand control in children with DCD. According to Larkin and Hoare (1991), a substantial number of children with DCD have difficulty tracking the path of a moving ball, especially when it is in the air. Even when the ball is rolling along the ground, their ability to predict the arrival time of the object is impaired, often responding too late or responding too early and not detecting last-minute changes in its trajectory if it hits an obstruction on the ground. In some cases problems with visual tracking might be due to an attentional problem or an inability to maintain focus on the moving ball. It is difficult to tease apart the overlapping problems of tracking difficulties and attention difficulties as they interact with each other. Some children can track and receive a ball if it is moving directly towards them; however, if it is coming from the side or a different direction they are unable to reposition their body to get behind and in line with the ball for catching. Timing problems can occur with the movement to the ball and with the fine motor act of catching. Some children snatch at the ball too early or respond too late, allowing the ball to pass through their hands and their catch is a very inefficient 'hugging to the chest'. Larkin and Hoare (1991) identify the following common problems: inability to maintain focus on the ball, inability to predict the flight of the ball, and a poor understanding of the speed and trajectory relationship of a moving object. Children have a delayed pickup of the flight path, and poor control of posture in terms of the positioning of the feet and the movement of the feet in relation to the movement of the ball. Their movement is slow if they do attempt to adjust to the ball, or their hands are not altered in response to the ball's position. The hands are often rigidly cupped or fingers spread apart. Some children close their eyes or turn their heads as the ball approaches and this impacts on their hand positioning. Often the children do not make appropriate adaptations to balls that are lower than hip height or higher than shoulder height or even straight out in front of the chest. They reach out with stiff arms to contact the ball instead of allowing the ball to contact the hands and 'give' on impact, and closure of the hands is too slow and the ball falls out. Sometimes the ball is caught in the fingertips as the grasp is made too early or trapped against the chest. The children do not show a shift of weight with the follow-through that matches the momentum of the ball.

6. Practical applications

An enriched movement environment, where physical activity is encouraged, will promote the development of the neuro-muscular and cardio-respiratory systems that support movement in a growing child. Early intervention is important for children with motor co-ordination difficulties in order to facilitate a positive developmental pathway. Our view is that their developmental pathways appear to be different, not merely delayed, and as inefficient motor patterning develops, it is important to teach these children how to perform movement skills efficiently. In turn, having more efficient movement will impact further on children's motor development by giving them the opportunity for further learning through movement experiences.

Various interventions are used in an effort to assist children with co-ordination difficulties. The theoretical or professional orientation of the teacher or clinician generally influences the approach taken, although some practitioners combine a variety of the more formalised approaches. The process-orientated approach typically used by occupational therapists and psychologists (Ayres, 1972; Kephart, 1960; Laszlo and Bairstow, 1985) focuses on the underlying processes of movement control such as sensory reception, perception and integration. The assumption is that improving these underlying processes will generalise to improved performance in other functional tasks such as dressing and handwriting. Another approach could be classified as the 'task-based' or 'task-orientated' approach. In this particular approach, typically used by physical educators and movement specialists, the focus is on the motor skills the child needs to perform at school and at home. So the focus is on the task rather than the sensory underpinning of movement. With the task-oriented approach, activities such as learning to run, descend stairs, throw, catch, ride a bike and swim efficiently are the basis of the programmes (for a review see Larkin and Parker, 2002). Recently there have been several reviews on the relative merits and limitations associated with particular approaches (Miyahara, 1996; Pless and Carlsson, 2000; Sigmundssen *et al.*, 1999; Sugden and Chambers, 2000) and the task-oriented approach appears to be gaining popularity.

The process-oriented approach has often been linked to improved academic development; however, the evidence has been equivocal. In a more recent review, Polatjako *et al.* (1992) confirmed the report by Kavale and Mattson (1983) that perceptual motor programming did not significantly improve learning abilities in children with learning disabilities who underwent sensory process or perceptual motor training. Polatjako *et al.* reported that the research 'does not support sensory integration treatment as an effective treatment for academic problems of learning disabled children. The real question is not how effective is the program but for whom is the program effective' (p. 339).

Certainly, one of the difficulties that is common to many studies looking at the 'sensory integration therapy' is how best to assess the children's performance using measures that are sufficiently sensitive to show change. Although it is common to compare different treatment groups to assess the value of interventions, there are, typically, wide individual differences in the degree of gain achieved with treatment. A group design assumes that individuals will respond in a similar manner and in a similar time frame. Our research in learning a basic motor skill shows that this does not occur. Consequently group average changes might not be the most relevant approach to detect improvement (Larkin and Parker, 1998).

Recently Leemrijse *et al.* (2000) used single case studies to compare sensory integration treatment to Le Bon Départ (LBD) treatment for children with developmental co-ordination disorder. Multiple measures were used to assess improvement – the Movement ABC test, a praxis test, a rhythm test, and visual analogue scales. The LBD programme resulted in significant improvement in the rhythm scores compared to sensory integration, a result that is not surprising given that the LBD methodology focuses on rhythm. Leemrijse *et al.* (2000) concluded that LBD contributed to improvements in problems with the underlying rhythm and timing processes of these children. Generally, children showed improvement after treatment but some motor problems remained in some children. The amount of improvement was greater following intervention with both the LBD and sensory integration than it was after just one programme. Importantly, these researchers indicated the need to match intervention to the specific needs of the child; for example, to differentiate the children with DCD who would most benefit from rhythm training in LBD from others who might respond to other interventions.

The task-specific approach can vary quite markedly (Revie and Larkin, 1993b; Wright and Sugden, 1998). Our task-specific approach is influenced by our background in motor learning and control, motor development, biomechanics, exercise psychology and exercise physiology. It focuses mostly on learning fundamental movement skills, especially locomotor skills, such as running and jumping, and object control skills such as kicking, throwing or hitting. Ideally the child gets to select at least one of the skills to be learned. For example, we currently have a child learning to hit using the game of T-ball as the context. Initially the child will learn to hit the ball in a closed environment, with the ball on the batting tee. At this stage, we focus on teaching correct stance, focus, backswing and follow-through technique so that the child develops an efficient style that looks good. Once this task is achieved, we can expand on the skill so that the child learns to use it in open environments, such as with a tossed ball and with the base running element added. These variations have to be explicitly taught so that they become added to the child's movement repertoire. Where possible, the choice of the specific skill taught is linked to family interests and cultural context. Because of the difficulties with fitness in these children, the teacher focuses on those elements of fitness specific to the task and important to its performance. With the hitting example above, abdominal strength, trunk flexibility, and arm and shoulder strength would be targeted. Thus task-specific fitness becomes part of the overall programme. Our task specific approach relies heavily on a multi-level approach by a teacher who is well versed in movement observation and intervention. It incorporates elements of many intervention approaches. For example, we do draw on aspects of the process-oriented approach (Ayres, 1972; Laszlo and Bairstow, 1985). We assist the learner to identify relevant sensory information, but this is done within the context of the specific task; for example, in feeling the twist of the trunk, and glueing eyes to the ball. Where appropriate, elements learned in one task are explicitly carried over to other related tasks. Likewise in our task-specific approach, where appropriate, we use problem-solving strategies and guided discovery that are a major focus of the Cognitive Orientation to daily Occupational Performance (COOP) approach (Miller *et al.*, 2001). This task-specific approach can be effectively used in the physical education class by a thoughtful and well-prepared teacher.

How successful is regular physical activity for children with movement difficulties? Thompson and colleagues (Thompson *et al.*, 1994) conducted a behaviour observation study of 28 children who were taught gymnastics, track and field, fitness work, dancing and basic games at school. Children's behaviour in the physical education class was observed over a period of months and coded as appropriate, inappropriate, off-task or not motor engaged (activity that was not directly leading to learning the focus skill). Thompson *et al.* highlighted the fact that the children with movement difficulties were, first, significantly less successful at the assigned motor tasks when compared to their peers in the same lesson. Second, more often they were not contributing to all the motor learning goals of the lesson as they were more frequently observed not doing any motor tasks, misbehaving, or doing a different motor task than that assigned. The off-task behaviour may in part relate to the difficulty that they have with mastery of motor tasks and their lower success in completing the set activities in the PE class. Pless and Carlsson (2000) suggest that intervention with these children might be more successful in smaller groupings; however, Wright and Sugden (1998) reported quite positive results with a class-based intervention using a task-oriented approach. It seems that successful participation in the physical education class would benefit from additional teacher support or additional individual or small group activity similar to that provided in the treatment of other learning disabilities.

In summary, children with movement difficulties are a heterogeneous group who require careful evaluation to determine their profile of difficulties and strength, in order that the needed social and physical support to reach their optimal potential is provided. Without this support they are at risk of early withdrawal from physical activity with its attendant health and psychosocial problems. Clearer profiling of these children's abilities would enable them to be directed towards physical activities that draw on their relative strengths rather than their weaknesses. Motivational strategies, encouraging participation together with positive social support and skilled teaching, provide an environment conducive to motor learning despite difficulties with motor control. It is our responsibility as physical educators to avoid practices that have a negative effect, and instead provide as enriched a movement environment as possible for children with motor learning difficulties.

References

American Psychiatric Association (1987) *Diagnostic and Statistical Manual of Mental Disorders*, 3rd edn, revised. Washington, DC: Author.

American Psychiatric Association (1994) *Diagnostic and Statistical Manual of Mental Disorders*, 4th edn. Washington, DC: Author.

Armitage, M. (1993) Laterality and motor asymmetry: a comparison between poorly and normally coordinated children. Unpublished masters thesis, The University of Western Australia, Crawley, Australia.

Armitage, M. and Larkin, D. (1993) Laterality, motor asymmetry and clumsiness. *Human Movement Science*, 12, 155–77.

Arnheim, D.D. and Sinclair, W.A. (1979) *The Clumsy Child: A Program of Motor Therapy*, 2nd edn. St Louis: Mosby.

Ayres, A.J. (1972) *Sensory Integration and Learning Disorders*. Los Angeles: Western Psychological Services.

Beyer, R. (1999) Motor proficiency of boys with attention deficit hyperactivity disorder and boys with learning disabilities. *Adapted Physical Activity Quarterly*, 16, 403–14.

Bouffard, M., Watkinson, E.J., Thompson, L.P., Causgrove Dunn, J.L. and Romanow, S.K.E. (1996) A test of the activity deficit hypothesis with children with movement difficulties. *Adapted Physical Activity Quarterly*, 13, 61–73.

Bruininks, R.H. (1978) *Bruininks–Oseretsky Test of Motor Proficiency Examiners. Manual.* Circle Pines, MI: American Guidance Service.

Burton, A.W. and Miller, D.E. (1998) *Movement Skill Assessment*. Champaign, IL: Human Kinetics.

Cantell, M.H., Smyth, M.M. and Ahonen, T.P. (1994) Clumsiness in adolescence: educational, motor and social outcomes. *Adapted Physical Activity Quarterly*, 11, 115–29.

Cantell, M. and Kooistra, L. (2002) Long-term outcomes of developmental coordination disorder. In S.A. Cermak and D. Larkin (eds), *Developmental Coordination Disorder* (pp. 23–38). Albany NY: Delmar.

Cermak, S.A., Gubbay, S.S. and Larkin, D. (2002) What is Developmental Coordination Disorder? In S.A. Cermak and D. Larkin (eds), *Developmental Coordination Disorder* (pp. 2–22). Albany NY: Delmar.

Chng, V. (1996) The effects of varying pacing demands on self-paced hand tapping: a developmental comparison between normal and developmental co-ordination disorder (DCD) children. Unpublished honours thesis, The University of Western Australia.

Chow, S.M.K., Henderson, S.E. and Barnett, A.L. (2001) The movement assessment battery for children: a comparison of 4-year-old to 6-year-old children from Hong Kong and the United States. *American Journal of Occupational Therapy*, 55, 55–61.

Cratty, B.J. (1994) *Clumsy Child Syndromes: Descriptions, Evaluation and Remediation.* Chur, Switzerland: Harwood.

Denckla, M.B. (1974) Development of motor coordination in normal children. *Developmental Medicine and Child Neurology*, 16, 729–41.

Dewey, D. and Kaplan, B.J. (1994) Subtyping of developmental motor deficits. *Developmental Neuropsychology*, 10, 265–84.

Dyspraxia Foundation (1998) Members' questionnaire – June, 1997 awareness and diagnosis (http://www.emmbrook.demon.co.uk/dysprax/report.html).

Fitzpatrick, D. (2000) The experience of physical awkwardness, a reflective retrospective view – a hermeneutic phenomenological study. Paper presented at the North American Federation of Adapted Physical Activity 2000 Symposium, November, New Orleans, Louisiana.

Greene, L.S. and Williams, H.G. (1993) Age-related differences in timing control of repetitive movement: application of the Wing–Kristofferson Model. *Research Quarterly for Exercise and Sport*, 64, 32–8.

Geuze, R.H. and Kalverboer, A.F. (1987) Inconsistency and adaptation in timing of clumsy children. *Journal of Human Movement Studies*, 13, 421–32.

Geuze, R.H. and Kalverboer, A.F. (1993) Bimanual rhythmic co-ordination in clumsy and dyslexic children. In S.S. Valenti and J.B. Pittenger (eds), *Studies in Perception and Action II*. Posters presented at the VIIth International Conferences on Event Perception and Action (pp. 24–28). Hillsdale, NJ: Lawrence Erlbaum.

Geuze, R.H. and Kalverboer, A.F. (1994) Tapping a rhythm: a problem for children who are clumsy and dyslexic. *Adapted Physical Activity Quarterly*, 11, 203–13.

Gubbay, S.S. (1975) *The Clumsy Child a Study in Developmental Apraxic and Agnosic Ataxia.* London: W. B. Saunders.

Hands, B. and Larkin, D. (2002) Physical fitness and developmental coordination disorder. In S.A. Cermak and D. Larkin (eds), *Developmental Coordination Disorder* (pp. 172–84). Albany, NY: Delmar.

Hands, B., Larkin, D. and Parker, H. (2000) Fitness levels in children with low motor competence. Paper presented at the 2000 Pre-Olympic Congress, September, Brisbane, Australia.

Harter, S. (1985) *Manual for the Self-perception Profile for Children.* Denver: University of Denver.

Harvey, B. and Reid, G. (1997) Motor performance of children with attention-deficit hyperactivity disorder: a preliminary investigation. *Adapted Physical Activity Quarterly*, 14, 189–202.

Henderson, L., Rose, P. and Henderson, S. (1992) Reaction time and movement time in children with a developmental co-ordination disorder. *Journal of Child Psychology and Psychiatry*, 33, 895–905.

Henderson, S.E. and Sugden, D.A. (1992) *Movement Assessment Battery for Children Manual.* Sidcup, Kent: Psychological Corp.

Hennessey, S.M. (1998) External pacing constraints on repetitive tapping in children with developmental co-ordination disorder. Unpublished honours thesis, The University of Western Australia, Crawley, Australia.

Hoare, D. (1991) Classification of movement dysfunction in children: descriptive and statistical approaches. Unpublished doctoral dissertation, The Universtity of Western Australia, Crawley, Australia.

Hoare, D. (1994) Subtypes of developmental co-ordination disorder. *Adapted Physical Activity Quarterly,* 11, 158–69.

Hoare, D. and Larkin, D. (1988) Movement differences between poorly coordinated boys and their well coordinated peers. Paper presented at the XXIVth International Congress of Psychology, August, Sydney, Australia.

Huh, J., Williams, H. and Burke, J. (1998) Development of bilateral motor control in children with developmental co-ordination disorders. *Developmental Medicine and Child Neurology,* 40, 474–84.

Hummelshoj, T. (1999) Motor timing abilities in attention deficit hyperactivity disorder (ADHD) subtypes. Unpublished honours thesis, The University of Western Australia, Crawley, Australia.

Kadesjo, B. and Gillberg, C. (1999) Developmental co-ordination disorder in Swedish 7-year-old children. *Journal of the American Academy of Child and Adolescent Psychiatry,* 38, 820–8.

Kadesjo, B. and Gillberg, C. (2001) The comorbidity of ADHD in the general population of Swedish school-age children. *Journal of Child Psychology and Psychiatry,* 42, 487–92.

Kaplan, B.J., Wilson, B., Dewey, D. and Crawford, S. (1998) DCD may not be a discrete disorder. *Human Movement Science,* 17, 471–90.

Kavale, K. and Mattson, P.D. (1983) 'One jumped of the balance beam': meta-analysis of perceptual–motor training. *Journal of Learning Disabilities,* 16, 3, 167–73.

Keogh, J.F. (1968) Incidence and severity of awkwardness among regular school boys and educationally subnormal boys. *Research Quarterly,* 39, 806–8.

Kephart, N.C. (1960) *The Slow Learner in the Classroom.* Columbus, OH: Merrill.

Kirby, A. and Drew, S. (1999) Is DCD a diagnosis that we should be using for adults? Is clumsiness the issue in adults and adolescents? Paper presented at the 4th Biennial Workshop on Children with Developmental Co-ordination Disorder: From Research to Diagnostics and Intervention, Groningen, The Netherlands.

Larkin, D. and Hoare, D. (1991) *Out of Step.* Perth: Active Life Foundation, University of Western Australia.

Larkin, D. and Parker, H. (1997) Physical self-perceptions of adolescents with a history of developmental coordination disorder. Poster presentation at NASPSPA, May, Denver, USA.

Larkin, D. and Parker, H.E. (1998) Teaching children to land softly: Individual differences in learning outcomes. *ACHPER Healthy Lifestyles Journal,* 45, 2, 19–24.

Larkin, D. and Parker H.E. (1999) Physical activity profiles of adolescents who experienced motor learning difficulties. In D. Drouin, C. Lepine and C. Simard (eds), *Proceedings of the 11th International Symposium for Adapted Physical Activity* (pp. 175–81). Quebec, Canada.

Larkin, D. and Parker, H. (2002) Task specific intervention for children with DCD: a systems view. In S.A. Cermak and D. Larkin (eds), *Developmental Coordination Disorder* (pp. 234–47). Albany NY: Delmar.

Larkin, D. and Revie, G. (1994) *Stay in Step: A Gross Motor Screening Test for Children K-2*. Sydney: Authors.

Larkin, D. and Rose, B. (1999) Use of the McCarron Assessment of Neuromuscular Development for identification of developmental coordination disorder. Paper presented at the 4th Biennial Workshop of Children with Developmental Coordination Disorder: From Research to Diagnostics and Intervention, October, Groningen, The Netherlands.

Larkin, D., Parker, H.E., Hands, B., Houghton, S. and Hummelshoj, T. (2000) Motor performance of children with ADHD. Poster presentation at the AIESEP Conference, August, Yeppoon, Qld., Australia

Laszlo, J. and Bairstow, P. (1985) *Perceptual–Motor Behaviour: Developmental Assessment and Therapy*. Eastbourne: Holt, Rinehart and Winston.

Leemrijse, C., Meijer, O.G., Vermeer, A., Ader, H.J. and Diemel, S. (2000) The efficacy of the Le Bon Départ and Sensory Integration treatment for children with developmental co-ordination disorder: a randomized study with six single cases. *Clinical Rehabilitation*, 14, 247–59.

Losse, A., Henderson, S.E., Elliman, D., Hall, D., Knight, E. and Jongmans, M. (1991) Clumsiness in children: Do they grow out of it? A 10-year follow-up study. *Developmental Medicine and Child Neurology*, 33, 55–68.

Lundy-Ekman, L., Ivry, R., Keele, S. and Woollacott, M. (1991) Timing and force control deficits in clumsy children. *Journal of Cognitive Neuroscience*, 3, 370–7.

Maeland, A.F. (1992) Identification of children with motor co-ordination problems. *Adapted Physical Activity Quarterly*, 9, 330–42.

McCarron, L.T. (1982) *MAND McCarron Assessment of Neuromuscular Development*, revised edn. Dallas, TX: Common Market Press.

Macnab, J.J., Miller, L.T. and Polatajko, H.J. (2001) The search for subtypes of DCD: is cluster analysis the answer? *Human Movement Science*, 20, 49–72.

Manitoba Department of Education (1980) *Manitoba Physical Fitness Performance Test Manual and Fitness Objectives*. Ottawa, Ontario: CAPHER.

Miller, L.T., Polatajko, H.J., Missiuna, C., Mandich, A.D. and Macnab, J.J. (2001) A pilot trial of a cognitive treatment for children with developmental co-ordination disorder. *Human Movement Science*, 20, 183–210.

Miyahara, M. (1994) Subtypes of students with learning disabilities based upon gross motor functions. *Adapted Physical Activity Quarterly*, 11, 368–82.

Miyahara, M. (1996) A meta-analysis of intervention studies on children with developmental co-ordination disorder. *Corpus Psyche et Societas*, 3, 11–18.

Miyahara, M. and Register, C. (2000) Perceptions of three terms to describe physical awkwardness in children. *Research in Developmental Disabilities*, 21, 367–76.

Miyahara, M, Tsujii, M., Hanai, T., Jongmans, M., Barnett, A., Henderson, S.E., Hori, M., Nakanishi, K. and Kageyama, H. (1998) The Movement Assessment Battery for Children: a preliminary investigation of its usefulness in Japan. *Human Movement Science*, 17, 679–97.

Morris, P.R. and Whiting, H.T.A. (1971) *Motor Impairment and Compensatory Education*. London: G. Bell and Sons.

O'Beirne, C., Larkin, D. and Cable, T. (1994) Co-ordination problems and anaerobic performance in children. *Adapted Physical Activity Quarterly*, 11, 141–9.

Parker, H.E., Larkin, D. and Chow, C.L. (in preparation) Timing control of children with developmental coordination disorder (DCD) in self-paced hand tapping.

Parker, H.E., Larkin, D. and Wade, M.G. (1997) Are motor timing problems subgroup specific in children with developmental coordination disorder. *Australian Educational and Developmental Psychologist*, 14, 35–42.

Peters, J.M., Barnett, A.L. and Henderson, S.E. (2001) Clumsiness, dyspraxia and develop-mental co-ordination disorder: how do health and educational professionals in the UK define the terms? *Child: Care, Health and Development*, 27, 399–412.

Pless, M. and Carlsson, M. (2000) Effects of motor skill intervention on developmental co-ordination disorder: A meta-analysis. *Adapted Physical Activity Quarterly*, 17, 381–401.

Polatajko, H., Kaplan, B. and Wilson, N. (1992) Sensory integration treatment in children with learning disabilities: its status 20 years later. *Occupational Therapy Journal of Research*, 12, 323–41.

Pryzysucha, E. and Taylor, J. (2000) A comparison of balance performance between boys with and without developmental coordination disorder. Poster presented at the North American Federation of Adapted Physical Activity 2000 Symposium, New Orleans, Louisiana.

Pyke, J.E. (1986) *Australian School Fitness Test for Students Aged 7–15*. Parkside, South Australia: ACHPER Publications.

Rasmussen, P. and Gillberg, C. (2000) Natural outcomes of ADHD with developmental co-ordination disorder at age 22 years: a controlled longitudinal, community-based study. *Journal of the American Academy of Child and Adolescent Psychiatry*, 39, 1424–31.

Raynor, A.J. (1989) The running pattern of seven year old children – coordination and gender differences. Unpublished honours thesis, The University of Western Australia, Crawley, Asutralia.

Raynor, A.J. (1998) Fractionated reflex and reaction times in children with developmental co-ordination disorder. *Motor Control*, 2, 114–24.

Raynor, A.J. (2001) Strength, power, and coactivation in children with developmental co-ordination disorder. *Developmental Medicine and Child Neurology*, 43, 676–84.

Revie, G. and Larkin, D. (1993a) Looking at movement problems: Problems with teacher identification of poorly co-ordinated children. *ACHPER National Journal*, 40, 4–9.

Revie, G. and Larkin, D. (1993b) Task specific intervention with children reduces movement problems. *Adapted Physical Activity Quarterly*, 10, 29–41.

Riggen, K.J., Ulrich, D. and Ozman, J.C. (1990) Reliability and concurrent validity of the Test of Motor Impairment – Henderson Revision. *Adapted Physical Activity Quarterly*, 7, 249–58.

Rosblad, B. and Gard, L. (1998) The assessment of children with developmental co-ordination disorders in Sweden: a preliminary investigation of the suitability of the Movement ABC. *Human Movement Science*, 17, 711–19.

Rose, B., Larkin, D. and Berger, B.G. (1994) Perceptions of social support in children of low, moderate, and high coordination. *ACHPER Healthy Lifestyles Journal*, 41, 18–21.

Rose, B., Larkin, D. and Berger, B. (1997) Co-ordination and gender influences on the perceived competence of children. *Adapted Physical Activity Quarterly*, 14, 210–21.

Rose, B., Larkin, D. and Berger, B. (1998) The importance of motor coordination for children's motivational orientations in sport. *Adapted Physical Activity Quarterly*, 15, 316–27.

Rose, B., Larkin, D. and Berger, B. (1999) Athletic anxiety in boys and girls with low and high levels of coordination. *ACHPER Healthy Lifestyles Journal*, 46, 10–14.

Schoemaker, M.M. and Kalverboer, A.F. (1994) Social and affective problems of children who are clumsy: How early do they begin? *Adapted Physical Activity Quarterly*, 11, 130–40.

Sigmundsson, H., Pedersen, A.V., Whiting, H.T.A. and Ingvaldsen, R.P. (1998) We can cure your child's clumsiness: a review of intervention methods. *Scandinavian Journal of Rehabilitative Medicine*, 30, 101–6.

Smyth, M.M. and Anderson, H.I. (2000) Coping with clumsiness in the school playground: social and physical play in children with co-ordination impairments. *British Journal of Developmental Psychology*, 18, 389–413.

Smyth, T.R. and Glencross, D.J. (1986) Information processing deficits in clumsy children. *Australian Journal of Psychology*, 38, 13–22.

Stott, D.H., Moyes, F.A. and Henderson, S.E. (1984) *The Test of Motor Impairment – Henderson Revision*. Guelph, Ontario: Brook Educational Publishing.

Sugden, D.A. and Chambers, M.E. (1998) Intervention approaches and children with developmental coordination disorder. *Pediatric Rehabilitation*, 2, 139–47.

Tan, S.K., Parker, H. and Larkin, D. (2001) Concurrent validity of motor tests used to identify children with motor impairment. *Adapted Physical Activity Quarterly*, 18, 168–82.

Thompson, L.P., Bouffard, M., Watkinson, E.J. and Causgrove Dunn, J.L. (1994) Teaching children with movement difficulties: Highlighting the need for individualized instruction in regular education. *Physical Education Review*, 17, 2, 152–9.

Ulrich, D.A. (2000) *TGMD-2 Test of Gross Motor Development*, 2nd edn, examiner's manual. Austin, TX: Pro-ed.

Volman, M. and Geuze, R. (1998) Relative phase stability of bimanual and visuomanual rhythmic co-ordination patterns in children with a Development Co-ordination Disorder. *Human Movement Science*, 17, 541–72.

Wann, J.P., Mon-Williams, M. and Rushton, K. (1998) Postural control and co-ordination disorders: the swinging room revisited. *Human Movement Science*, 17, 491–513.

Williams, H. (2002) Motor control in children with developmental co-ordination disorder. In S.A. Cermak and D. Larkin (eds), *Developmental Co-ordination Disorder* (pp. 117–37). Albany NY: Delmar.

Williams, H. and Woollacott, M. (1997) Charactersitics of neuromuscular responses underlying posture control in clumsy children. In J. Clark and J. Humphrey (eds), *Motor Development: Research and Reviews*, 1, 8–23.

Williams, H. and Burke, J. (1998) Development of bilateral motor control in children with developmental co-ordination disorders. *Developmental Medicine and Child Neurology*, 40, 474–84.

Williams, H., Woollacott, M. and Ivry, R. (1992) Timing and motor control in clumsy children. *Journal of Motor Behavior*, 24, 165–72.

World Health Organisation (1992) *The ICD-10 Classification of Mental and Behavioural Disorders. Clinical Descriptions and Diagnostic Guidelines*. Geneva: World Health Organization.

Wright, H.C. and Sugden, D.A. (1996) The nature of developmental co-ordination disorder: Inter- and intragroup differences. *Adapted Physical Activity Quarterly*, 13, 357–71.

Wright, H.C. and Sugden, D.A. (1998) A school based intervention programme for children with developmental co-ordination disorder. *European Journal of Physical Education*, 3, 35–50.

9 Perceptual–motor behaviour in children with Down syndrome

*Dominic A. Simon, Digby Elliott and
J. Greg Anson*

1. Introduction

Children born with Down syndrome possess three 21st chromosomes in every cell of their body (cf. mosaicism). The syndrome is present in approximately one in every 800 live births, and is associated with a number of anatomical and physiological abnormalities that impact on both physical and cognitive development. In this chapter, we review studies from our own laboratories and elsewhere designed to examine perceptual–motor behaviour in this unique group of people. Our focus is on the control of goal-directed upper limb movements. Of interest is determining the similarities and differences between persons with Down syndrome and normally developing children, and what the implications of any differences are for understanding perceptual–motor behaviour in different movement contexts.

It is well known that children and young adults with Down syndrome require more time to both initiate and complete simple, goal-directed upper limb movements than nondisabled persons of a similar chronological age (see Anson and Mawston, 2000, and Welsh and Elliott, 2000 for a review). There is less agreement as to whether a disadvantage, or at least a difference, exists when children with Down syndrome are compared to other persons of a similar developmental age. The answer to this question, as well as a description of any developmental differences that might exist between children with Down syndrome and normally developing children, provides the basis for understanding how persons with Down syndrome perform simple reaching and aiming movements such as the ones involved in preparing or eating a meal, using a keyboard, and performing various personal care activities. This understanding is necessary if we are to structure educational programmes that will optimise motor skill acquisition and development.

2. Movement preparation and response initiation

Simple reaction time

In perceptual–motor behaviour, movement preparation and response initiation are frequently described from an information-processing perspective (Schmidt and Wrisberg, 1999). This behavioural perspective views the human (or animal) as an active processor of information. In the case of a single response, such as a discrete goal-directed upper limb movement, the response begins with an input (stimulus information – a signal to tell the individual to 'go!'). The response ends when the moving limb achieves its outcome (e.g. hitting a target or grasping an object).

The time between presentation of the stimulus information and initiation of the movement is a measure of the speed of information-processing or reaction time. This duration is substantially longer than the time needed for the brain (and central nervous system) to simply pass along the information to muscles to begin a movement. Even fast reaction times on the order of 110 ms (see, for example, Anson and Bird, 1993) are more than twice as long as the estimated minimal biological delay between stimulus onset and muscle activation (Fetz *et al.*, 1989). Thus, reaction time in its simplest form appears to include more events than are due to transmission of action potentials from sensory receptor to muscle alone. From a behavioural perspective these events are described as three stages of information-processing that occur between stimulus onset and movement: stimulus detection, response selection, and response programming.

When two or more responses are possible, information-processing (implicitly, reaction time) involves all three stages. Reaction time under these conditions is called choice reaction time – the performer can only select the appropriate response when the stimulus is presented. By contrast, when only one response is possible it is believed that the stimulus identification and response selection stages of information-processing can be completed before the stimulus occurs. Therefore, only response programming needs to be completed when the stimulus is presented. In this situation the delay due to information-processing is called simple reaction time. In simple reaction time, much of the movement preparation can be completed before the stimulus. Thus simple reaction time provides a relatively 'clean' measure of how long the neuromotor system takes to activate the appropriate muscles and start the movement. A caveat is warranted at this point. It is easy to assume that information-processing during simple reaction time is a description of the work of the brain, specifically the premotor, supplementary motor and motor cortical areas plus their spinal cord and muscle connections. While it is generally accepted that movement is controlled hierarchically by a hierarchically organised neuromotor system, it is timely to note an observation by John Rothwell:

> ... it is a thorny problem of motor control as to what details are specified where and when in the chain of command producing a movement.
>
> (Rothwell, 1994, p. 4)

Notwithstanding that caveat, simple reaction time is a tool frequently used to examine the integrity of information-processing delays in humans. It is particularly useful in providing comparative measures of functional information-processing between participants representing 'control' populations and participants from clinical populations such as Down syndrome and Developmental Co-ordination Disorder.

At the start of a 100m race the sprinter is in the blocks. At this point the sprinter knows exactly what response is required – initiate movement as quickly and accurately as possible when the gun sounds. The only uncertainty is the exact time at which the gun will sound, and with practice even this uncertainty is minimised as sprinters become familiar with the starter's sequence. Technically, the sprinter cannot initiate movement before the gun sounds without penalty, so a true reaction time situation exists. Furthermore, because event uncertainty and temporal uncertainty are minimised before the stimulus occurs, the sprint start represents a classic example of a simple reaction time response.

By definition, simple reaction time is the time from stimulus onset until the initiation of movement as detected by some form of sensing device such as an electromechanical or infrared switch, force transducer, accelerometer or potentiometer. The choice of sensing device can be important – accelerometers and potentiometers are generally more sensitive and accurate than electro-mechanical switches that often have 'slop' or 'play' in them making the measure of reaction time more variable. With regard to measurement of information-processing, when electromechanical switches are used, between 30 per cent and 40 per cent of reaction time is taken up by time for muscle activation and switch delay. This proportion is less when potentiometer signals form the basis of measurement of reaction time, and less still when accelerometer signals are used. In real terms muscle activation time and switch delay are not part of the information-processing event duration.

A more accurate representation of information-processing delay is obtained when reaction time is fractionated using electromyography (EMG). This form of fractionation allows simple reaction time to be separated into two components. The first component, called premotor time, is the duration between stimulus onset and the onset of activation of the focal muscle initiating the movement. The second component, called motor time, is the duration between onset of muscle activation and the initiation of movement. Motor time is calculated by subtracting the premotor time from reaction time. Premotor time is a measure of central delay in the neuro-muscular system and is thus a more accurate measure of information-processing. Motor time is a measure of peripheral delay that includes both muscle activation duration and switch delay.

Individuals with Down syndrome demonstrate longer simple reaction time than chronologically-matched young adult participants without Down syndrome (see, for example, Anson, 1992; Anson and Mawston, 2000). And when individuals with Down syndrome are matched with others on mental function, people in the Down syndrome group show lengthened simple reaction time (Berkson, 1960; Kerr and Blais, 1987, 1988; Davis *et al.*, 1991). In spite of frequent observations of lengthened simple reaction time in persons with Down syndrome, a wholly satisfactory explanation remains elusive. Three potentially contributing factors include hypotonia, differences in central versus peripheral processing, and differ-ences in the order or sequence of limb segments during initiation of goal-directed upper limb movements.

Hypotonia refers to the absence or markedly reduced levels of electrical activity in a muscle. The muscle appears as floppy or lacks 'tone'. Hypotonia has frequently been linked to Down syndrome specifically, to infants with Down syndrome, through the term 'floppy baby syndrome' (Wisniewski *et al.*, 1988). Anwar and Hermelin (1979) associated lengthened reaction time with hypotonia, but recent research has cast doubts on a causative relationship between hypotonia and reaction time. For example, Shumway-Cook and Woollacott (1985) reported that stretch-reflex activity in young individuals with Down syndrome was normal. Further evidence from experiments in which changes in joint stiffness were investigated also argued against the presence and influence of hypotonia in Down syndrome (Davis and Kelso, 1982; Davis and Sinning, 1987).

Although hypotonia does not seem to be a satisfactory explanation for lengthened simple reaction time in Down syndrome (Latash, 1992), there is evidence that the activation pattern within muscles is different. Anson and Mawston (2000) described the pattern of activity in muscles of young people with Down syndrome who were performing an upper limb reaction time task – to hit a styro-foam target with the right index finger, as fast as possible on detecting an imperative auditory stimulus. For participants in the control group, the patterns of muscle activation featured brief bursts of activity in the principal agonist muscles. In contrast, the electromyograms for individuals with Down syndrome showed multiple bursts, initially of low amplitude, that increased in amplitude slowly, but only after the movement had been initiated. One possible explanation is that while the action potentials from the alpha motor neuron to muscle were sufficient to depolarise the motor endplate, the conduction of the action potentials through the muscle fibre was both attenuated and delayed. This is unlikely to have resulted in hypotonia as there was ample evidence of heightened electrical activity in the muscles that were investigated.

Within the context of this discussion, central processing refers to the series and sequences of events in simple reaction time that occur between the onset of an imperative stimulus and the onset of significant change in muscle activity as measured by surface electromyography. The measured duration of these events is premotor time (PMT). In reality, central processing includes events and time before the imperative stimulus, from the moment that a participant begins the cognitive process of movement preparation, perhaps coincident with a warning signal. Utilisation of electroencephalography and pre-trigger data capture would provide a means to measure this central processing, but is beyond the scope of the present discussion.

Peripheral processing includes the events of muscle activation up until the time at which onset of movement occurs as detected, for example, by a switch or accelerometer. The measured duration of peripheral processing is called motor time (MOT). It is usually calculated by subtracting the PMT of the principal agonist muscle from the reaction time. Depending on the sensitivity and resolution of the reaction-time-measuring device, MOT would be expected to represent about 30 per cent to 40 per cent of the reaction time interval. The utilisation of electro-myography to separate the central and peripheral components of reaction time results in fractionated reaction time.

In our laboratory a typical reaction time experiment involves the production of a discrete goal-directed upper limb movement in response to an imperative auditory stimulus. Sometimes the extent of the movement is delimited by a large styrofoam target but accuracy is not a limiting feature. Electromyograms are recorded from the principal agonist muscles (anterior deltoid, biceps and extensor indicis). Participants are seated in a dental chair that provides optimal postural support and permits focused evaluation of performance of the involved upper limb. Participants usually receive a block of 20–25 trials in each experimental condition.

Results are presented in terms of mean fractionated reaction time (SRT, PMT, MOT). A consistent finding (see, Anson, 1992; Anson and Mawston, 2000) has been the not too surprising observation that for individuals with Down syndrome SRT is longer. Sometimes, time taken to initiate the movement is as much as double that in chronologically age-matched and gender-matched adult participants. Delays are greater in both central and peripheral components of SRT. Within the central component, the increased delay (increase in PMT) is not associated with slower nerve conduction velocity, which has been reported to be normal (Mawston and Anson, 1994). However, when attention to performing the task at hand was assessed on a trial-by-trial basis, there was a substantial difference between the performances of the control group and the Down syndrome group. Attention was measured, albeit crudely, by counting (from recorded video tape) the number of times the participant glanced away from the target during the movement preparation interval. The movement preparation interval was the period between the verbally presented 'Ready' command, and an imperative auditory stimulus. The number of off-task glances per second was computed as a measure of inattention. Participants in the control group maintained focused attention on the target in 99 per cent of trials whereas the score for the Down syndrome group was 24 per cent on task. When the 25 per cent fastest and 25 per cent slowest trials for the Down syndrome group were extracted, diminished attention (measured by off-task glancing) was observed with greater frequency in the slowest 25 per cent of trials. In the Down syndrome group, fluctuation in attention may have contributed to both increased variability and increased delay in central processing.

Individuals with Down syndrome also demonstrated a longer MOT component of SRT than their chronologically age-matched and gender-matched controls. Inspection of EMG records indicated that the rate of change in onset of activation of agonist muscles was much lower (ramp-like) than observed in control participants, where the change in EMG was rapid (step-like). Also, in Down syndrome the measured SRT frequently occurred after the initial burst of muscle activation, whereas in control participants SRT was most often synchronised with the initial burst of muscle activity (Anson and Mawston, 2000). While several characteristics of increased central and peripheral processing delays in Down syndrome have been described, the specific cause of these characteristics awaits the outcome of further research.

Part of the instrumentation in our studies of simple reaction time in Down syndrome involves measuring reaction time at different anatomical points on the upper limb segments. Usually SRT is measured at the tip of the index finger and at the elbow. Multiple measures of reaction time permit examination of the order of limb segment displacement during movement initiation. For rapid discrete goal-directed upper limb movements, the order of segment initiation would be predicted to be proximal-to-distal (De Lussanet and Alexander, 1997; Karst and Hasan, 1991). That is, shoulder flexion should precede elbow flexion and index finger extension in initiating propulsion of the upper limb toward the target. Indeed, in results from the data of control participants in previous experiments (Anson, 1992; Anson and Mawston, 2000) a proximal-to-distal pattern was clearly evident (see figure 9.1). A quite different picture emerged from the results for individuals with Down syndrome, as shown in figure 9.2.

After completing several experiments on reaction time and Down syndrome, one of the earliest and most robust results has been the frequent observation of a distal-to-proximal pattern of segment activation associated with movement initiation (Anson, 1989; Anson and Davis, 1988). Kinematically, this was revealed in reaction times being faster at the index finger than at the elbow. Physiologically, this observation was supported by the measurement of premotor time that indicated extensor indicis muscle was activated before anterior deltoid. Collectively, the SRT and PMT results remain a puzzle yet to be solved. Some explanations can be ruled out. The distal-to-proximal pattern is not a consequence of reliance on visual feedback of the hand or finger during movement preparation and initiation (Anson and O'Connor, 1989). It is not due to diminished attention, as the pattern remained, independent of the frequency of off-task glancing (Mawston and Anson, 1994). The pattern does not occur less frequently with extended practice (Anson and Gorely, 1990). And the distal-to-proximal pattern does not appear to be related to or affected by specific experimenter-imposed 'react fast' or 'move fast' strategies for response preparation and initiation (Anson et al., 1994). Furthermore, the distal-to-proximal pattern is not selectively associated with slower or faster reaction times within blocks of trials performed by individuals with Down syndrome (Anson and Mawston, 2000).

At this time we cannot offer an entirely satisfactory explanation for the distal-to-proximal results. It is possible that they are associated with the general experimental/laboratory procedures. Evaluating upper limb performance responses within a setting of the tasks by daily living activities might be one way to assess the task-specific hypothesis. It is possible that a task that might be perceived by those with Down syndrome as more meaningful or intrinsically rewarding could affect the reaction time outcome. At this time we are not aware of any functional advantage to distal-to-proximal initiation of rapid discrete goal-directed upper limb reaching movements.

Because we cannot offer a satisfactory explanation for the distal-to-proximal pattern, practical implications for motor learning should be considered with the qualification caveat emptor. One suggestion might be to employ strategies that focus on the task outcome rather than adherence to standard form. If the task involves reaching for an object, encourage the individual to 'capture' the object as quickly as possible. Successful task completion would focus on the outcome, the product if you like, and less on differences in effector sequencing.

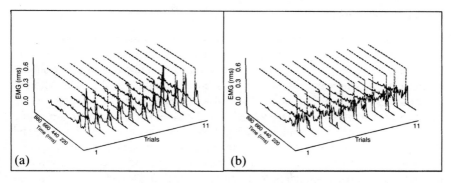

Figure 9.1 Reaction time measures from two switches (elbow and index finger) for one participant in the control group illustrate a synchronous onset of movement. However, EMG recordings from two agonist muscles clearly show a proximal-to-distal pattern of muscle activation. (a) Simple RT (elbow = dashed; finger = dotted) and EMG (RMS) for each of 11 trials for the control participant show consistent trial-to-trial performance in the pattern of proximal muscle activation (anterior deltoid). (b) From the same participant in figure 1a. Data are the same, but EMG (RMS) is from the distal muscle (extensor indicis). [Reprinted by permission from J.G. Anson and G.A. Mawston, 2000, Patterns of muscle activation in simple reaction-time tasks. In D.J. Weeks, R. Chua and D. Elliott (eds), *Perceptual–Motor Behavior in Down Syndrome* (pp. 3–24). Champaign, IL: Human Kinetics.]

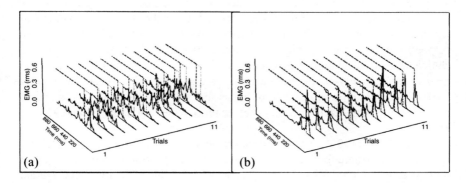

Figure 9.2 For an individual with Down syndrome, the reaction time and EMG measures tell a different story from that in the control group. Reaction time measured at the finger is consistently shorter (faster) than reaction time measured at the elbow. This distal-to-proximal pattern is corroborated by the EMG recordings that show activation of the distal muscle to precede that of the proximal muscle. (a) Simple RT (elbow = dashed; finger = dotted) and EMG (RMS) for each of 11 trials for one participant with Down syndrome (chronologically age-matched to the control participant whose data appear in Figure 9.1). EMG (RMS) data are from the proximal muscles (anterior deltoid) and show consistent timing, exemplified by the large range of differences between the RT measures at the finger and elbow. (b) From the same participant in Figure 9.2a. RT data are the same, but EMG (RMS) is from the distal muscle (extensor indicis). [Reprinted by permission from J.G. Anson and G.A. Mawston, 2000, Patterns of muscle activation in simple reaction-time tasks. In D.J. Weeks, R. Chua and D. Elliott (eds), *Perceptual–Motor Behavior in Down Syndrome* (pp. 3–24). Champaign, IL: Human Kinetics.]

Choice reaction time

Choice reaction time is a measure of the time taken to initiate a response when a stimulus indicates which of multiple responses is to be performed. In a typical laboratory situation presentation of a light might signal that one response should be performed, whereas presentation of a buzzer might signal that a different response should be performed. In the real world people are faced with making rapid choices of which response to make all the time. For example, if something were to fall out when opening the refrigerator door, one would wish to respond differently if the item were a raw egg, than if it were a plastic bottle of ketchup.

As in the simple reaction time paradigm, one has first to detect that a stimulus has occurred before responding to it, but unlike the simple case, choice reaction time does not allow one to pre-prepare the specific response that is to occur. Common factors that may be manipulated in a choice reaction time task are the number of response alternatives, the similarity of the responses that are to be decided amongst, and the probability that a given stimulus will be presented.

Generally, the relationship between reaction time and the number of response alternatives follows a log-linear relationship, known as Hick's law (also the Hick–Hyman law, see e.g. Schmidt and Lee, 1999, for a review). The essence of the relationship is that reaction time increases by a fixed amount every time the number of response alternatives is doubled. Hence the additional time it takes to respond to four choices, as compared to two choices, is the same as the increase when one shifts from four choices to eight. It should be noted that the Hick's law relationship can break down under conditions of extended practice and when stimulus response compatibility is extremely high (Leonard, 1959). In these situations additional choices often have no impact on reaction times. In investigations of choice reaction time in intellectually-challenged participants, it has been shown that the slope of the Hick's law relationship tends to be higher than for chronologically age-matched controls from the general population, but the form of the relationship holds (Vernon, 1986).

LeClair *et al.* (1993) investigated the influence of advance movement information in a study where the task was to move as fast as possible to press one of four buttons using whichever hand corresponded with the side of the illuminated target button. Advance cue information was provided by illuminating one, two, or four buttons prior to the movement stimulus, thereby making the task either a simple (one possible target), or a choice (two or four possible targets) reaction time task. Le Clair *et al.* compared groups of people with Down syndrome, with undifferentiated intellectual challenges, and from the general population, all matched for chronological age. The Down syndrome and the undifferentiated intellectually-challenged participants showed similar RT results and were both slower than those from the general population. Overall, however, there was no interaction between group and choice condition, suggesting that the impact of increasing the number of response alternatives was effectively the same for all three groups: more choices yielded longer RTs.

In a follow-up experiment LeClair and Elliott (1995) employed a similar paradigm in which adult participants were to move their preferred index finger from a home position, located on the midline to one of two target button lights. These targets were located forward of the home button and either side of the midline. Participants were again from three different groups: Down syndrome, undifferentiated intellectually-challenged, and general population. Pre-cue information was presented so that either one or both targets were signaled, but in the one-button case the accuracy of the pre-cue was manipulated to be correct on 80 per cent of trials. Mode of pre-cueing was either visual (one or both targets were illuminated) or verbal (one or both of the targets were named), while the actual movement cue was always visual. Manipulating the pre-cue accuracy enabled evaluation of the degree to which the participants could use advance information about the probability of the response, and the visual versus verbal pre-cue manipulation was intended to see if the nature of the cue had a similar impact on the three groups.

The results indicated that for all groups RT decreased with increasing certainty of the correct stimulus. However, the group with Down syndrome stood out from the other two groups. While all three groups reacted more quickly after a visual rather than a verbal cue, the difference between cue conditions was largest for those with Down syndrome in the most reliable cue condition (80 per cent). Overall, all three groups benefited equally from the visual advanced cue information but the group with Down syndrome did not show as much benefit as the other two groups when the pre-cue was verbal. This result is consistent with a more general research finding that people with Down syndrome have greater difficulty in processing auditory/verbal information compared to visual information (e.g. Elliott *et al.*, 1990).

In investigating a model of atypical cerebral organisation proposed to account for unusual dichotic listening data in Down syndrome (Elliott *et al.*, 1987), Welsh and Elliott (2001) had participants perform a two-choice rapid movement task. On each trial the movement direction, either toward or away from the body along the midline, was cued either visually (either the target was illuminated directly, or lights adjacent to the start position signaled the target) or auditorally (the colour of the target button was presented via headphones to both ears simultaneously). Adult participants with Down syndrome were not reliably slower in mean RT than a group of chronologically age-matched participants with undifferentiated intellectual challenges, though both groups were slower than a group of participants from the general population. There was also a main effect of stimulus condition such that the verbal condition elicited the shortest reaction times. However, while the non-challenged group did not differ across stimulus conditions, for the Down syndrome and undifferentiated intellectually-challenged groups, the indirect mapping condition had longer RTs than the verbal or direct mapping conditions. Notably, the greater difficulty in responding to verbal stimuli over visual stimuli found by others (e.g. LeClair and Elliott, 1995, see above) was not replicated in this particular experiment. Further research is needed to determine the conditions under which verbal stimuli do and do not lead to RT disadvantages compared to visual stimuli.

In work on motor skill acquisition by Kerr and Blais (1985), young adult males with Down syndrome (mean chronological age around 18 years), undifferentiated intellectually-challenged and general population (high school and elementary school) participants (matched in turn for each of chronological and functional age) performed repeated trials of a pursuit-tracking task. The task involved repeatedly turning a steering-wheel apparatus, similar to that on an airplane, so as to bring a pointer in line with whichever of five target lights was illuminated. The pointer had to be moved into the target area for a period of 200 ms and then a new light would illuminate, prompting the appropriate movement to bring the pointer into the area of this next target. The task could thus be characterised as involving discrete rapid movements with uncertainty about direction and extent of movement. Due to the spatial arrangement of the target positions, the probability of the next movement being towards the left or the right was position-dependent (e.g. if at the extreme left, the probability of moving to the right was 100 per cent, if in the central position, left and right movements were equally probable – beyond this, the distance of the next movement would, of course, also vary). Eight trials, consisting of 100 movements each, were completed by each participant, and individual movements were broken down according to directional probability, distance etc. For correct RT measures (i.e. movement begun in the correct direction), it was found that when persons with Down syndrome were matched for functional age they were significantly slower than their general population counterparts. The RTs of undifferentiated intellectually-challenged participants fell between, but did not differ from, the other two groups. When matched for chronological age the Down syndrome and undifferentiated intellectually-challenged participants did not differ but were both significantly slower than the control participants. When directional probability was considered the undifferentiated intellectually-challenged and control participants showed their shortest RTs for the 100 per cent direction (i.e. moving from the end points). The Down syndrome group, on the other hand, moved fastest in the lowest probability condition. Further analysis suggested that this effect may have been an artifact of the Down syndrome group simply making earlier movements when the target was adjacent to the starting position, but either way the fact remains that Down syndrome participants were apparently not using the advance information inherent in the task in the same way as the undifferentiated intellectually-challenged and control groups. The fact that participants with Down syndrome had fewer errors than the other groups, particularly in the lowest probability condition, coupled with their having the overall longst RTs, might reflect use of a qualitatively different strategy for the task than that used by the other two groups.

In a follow-up experiment using the same task, Blais and Kerr (1986) found that RTs tended to increase with decreased certainty of directional probability for undifferentiated intellectually-challenged and control participants. However, the Down syndrome group, although slower overall than the other groups, once again showed their shortest RTs for the lowest directional probability. The movements with highest directional probability were next fastest, and intermediate directional certainty movements (50 per cent and 75 per cent – which did not differ) were slowest. Thus a form of inverted U relationship obtained between RT and directional probability for participants with Down syndrome. Errors in directional initiation were lowest in the Down syndrome group. The authors suggest that the participants with Down syndrome may have been more reflective in their approach to the task than those in the other groups; however, the form of the relationship between directional probability and RT does not fit a general trend towards reflectivity in this population.

A further study (Kerr and Blais, 1987) using the same discrete movement-tracking task, indicated that with practice, children and adults with Down syndrome not only brought their RTs down to the range of the general population, but their ability to utilise directional probability also became similar to that of the other groups. Thus Kerr and Blais suggest that the apparent differences for those with Down syndrome seen in their earlier studies may be attributable not to a limitation in processing ability, but more to their being in a different (i.e. earlier) stage of learning. To the extent that such an improvement might be generalisable across different tasks involving rapid selection between response alternatives, this latter result is encouraging. It suggests that at least some of the identifiable difficulties observed in Down syndrome compared with the general population may be attenuated or even removed by practice. Interestingly, Kerr and Blais (1988) found that when they provided some pre-training about the probability structure of their experimental task, participants with Down syndrome improved their performance, but on the MT rather than the RT component. One of the research challenges in this field lies in exploring the extent to which such practice benefits are observable in tasks other than the one used by Kerr and Blais.

In summary, the work on choice RT in Down syndrome indicates that people with Down syndrome are usually slower in reacting than the general population, and sometimes slower than other intellectually-challenged groups. They have shown longer RT in responding to verbal rather than visual stimuli (e.g. LeClair and Elliott, 1995), though not always (Welsh and Elliott, 2001), and the precise conditions under which modality of stimulus (visual or verbal) influences choice reaction times remain to be determined. Although, in keeping with Hick's law, people with Down syndrome show a standard increase in RT when the number of response alternatives increases, the increase is more rapid than in the general population (Vernon, 1986). They apparently benefit from compatible stimulus response mapping in a manner consistent with the rest of the population (Welsh and Elliott, 2001). In addition persons with Down syndrome seem less able to utilise probability information inherent in movement tasks, but are able to benefit greatly from practice to the point where choice RT performance does not differ reliably either in magnitude or apparent strategy from the general population (Blais and Kerr, 1986; Kerr and Blais, 1985, 1987). Perhaps some of the most important practical questions still open that relate to choice reaction time in Down syndrome concern the generalisability of the practice effect found by Kerr and Blais (1987). If such findings can be replicated with other tasks requiring choice RT, then it may be that people with Down syndrome are not limited to the abilities apparent in a 'snapshot' experiment where only immediate performance is considered. Indeed they may well be able to achieve 'normal' levels of performance with sufficient practice. The fact that of the experiments described in this section, only those by

Kerr and Blais included younger participants begs the question of whether older people with Down syndrome can derive the same practice benefits as younger individuals.

3. Movement execution: visual and kinesthetic regulation

For over a century (Woodworth, 1899), researchers have been interested in the relative contribution of advance planning and the on-line regulation to the control of simple goal-directed movement. Based on a between-task comparison of rapid finger-tapping and pursuit rotor performance, Frith and Frith (1974) suggested that clumsiness in adults with Down syndrome was due to an inability to develop central control of their upper limb movements. This 'motor programming' problem was thought to make a person with Down syndrome overly dependent on response-produced visual and kinesthetic feedback for the on-line regulation of movement.

Anwar (1981; Anwar and Hermelin, 1979) examined this hypothesis directly by comparing the reaching performance of children with Down syndrome to other disabled and nondisabled children under conditions of reduced and augmented visual feedback. Although the children with Down syndrome did not perform as well as typically developing children of the same chronological age, they were not any more disadvantaged under conditions of reduced visual feedback than other intellectually-challenged children. Moreover, their performance in both conditions was similar to the performance of typically developing children of a similar mental age. These results indicate that slowness and movement error in persons with Down syndrome cannot be attributed solely to problems with motor programming.

Henderson *et al.* (1981) compared the tracking and drawing performance of children with Down syndrome to other intellectually-challenged and non-challenged children of a similar mental age. They reported that while the children with Down syndrome had no difficulty with the spatial components of these tasks, they were impaired, relative to other participants, on the temporal aspects of tracking. This difficulty could arise from either the inability to process and utilise predictable environmental information, or trouble timing the onset of muscular forces. The former conclusion is consistent with work by Kerr and Blais (1985, see above). However, the latter explanation coincides with the results of a catching study conducted by Planinsek (see Savelsbergh *et al.*, 2000) that indicated that children with Down syndrome are slow in timing the grasp of the ball.

In recent years, the development of high-speed optoelectric movement analysis systems has made it possible for us to monitor the trajectories of simple aiming, reaching and tracking movements. By examining how these trajectories change with the task requirements, we can gain important insights into how these movements are controlled (Elliott and Carson, 2000). Recently these techniques have been used to study the control of upper limb movements in children and young adults with Down syndrome.

Judith Charlton and her colleagues (Charlton *et al.*, 1996, 1998) have used two- and three-dimensional movement analysis techniques to study reach-to-grasp actions in 8- to 10-year-old children with Down syndrome. As well as manipulating the characteristics of the object being grasped, they varied the task goals. For example, an object could simply be picked up, grasped and placed in another position, or picked up and thrown into a container (see Marteniuk *et al.*, 1987). These task variations were introduced to determine how well children with Down syndrome are able to develop and generalise internal representations for prehension to task-specific movement requirements.

Prehension movements are composed of two interrelated components (Jeannerod, 1981, 1984). The transport or reach component of the movement brings the hand into the vicinity of the target object, while actually grasping the object requires a manipulative component in which the fingers open and then close around the object. The transport portion of the movement involves determining the object's position in three-dimensional space, translating that position to a body-centred frame of reference and then specifying the timing and intensity of the muscular forces required to move the limb to the target area. How the limb trajectory toward the target object unfolds can depend on what the performer is required to do with the object once it has been acquired (Marteniuk *et al.*, 1990). The grasp component of a prehension movement depends not only on the task required, but also the intrinsic characteristics of the object, such as the size, shape, weight and surface texture (see Jeannerod and Marteniuk, 1992 for a review).

With respect to the transport component of the movement, children with Down syndrome took longer to reach the objects and achieved lower peak velocities than control participants of a similar chronological age. While their mean performance was similar to typically developing children of similar mental age (i.e. younger children), 8- to 10-year-olds with Down syndrome exhibited greater trial-to-trial variability in their movement trajectories. Although the movement trajectories of all the children were affected by the object's characteristics and the task requirements, the children with Down syndrome and the developmentally younger control participants spent a greater proportion of the overall movement decelerating the limb than the 8- to 10-year-old control subjects. The developmentally younger participants also exhibited more discontinuities in their trajectories during deceleration (see also Kulatunga-Moruzi and Elliott, 1999), particularly so when the precision requirements of the task were high (Charlton, Ihsen and Lavelle, 2000). Long deceleration times and irregularities in the trajectory, as well as greater trial-to-trial variability, are typically associated with the use of visual and kinesthetic response-produced feedback to correct error in the initial movement impulse (Chua and Elliott, 1993; Hodges *et al.*, 1995; see figure 9.3). Of course, a dependence on feedback could reflect initial difficulty in organising a movement to meet the task requirements (e.g. Frith and Frith, 1974).

In the work by Charlton *et al.*, the grasp behaviour of children with Down syndrome generally mirrored the performance of chronologically younger children. Specifically, while they scaled their grasp aperture to the size of the object, they were more likely to employ a whole hand grasp than the more precise pincer grasp as they were grasping very small objects. However, Savelsbergh *et al.* (2000) point out that grasping patterns often depend on the ratio of hand size and object size.

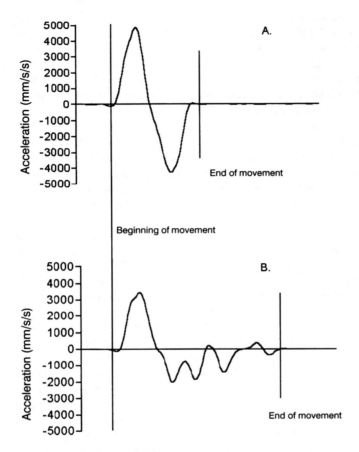

Figure 9.3 Typical acceleration profiles for a single rapid aiming movement for (A) a participant without developmental disability and (B) a participant with Down syndrome (e.g. Hodges *et al.*, 1995). [Reprinted by permission from T.N. Welsh and D. Elliott, 2000, Preparation and control of goal-directed limb movements in persons with Down syndrome. In D.J. Weeks, R. Chua and D. Elliott (eds), *Perceptual–Motor Behavior in Down Syndrome* (pp. 49–70). Champaign, IL: Human Kinetics.]

Children with Down syndrome have a smaller average hand size than their normally developing peers, and for this reason alone can be expected to exhibit grasp patterns similar to younger children (Savelsbergh, Van der Kamp and Davis, 2001).

While most of our work on reaching and aiming has been with adults, it is clear that persons with Down syndrome are slower in reaching target objects because of the time they spend decelerating the limb, and making adjustments to the movement trajectory as they approach the target. We found this pattern of performance regardless of whether on-line visual information about the position of the limb and the target was available or not (Hodges *et al.*, 1995). Interestingly, while eliminating vision on movement initiation decreased aiming precision in all participants, the performance of intellectually-challenged participants without Down syndrome was more disrupted than the aiming of adults with Down syndrome and non-challenged adults. Because there were few differences between the two intellectually-challenged groups for the initial movement impulse, the superior performance of persons with Down syndrome in the no-vision condition seems to be associated with their ability to use kinesthetic information more effectively.

In summary, it seems that while there may be some small motor control differences related to timing the onset and offset of muscular force, children with Down syndrome perform most visual–motor tasks in a manner equivalent to chronologically younger children. Specifically, they are slower in executing simple goal-directed movements, partly because they are more dependent on response-produced feedback than other children of a similar chronological age. It also appears to be the case that children with Down syndrome do not spontaneously make use of task and environment information that has the potential to facilitate anticipatory behaviour. It remains to be seen whether or not feedforward strategies can be acquired with practice (see Elliott, 1990 for a review).

4. Verbal mediation in the control of upper limb movements

Motor control

Although persons with Down syndrome perform visually-directed aiming movements in a manner similar to developmentally younger children, their ability to organise and execute simple movements on the basis of verbal direction is impaired relative to their peers of a similar mental age. For example, Elliott *et al.* (1990) have shown that young adults with Down syndrome have difficulty reproducing sequences of oral and manual gestures when these gestures are cued with verbal instruction, as opposed to being demonstrated. Relative to other intellectually-challenged persons, this verbal–motor problem becomes more pronounced as the number of the elements in the movement sequence is increased. This difficulty is not a verbal memory/processing problem, because persons with Down syndrome are able to correctly point to pictures of other individuals performing the same movements when they are verbally cued. Rather, persons with Down syndrome appear to have difficulty using the verbal information to structure the appropriate movement (see Le Clair and Elliott, 1995 and the reaction time work discussed earlier).

Part of the verbal–motor integration problem experienced by persons with Down syndrome may be due to a unique pattern of brain organisation in this group. A number of dichotic listening studies have demonstrated that children (e.g. Hartley, 1981; Pipe, 1983) and adults (e.g. Elliott and Weeks, 1993) with Down syndrome display a left ear–right hemisphere advantage for the perception of speech sounds, while for most of us there is a right ear–left hemisphere advantage (see Elliott *et al.*, 1994). In spite of this apparent reversed cerebral specialisation for speech perception, persons with Down syndrome generally are left-hemisphere-specialised for the organisation and control of movement, including speech movements (Elliott *et al.*, 1987; Heath and Elliott, 1999). It is our contention (see Chua *et al.*, 1996; Heath *et al.*, 2000) that this dissociation between functional systems (i.e. speech perception and movement organisation) that are normally subserved by the same cerebral hemisphere (the left) leads to a breakdown in communication during the performance of tasks that require both verbal decoding and movement organisation. The degradation of information during interhemispheric communication may be compounded by the fact that children and adults with Down syndrome have a thinner corpus callosum (Wang *et al.*, 1992) in the area associated with semantic communication. In terms of atypical cerebral specialisation, it is interesting that the persons with Down syndrome who exhibit the most pronounced right ear advantage for the perception of speech sounds also display the greatest verbal–motor difficulties (Elliott and Weeks, 1993).

Motor learning

Motor learning is a field devoted to investigating the impact of various forms and amounts of practice on the ability to perform motor skills. The emphasis is not generally on immediate capability, which may be heavily influenced by temporary factors, but rather on the relatively permanent changes in skill level brought about by practice. A beginner golfer who goes to the range and has close supervision while under the immediate tutelage of the club pro may perform very well while the pro is standing right there correcting every little nuance of the swing. When the golfer first goes to the range by herself and attempts to replicate her performance she may do very much worse. A key to investigating the influences of various factors on motor learning is to assess performance at some delay after practice has taken place. Sometimes, transfer to a related task is assessed to determine the generalisability of the learning. Usually, extrinsic sources of feedback, such as verbal reports from the instructor, are removed at test. It is only when such feedback-free, delayed tests of learning are conducted, that the immediate *performance* effects seen during practice can be dissociated from the relatively long-term *learning* effects seen at a delay (Salmoni *et al.*, 1984; Schmidt and Lee, 1999). The necessity for such delayed tests is exemplified by practice interventions that have essentially opposite effects on immediate performance and longer-term learning. A good example is the contextual interference effect (Shea and Morgan, 1979). Here repeated practice of a given movement (blocked practice) leads to a higher level of performance, than does interspersing trials of different movements between practice trials (random practice). However, when assessed at a delay, random practice is generally shown to have supported better learning.

In assessing motor learning in Down syndrome the focus should not necessarily be on the absolute levels of performance. Across a wide spectrum of skills, people with Down syndrome show performance that is less accurate, or less quick, than matched controls. Thus, demonstrating differences in absolute performance levels may not be terribly enlightening with regard to motor learning (except, perhaps, where extended practice leads their performance to come in line with that of controls from the wider population – see, Kerr and Blais, 1987, above). Of interest in assessing practice methods for people with Down syndrome is whether the form of benefit is the same as, or different from, that seen in the wider population. If similar effects occur as are seen in the mainstream motor learning literature, then it seems reasonable to apply the same practice methods for those with Down syndrome as for other learners. If, however, people with Down syndrome show qualitatively different responses to manipulations of practice conditions when compared to control participants, then it would be appropriate to structure the learning environment more specifically for those with Down syndrome.

Edwards *et al.* (1986) investigated the influence of contextual interference on senior high school children (approx. mean age = 18 years) with Down syndrome and children matched for mental age (approx. mean = 5 years) as they learned a coincident timing task. A Bassin timer apparatus was set up so that successive lights were illuminated to create apparent motion of a light toward the participant. The task was to move 20 cm from a start position to knock down a barrier adjacent to the Bassin apparatus so that, as closely as possible, the barrier was knocked down coincident with the arrival of the apparent motion of the light at a predetermined point. The apparent speed of approach of the light was varied across four levels, and for different participants trials of the different speeds were arranged in a blocked fashion (all trials of a given speed were completed before moving on to the next speed), or a random fashion (successive trials varied in speed, in an unpredictable fashion). Practice proceeded for 64 trials, with each trial followed by feedback. After a 10-min retention interval, eight transfer trials at each of three new approach speeds were performed. The transfer speeds were selected so that one was inside the range of practised speeds, while the other two were from outside that range: one slower, the other faster.

The results were not clear-cut, perhaps owing to the task chosen. Interestingly, for the participants with Down syndrome, random practice was better for immediate performance than was blocked, a result rather inconsistent with the standard contextual interference effect. For transfer, also, the advantage was for random practice in the Down syndrome participants. Strong conclusions based on these results would be ill advised however, as the non-challenged participants did not show a clear example of the effects of practice schedule on acquisition performance and transfer. It was certainly not the case, however, that random practice made for inferior learning in the Edwards *et al.* study. On that basis then, it seems sensible to use a random rather than a blocked schedule in practice for people with Down syndrome, as any effects that occur seem to be positive. Further investigation of the role of the influence of contextual interference (and other practice manipulations) on learning in Down syndrome is clearly important. Teachers, coaches and vocational instructors need to be aware of what practice techniques do and do not facilitate improved learning in the Down syndrome population.

In a study by Elliott *et al.* (1991), adult participants with and without Down syndrome practised a three-element movement sequence that was to be completed as quickly as possible. The movement sequence was cued prior to each trial. Once practice trials had been performed and a short rest taken, retention performance was assessed without verbal cueing, and then transfer to the non-dominant hand was also assessed. Measures of reaction time revealed that the persons with Down syndrome were slower to initiate movements during acquisition than control participants while a group of undifferentiated intellectually-challenged individuals performed between, but did not differ reliably from, the other two groups. At the start of retention, however, and unlike the other two groups, persons with Down syndrome showed a sharp increase in RT compared with the end of practice. There was some recovery from this increase as retention trials proceeded, but the Down syndrome group remained slower than the other groups throughout retention. Transfer RTs indicated that the control group was faster than the two mentally handicapped groups, which did not differ reliably. Complete transfer occurred for the Down syndrome and control group, whereas the undifferentiated intellectually-challenged groups showed a small deterioration. For movement time data, throughout practice and retention the control group performed the sequence faster than the other two groups, which did not differ. In transfer, the Down syndrome slowed down, as did the undifferentiated intellectually-challenged group, while the control group maintained MT. The authors suggested that the Down syndrome participants suffered more from the removal of verbal cueing than did the other groups because of the difficulty that they have in organising movements based on verbal direction – made even more difficult when the sequence not only has to be translated from verbal cue to action, but, in the case of the retention trials, remembered aa well. This study did not include different cue types for comparison with the verbal mode, but a more recent study (Maraj *et al.*, 2000) allowed for such a comparison.

Maraj *et al.* (2000) had children and adults, with and without Down syndrome, practice manipulating a computer mouse so that the cursor moved from a home position to each of three targets that were arranged vertically on the screen. The order of the targets (e.g. middle, top, bottom) was cued for each trial, either visually (the cursor moved to each of the targets in turn) or verbally. The goal was to make the appropriate sequence of movements as fast as possible. Participants with Down syndrome were slower to initiate their movements during practice than undifferentiated intellectually-challenged persons who in turn were slower than control participants. Persons with Down syndrome performed better when the cues were provided visually rather than in the verbal situation. In contrast with the results of Elliott *et al.* (1991), participants with Down syndrome were not slower than the other groups in initiating their movements at delays of 1 and 24 hours regardless of whether they had been trained visually or verbally. Those with Down syndrome were also just as quick to initiate their movements in transfer trials (i.e. cueing modality was not that used in practice). For movement time, participants with Down syndrome took longer to complete movements in the verbal than in the visual condition during acquisition. In retention, movement times were longer in the verbal than the visual condition. At the 1-hour delay those with Down syndrome did not differ from the undifferentiated intellectually-challenged group, but at 24 hours they showed a dramatic increase in MT. Thus, increased delay seemed to make an already difficult processing mode even more difficult. Also, in transfer, performance was relatively easy under verbal conditions when it had been practised under visual conditions, especially so for children and adults in the Down syndrome group. Overall the retention and transfer results indicated that, whether the criterion test cueing conditions were verbal or visual, practice under visual cueing conditions yielded superior learning.

Together with work by Elliott *et al.* (1990) indicating that persons with Down syndrome exhibit more errors when sequencing actions based on verbal rather than visual cueing, these results suggest that, as far as possible, visual rather than verbal instructions should be provided for Down syndrome learners. So far the efficacy of combined visual *and* verbal cueing has not been investigated. As such, it is unclear whether such a combination would be better or worse for learning than visual cueing alone. There are clearly many important questions yet to be answered regarding motor learning in Down syndrome. The extent to which learning in this population operates in a predictable fashion and how that differs qualitatively from the rest of the population represents an open area of research.

5. Development versus differences

For many years, researchers have argued as to whether perceptual–motor and cognitive problems in persons with Down syndrome and other intellectually challenging conditions can best be understood from a developmental or difference perspective. The developmental model has generally been associated with a greater degree of optimism. This is because development is viewed as a life-long process. Thus, although perceptual–motor and cognitive changes may proceed slowly, they proceed nonetheless. While a developmental model does a reasonable job of describing some behaviour in persons with Down syndrome, it is naive to believe that there will not be some perceptual–motor and cognitive differences in this genetically unique group. We have described several of those differences in this chapter. It is not the case that differences between children with Down syndrome and other children simply constrain behaviour. Rather, children and adults with Down syndrome develop unique ways of dealing with the environment in order to make the most efficient use of the perceptual–motor and cognitive tools they have available.

As Latash and Anson (1996) suggest, 'normal movements' in atypical populations may reflect an entirely different benchmark of 'normality'. In this regard the greater degree of optimism associated with the developmental model might be misleading because the expected observations of progression are drawn from data from a different 'normality' model. In contrast, a model that views persons with Down syndrome as different from other persons would encourage an emphasis on comparisons of performance within the population based on the intrinsic characteristics of persons with the syndrome. For example, the motor behaviour of persons with Down syndrome is often described as clumsy. 'Clumsiness' is a term used to describe movements that appear different from and less efficient than those seen in the population at large. For the person with Down syndrome, 'clumsy' movements may be the outcome of a central nervous system that understands its functional limits and 'prefers' safe movement outcomes to total failure. Perhaps, in reaction time response situations, slower reaction times observed in individuals with Down syndrome represent a compromise between successful task completion and increased risk of failure or loss of control if the emphasis is on 'as fast as possible' performance. From a 'differences' viewpoint, successful task completion (with slow reaction time) could be viewed as an adaptive response mediated by the central nervous system, not an 'abnormal' response. Alternatively, a developmental approach may imply unrealistic expectancies of continued (albeit slow) progress toward an inappropriately defined 'normality'.

In sum, whatever perspective is chosen to examine and evaluate perceptual–motor behaviour in persons with Down syndrome, it is important for scientists and practitioners to consider carefully both the content and context of the movement task environment. The transition from empirical, laboratory-based tasks and data to performance demands in 'real world' tasks is strongly encouraged.

References

Anson J.G. (1989) Effects of moment of inertia on simple reaction time. *Journal of Motor Behavior*, 21, 60–71.

Anson, J.G. (1992) Neuromotor control and Down syndrome. In J.J. Summers (ed.), *Approaches to the Study of Motor Control and Learning* (pp. 387–412). Amsterdam: North-Holland.

Anson, J.G. and. Bird, Y.N. (1993) Neuromotor programming: bilateral and unilateral effects on simple reaction time. *Human Movement Science*, 12, 37–50.

Anson, J.G. and Davis, S.A. (1988) Neuromotor programming and Down syndrome. *International Journal of Neuroscience*, 40, 82.

Anson, J.G. and Gorely, P.J. (1990) Down syndrome: movement control and performance variability. Paper presented at the Commonwealth and International Conference on Physical Education, Sport, Health, Dance, Recreation and Leisure, Auckland, New Zealand.

Anson, J.G., Lockie, R.M. and Mawston, G.M. (1994) Down syndrome: persistence of distal-to-proximal sequencing. Paper presented at the Second International Conference of Motor Control in Down syndrome, Chicago, IL.

Anson J. G. and Mawston, G.M. (2000) Patterns of muscle activation in simple reaction-time tasks. In R. Chua, D.J. Weeks and D. Elliott (eds), *Perceptual–Motor Behavior in Down Syndrome* (pp. 3–24). Champaign, IL: Human Kinetics.

Anson, J.G. and O'Connor, H.M. (1989) Down syndrome: Initiation of discrete rapid movements. *International Journal of Neuroscience*, 46, 36.

Anwar, F. (1981) Motor function in Down syndrome. In N.R. Ellis (ed.), *International Review of Research in Mental Retardation*: Vol 10 (pp. 107–38). New York: Academic Press.

Anwar, F. and Hermelin, B. (1979) Kinesthetic movement after-effects in children with Down syndrome. *Journal of Mental Deficiency Research*, 23, 287–97.

Berkson, G. (1960) An analysis of reaction time in normal and mentally retarded young men. III. Variation of stimulus and of response complexity. *Journal of Mental Deficiency Research*, 4, 69–77.

Blais, C. and Kerr, R. (1986) Probability information in a complex motor task with respect to Down syndrome. *Journal of Human Movement Studies*, 12, 183–94.

Charlton, J.L., Ihsen, E. and Lavelle, B.M (2000) Control of manual skills in children with Down syndrome. In R. Chua, D.J. Weeks and D. Elliott (eds), *Perceptual–Motor Behavior in Down Syndrome* (pp. 25–48). Champaign, IL: Human Kinetics.

Charlton, J.L., Ihsen, E. and Oxley, J. (1996) Kinematic characteristics of reaching and grasping in children with Down syndrome. *Human Movement Science*, 15, 727–43.

Charlton, J.L., Ihsen, E. and Oxley, J. (1998) The influence of context in the development of reaching and grasping: implications for assessment of disability. In J.P. Piek (ed.), *Motor Behavior and Human Skill. A Multidisciplinary Approach* (pp. 283–302). Champaign, IL: Human Kinetics.

Chua, R. and Elliott, D. (1993) Visual regulation of manual aiming. *Human Movement Science*, 12, 365–401.

Chua, R., Weeks, D.J. and Elliott, D. (1996) A functional systems approach to understanding verbal motor integration in individuals with Down syndrome. *Down Syndrome: Research and Practice*, 4, 25–36.

Davis, W.E. and Kelso, J.A.S. (1982) Analysis of 'invariant characteristics' in the motor control of Down syndrome and normal subjects. *Journal of Motor Behavior*, 14, 194–212.

Davis, W.E. and Sinning, W.E. (1987) Muscle stiffness in Down syndrome and other mentally handicapped subjects: a research note. *Journal of Motor Behavior*, 19, 130–44.

Davis, W.E., Ward, T. and Sparrow, W.A. (1991) Fractionated reaction times and movement times of Down syndrome and other adults with mental retardation. *Adapted Physical Activity Quarterly*, 8, 221–33.

De Lussanet, M.H.E. and Alexander, R.M. (1997) A simple model for planar arm movements: optimizing mechanical activation and moment-arms of uniarticular and biarticular arm muscles. *Journal of Theoretical Biology*, 184, 187–201.

Edwards, J.M., Elliott, D. and Lee, T.D. (1986) Contextual interference effects during skill acquisition and transfer in Down syndrome adolescents. *Adapted Physical Activity Quarterly*, 3, 250–8.

Elliott, D. (1990) Movement control in Down syndrome: a neuropsychological approach. In G. Reid (ed.), *Problems in Movement Control* (pp. 201–16). Amsterdam: North-Holland.

Elliott, D. and Carson, R.G. (2000) Moving into the new millennium: some perspectives on the brain in action. *Brain and Cognition*, 42, 153–6.

Elliott, D., Gray, S. and Weeks, D.J. (1991) Verbal cueing and motor skill acquisition for adults with Down syndrome. *Adapted Physical Activity Quarterly*, 8, 210–20.

Elliott, D. and Weeks, D.J. (1993) Cerebral specialization for speech perception and movement organization in adults with Down syndrome. *Cortex*, 29, 103–13.

Elliott, D., Weeks, D.J. and Chua, R. (1994) Anomalous cerebral lateralization and Down syndrome. *Brain and Cognition*, 26, 191–195.

Elliott, D., Weeks, D.J. and Elliott, C.L. (1987) Cerebral specialization in individuals with Down Syndrome. *American Journal of Mental Retardation*, 97, 237–71.

Elliott, D., Weeks, D.J. and Gray, S. (1990) Manual and oral praxis in adults with Down syndrome. *Neuropsychologia*, 28, 1307–15.

Fetz, E.E., Cheney, P.D., Mewes, K. and Palmer, S. (1989) Control of forelimb muscle activity by populations of corticomotoneuronal and rubromotoneuronal cells. *Progress in Brain Research*, 80, 437–49.

Frith, U. and Frith C.D. (1974) Specific motor disabilities in Down syndrome. *Journal of Child Psychology and Psychiatry*, 15, 293–301.

Hartley, X.Y. (1981) Lateralisation of speech stimuli in young Down syndrome children. *Cortex*, 17, 241–8.

Heath, M. and Elliott, D. (1999) Cerebral specialization for speech production in persons with Down syndrome. *Brain and Language*, 69, 193–211.

Heath, M., Elliott, D., Weeks. D.J. and Chua, R. (2000) A functional systems approach to movement pathology in persons with Down syndrome. In R. Chua, D.J. Weeks and D. Elliott (eds), *Perceptual–Motor Behavior in Down Syndrome* (pp. 305–20). Champaign, IL: Human Kinetics.

Henderson, S.E., Morris, J. and Frith, U. (1981) The motor deficit in Down syndrome children: A problem of timing? *Journal of Child Psychology and Psychiatry*, 22, 223–45.

Hodges, N.J., Cunningham, S.J., Lyons, J.L., Kerr, T.L. and Elliott, D. (1995) Visual feedback processing and goal-directed movement in adults with Down syndrome. *Adapted Physical Activity Quarterly*, 12, 176–86.

Jeannerod, M. (1981) Intersegmental co-ordination during reaching at natural visual objects. In J. Long and A. Baddeley (eds), *Attention and Performance IX* (pp. 153–68). Hillsdale, NJ: Erlbaum.

Jeannerod, M. (1984) The timing of natural prehension movements. *Journal of Motor Behavior*, 16, 235–54.

Jeannerod, M. and Marteniuk, R.G. (1992) Functional characteristics of prehension: from data to artificial neural networks. In L. Proteau and D. Elliott (eds), *Vision and Motor Control* (pp 197–232). Amsterdam: North-Holland.

Karst, G.M. and Hasan, Z. (1991) Timing and magnitude of electromyographic activity for two-joint arm movements in different directions. *Journal of Neurophysiology*, 66, 1594–604.

Kerr, R. and Blais, C. (1985) Motor skill acquisition by individuals with Down syndrome. *American Journal of Mental Deficiency*, 90, 313–18.

Kerr, R. and Blais, C. (1987) Down syndrome and extended practice of a complex motor task. *American Journal of Mental Deficiency*, 91, 591–7.

Kerr, R. and Blais, C. (1988) Directional probability information and Down syndrome: a training study. *American Journal on Mental Retardation*, 92, 531–8.

Kulantanga-Moruzi, C. and Elliott, D. (1999) Manual and attentional assymetries in goal-directed movements for adults with Down syndrome. *Adapted Physical Activity Quarterly*, 16, 138–54.

Latash, M.L. (1992) Motor control in Down syndrome: the role of adaptation and practice. *Journal of Developmental and Physical Disabilities*, 4, 227–61.

Latash, M.L. and Anson, J.G. (1996) What are 'normal movements' in atypical populations? *Behavioral and Brain Science*, 19, 55–94.

LeClair, D.A. and Elliott, D. (1995) Movement preparation and the costs and benefits associated with advance information for adults with Down syndrome. *Adapted Physical Activity Quarterly*, 12, 239–49.

LeClair, D.A., Pollock, B.J. and Elliott, D. (1993) Movement preparation in adults with and without Down syndrome. *American Journal on Mental Retardation*, 97, 628–33.

Leonard, J.A. (1959) Tactual choice reactions: I. *The Quarterly Journal of Experimental Psychology*, 11, 76–83.

Maraj, B.K.V., Li, L., Hillman. R., Jeansonne, J. and Ringenbach, S.D. (2003) Verbal and visual instruction in motor skill acquisition for persons with and without Down syndrome. *Adapted Physical Activity Quarterly*, 20, 57–69.

Marteniuk, R.G., Leavitt, J.L., MacKenzie, C.L. and Athenes, S. (1990) Functional relationships between grasp and transport components in a prehension task. *Human Movement Science*, 9, 149–76.

Marteniuk, R.G., MacKenzie, C.L., Jeannerod, M., Athenes, S. and Dugas C. (1987) Constraints on human arm movement trajectories. *Canadian Journal of Psychology*, 41, 365–78.

Mawston, G.A. and Anson, J.G. (1994) Down syndrome: Attention and neuromotor reaction time. *International Journal of Neuroscience*, 74, 148.

Pipe, M.E. (1983) Dichotic-listening performance following auditory discrimination training in Down syndrome and developmentally retarded children. *Cortex*, 19, 481–91.

Rothwell, J. (1994) *Control of Human Voluntary Movement*, 2nd edn. London: Chapman and Hall.

Salmoni, A.W., Schmidt, R.A. and Walter, C.B. (1984) Knowledge of results and motor learning: a review and critical reappraisal. *Psychological Bulletin*, 95, 355–86.

Schmidt, R.A. and Lee. T.D. (1999) *Motor Control and Learning: A Behavioral Emphasis*, 3rd edn. Champaign, IL: Human Kinetics.

Schmidt, R.A. and. Wrisberg, C.A. (1999) *Motor Learning and Performance*, 2nd edn. Champaign, IL: Human Kinetics.

Savelsbergh, G.J.P., Van der Kamp, J. and Davis, W.E. (2001) Perception–action coupling in grasping of children with Down syndrome. *Adapted Physical Activity Quarterly*, 18, 451–7.

Savelsbergh, G., Van der Kamp, J., Ledebt, A. and Planinsek, T. (2000) Information–movement coupling in children with Down syndrome. In D.J. Weeks, R. Chua and D. Elliott (eds), *Perceptual–Motor Behavior in Down Syndrome* (pp. 251–75). Champaign, IL: Human Kinetics.

Shea, J.B. and Morgan, R.L. (1979) Contextual interference effects on the acquisition, retention, and transfer of a motor skill. *Journal of Experimental Psychology: Human Learning and Memory*, 5, 179–87.

Shumway-Cook, A. and Woollacott, M.H. (1985) Dynamics of postural control in the child with Down syndrome. *Physical Therapy*, 65, 1315–22.

Vernon, P.A. (1986) Speed of information-processing, intelligence and mental retardation. In M.G. Wade (ed.), *Motor Skill Acquisition of the Mentally Handicapped* (pp. 113–29). Amsterdam: North-Holland.

Wang, P.P., Doherty, S. Hesselink, J.R. and Bellugi, U. (1992) Callosal morphology concurs with neurobehavioral and neuropathological findings in two neurodevelopmental disorders. *Archives of Neurology*, 49, 407–11.

Welsh, T.N. and Elliott, D. (2000) Preparation and control of goal-directed limb movements in persons with Down syndrome. In D.J. Weeks, R.Chua and D. Elliott (eds), *Perceptual–Motor Behavior in Down Syndrome* (pp. 49–70). Champaign, IL: Human Kinetics.

Welsh, T.N. and Elliott (2001) The processing speed of visual and verbal movement stimuli by adults with and without Down syndrome. *Adapted Physical Activity Quarterly*, 18, 156–7.

Wisniewski, K.E., Miezejeski, C.M and Hill, A.L. (1988) Neurological and psychological status of individuals with Down syndrome. In L. Nadel (ed.), *The Psychobiology of Down Syndrome* (pp. 315–43). Cambridge MA: MIT Press.

Woodworth, R.S. (1899) The accuracy of voluntary movements. *Psychological Review*, 3 (Monograph Suppl. 2), 1–119.

10 Discrete bimanual movement co-ordination in children with hemiparetic cerebral palsy

Bert Steenbergen, Andrea Utley,
David A. Sugden and
Pauline S. Thiemann

1. Introduction

The majority of tasks in daily life require that we use both our hands together, predominantly in an asymmetrical way, e.g. unscrewing a jar or a bottle, washing dishes, typing a text on a keyboard, tying a knot. These tasks impose specific spatio-temporal constraints on bimanual co-ordination. Stated differently, both hands have to work together such that they are well co-ordinated both in space and time. Apart from the specific constraints imposed by the task, there also exist spatial and temporal interactions between both hands. For instance, drawing circles with one hand and drawing lines with the other hand is quite difficult as a consequence of the influence of both hands on each other. Research into bimanual movements and the mutual influence of both hands is quite abundant. This is especially so for the effect of temporal constraints. Overall, the results show that there is a tendency for both hands to be synchronised in time, even if the hands perform different tasks. Research into the spatial influence between both hands has received far less attention.

When individuals are faced with the performance of discrete asymmetric bimanual tasks, i.e. movements that differ for each hand with respect to their spatio-temporal pattern, they often encounter (mutual) synchronisation tendencies (e.g. Franz *et al.*, 1991; Marteniuk *et al.*, 1984). That these tendencies can be overcome is elegantly shown by concert piano players, also evidencing the fact that this is only possible after extensive amounts of practice.

In the theoretical accounts of spatio-temporal interactions in bimanual control we can roughly distinguish two approaches: the information-processing approach (e.g. Marteniuk *et al.*, 1984) and the dynamical systems approach (e.g. Kelso *et al.*, 1979a; 1979b). Note that this polarisation by no means implies that these are the only two approaches that exist. However, much research into bimanual co-ordination has initially been instigated by one or other of these approaches. Still, combined approaches do exist as well (e.g. Boessenkool *et al.*, 1999). Recently, more neurobehavioural accounts of bimanual co-ordination are observed (e.g. Swinnen *et al.*, 1997; Swinnen *et al.*, 1998; Franz *et al.*, 1996).

In this chapter we will not explicitly take a stance for either one of the approaches. Rather, our aim is to provide an overview of the research on bimanual co-ordination in children with cerebral palsy that we will frame in the context of studies that examined bimanual co-ordination in adults and during development. In the first part of this chapter, we will review research on the temporal and spatial interactions between both hands when performing bimanual tasks, in the aforementioned three groups. From this review it will become clear that research on the spatial interactions between both hands has received only scant attention, and that this is particularly so in children with hemiparetic cerebral palsy. In the second part of this chapter we will present preliminary results of a study in which the effects of spatial constraints on semi-circle drawing is examined in children with hemiparetic cerebral palsy.

2. Bimanual co-ordination: temporal and spatial constraints

Healthy populations

One of the most obvious constraints on bimanual co-ordination is the temporal constraint. Picture a situation in which you are sitting at a dining table and want to start eating. Suppose you need a fork and spoon for this action (e.g. in the case of eating spaghetti), and the fork is close to your left hand at the left of the plate while the spoon that has to be picked up with your right hand lies further away at the top of the plate. While the pieces of cutlery lie at different distances of the corresponding hand, both hands arrive at virtually the same moment at the fork and spoon. In other words, both hands work very closely together in the temporal domain, although this is not strictly necessary in order to perform the task. Next to this temporal coupling, we may also observe coupling between the spatial trajectories of both hands. Chances are high that the trajectory of the left hand that reaches for the fork will deviate slightly to the right, whereas the trajectory of the right hand will deviate somewhat to the left. Are these observations merely anecdotal (in which case the story ends here), or are we facing systematic phenomena in the co-ordination of bimanual movements (which legitimises us to continue the story)?

The above example, reaching with both hands to objects placed at different distances, has been extensively studied by Kelso and co-workers (Kelso *et al.*, 1979a; 1979b; Kelso *et al.*, 1983). In their research, they made use of a lawful relationship between on the one hand *movement time* and on the other hand *object width* and *object distance,* that was discovered almost five decades ago by Fitts (Fitts, 1954). This lawful relationship has become known as Fitts' law and is formally expressed as $MT = a + b \log2(2A/W)$, where a and b are constants, A is object distance (or, amplitude), and B is object width. The expression $\log2(2A/W)$ is denoted as 'index of difficulty' (ID). Each specific task configuration (object location in space, object width) can be assigned a specific value of this index of difficulty on the basis of which predictions can be made about the time it takes to reach an object. Kelso (Kelso *et al.*, 1979a, 1979b, 1983) used this lawful relationship to compare unimanual and bimanual movement control in healthy adult subjects. Subjects had to reach for objects that differed in ID. In the unimanual movement conditions, movement time was a function of ID. However, when both hands had to reach for targets that differed in ID, Fitts' law was violated. Both hands reached the targets at virtually the same time. These data were interpreted as indicative of a co-ordinative structure type of control, whereby the two limbs are 'constrained to function as a single synergistic unit within which component elements vary in a related manner' (Kelso *et al.*, 1983, p. 369). The absolute synchrony that was found by Kelso *et al.* (1983) could however not be replicated when asymmetry in task demands (target size, movement amplitude, hurdle height) between both limbs was increased (e.g. Fowler *et al.*, 1991; Goodman *et al.*, 1983; Marteniuk *et al.*, 1984). For example, in a bimanual aiming task, Goodman *et al.* (1983) placed a hurdle in the movement path of one of the limbs. It was observed that the limb with the hurdle in its path altered its movement trajectory. However, the other limb that had no obstacle in its movement path also altered its movement trajectory. More importantly, the strict temporal synchrony between both limbs was not maintained under this condition.

While research into the temporal constraints on bimanual co-ordination is quite abundant, examinations into the spatial constraints on bimanual co-ordination are relatively scarce, despite the fact that these constraints are quite obvious. As an example of the latter consider the research by Franz *et al.* (1991). Their experiment aimed to unravel the spatial rules of bimanual co-ordination. Subjects in their study had to draw circles with one hand and lines with the other. Design of the experiment was more or less similar to Kelso's *et al.* (1979a). That is, both limbs had to draw both figures in isolation (unimanual conditions), and with both hands together, when figures were similar for both limbs (both circles or lines) and dissimilar among both limbs (circles with one hand and lines with the other and vice versa). In the latter conditions, the drawing traces of both hands became spatially similar. Circles tended to become more ellipsoid, while lines became more curved. In the bimanual equal conditions this was not the case. Circles and lines drawn in these conditions were comparable to those that were drawn in the unimanual conditions. Thus, when two figures of different spatial forms are drawn there exists spatial convergence (Franz *et al.*, 1991); that is, the tendency for the figures to look more like each other.

More recently, Swinnen (Swinnen *et al.*, 1997, 1998; Bogaerts and Swinnen, 2001) have explored the role of spatial constraints on bimanual co-ordination further by making an explicit distinction between *egocentric* and *allocentric* constraints. The egocentric constraint is defined with respect to the longitudinal axis of the body (intrinsic space co-ordinates). It refers to the phenomenon that movements requiring the simultaneous activation of homologous muscles are performed more accurately and consistently than movements involving nonhomologous muscles. Conversely, the allocentric constraint is defined with respect to extrinsic space co-ordinates. Here, particular categories of limb movements made in the same directions are produced more accurately and consistently than movements in different directions. Thus, egocentric constraints refer to intrinsic body co-ordinates. Here, symmetry is defined by, for example, moving both limbs in phase, in which case homologous muscles are activated in parallel. In contrast, allocentric constraints refer to an extrinsic frame of reference. Here, symmetry is defined as moving in the same direction in Euclidean space, such as moving both arms to the left, top etc. Studying the impact of both constraints in bimanual tasks may inform us about preferential patterns of the CNS for the control of bimanual co-ordination (cf. Swinnen *et al.*, 1997, 1998).

Swinnen *et al.* (1997) studied the role of allocentric and egocentric constraints on two-dimensional circular drawing movements. The results showed that accuracy and consistency of responding were enhanced in the in-phase mode as compared to the anti-phase mode, irrespective of movement direction and limb type. These findings underscore the eminent role played by egocentric constraints in bimanual co-ordination. Swinnen *et al.* (1998) confirmed the generalisability of the egocentric constraint across various co-ordination patterns, but at the same time provided evidence for the constraining effect of movement direction in extrinsic space (allocentric constraint). By the same token, Baldissera, Cavallari and Civaschi (1982) found that it is more difficult to make bimanual movements in different directions (as defined in the extrinsic co-ordinate axis; one limb moving up while the other moves down) than movements in the same direction. These authors argued that the spatial relationship between the limb movements (i.e. allocentric constraint) was more important for attaining co-ordinative stability as compared to particular patterns of muscle pairing (i.e. egocentric constraint).

In contrast to the egocentric constraints, the convergence and interference effects found for the allocentric constraints are not muscle-specific. This has been very convincingly shown in a study by Franz and Ramachandran (1998). When subjects in their study made circular motions by twirling the index finger of one hand while simultaneously drawing lines with the other hand, the circles become more line-like and the lines become more circle-like, similar to the convergence effects found by Franz *et al.* (1991). Notably, contrary to the Franz *et al.* (1991) study in which homologous muscle groups were used to produce the trajectories, in the Franz and Ramachandran (1998) study different sets of muscles were used to produce the task. More dramatically, the spatial convergence effect was even shown in the partial absence of muscles needed to perform the task. One subject, experiencing a vivid phantom limb experience after amputation of one limb, produced twirling motions of the index finger of his phantom limb while drawing linear motions by using his intact limb. Even in this subject, spatial interference was found, as measured in the line task. This effect was similar to the interference effect that was observed when subjects with two intact limbs performed the task (Franz and Ramachandran, 1998). Taken collectively, these results strongly indicate that spatial coupling is on the one hand abstract (not linked to specific muscles) and may even be independent of feedback (phantom limb). Hence, spatial coupling must be partially based upon central processes of planning and representation.

The role of allocentric constraints has received only minor attention in behavioural studies on bimanual co-ordination, despite the fact that ample evidence exists for direction as an important movement parameter coded in the various brain structures during the production of unilateral reaching movements. In neurophysiological studies, Georgopoulos and co-workers (Georgopoulos, 1991; Georgopoulos *et al.*, 1988; Georgopoulos *et al.*, 1993) found that the majority of cells have a directional preference. Movement in a specific direction is represented by a weighted sum of the directions signaled by a population of cells in the motor cortex (the 'population coding hypothesis'). These directional specifications interact through interhemispheric pathways as shown by Franz *et al.* (1996) in a study on bimanual line drawing in split brain patients. As a sporadic example of an advantage of a brain disorder on task performance, subjects with callotosomy did not show disruptions in the spatial characteristics of the drawings when drawing different shapes, in contrast to controls. However, temporal coupling was similar for both groups. These combined findings suggest that the spatial effects reflect interactions via the intact corpus callosum, whereas the temporal effects do not. This implies that spatial planning and representation of bimanual movements appear to depend on direct cortical interactions between the hemispheres, possibly through interhemispheric pathways (Franz *et al.*, 1996). Thus, the behaviourally observed deviations from preferred modes of interlimb co-ordination are indicative of neural encoding processes of spatial (direction) movement parameters in different regions of the brain, which are subject to interhemispheric exchange (cf. Bogaerts and Swinnen, 2001; Donchin *et al.*, 1999).

Development

From the foregoing it is clear that interhemispheric inhibition is a necessary pre-requisite for the sound performance of asymmetrical bimanual movements. The major fibre bundle connecting the two hemispheres, the corpus callosum, is one of the last structures to complete myelinisation (e.g. Farber and Knyazeva, 1991). Fagard *et al.* (2001) examined whether the development of interhemispheric com-munication was congruent with a behaviourally observed improvement in bimanual co-ordination. Performance on the bimanual task was assessed by having children (5–10 years and 3–7 years) drawing parallel and mirror lines. Interhemispheric co-ordination was indirectly assessed by comparing the latency of a manual response to a visual stimulus when the hemisphere perceiving the stimulus and the hemisphere controlling the manual response were the same (uncrossed con-dition) to the latency when they were different (crossed condition). In both age groups the crossed–uncrossed difference decreased with age, suggesting improve-ment in interhemispheric communication. This was paralleled by a progress in bimanual co-ordination, especially in those conditions that required the resistance to the attraction of mirror movements. Mirror movements are unintended move-ments of the contralateral hand and fingers that are associated with voluntary movements of the hand and fingers (e.g. Kutz-Buschbeck *et al.*, 2000; Carr *et al.*, 1993). For temporal constraints, a similar effect was shown. For children it is more difficult to perform rotary hand movements at different velocities (Fagard *et al.*, 1985). Additionally, Fagard (1987) showed that when both hands rotate with the same velocity, better performance is obtained with mirror-like movements compared to parallel movements. This performance difference decreased with age, as 9-year-old children were as competent for parallel movements as they were for mirror movements.

It has to be noted that mirror movements are a very common motor pattern in young children. In normal development these mirror movements gradually disappear during the first decade of life (e.g. Connolly and Stratton, 1968; Lazarus and Todor, 1987). However, in the next paragraph we will see that this is not the case during development in children with hemiparesis. There are two potential mechanisms that may promote the behaviourally observed mirror activity. First, there exists neural cross-talk at different levels of the nervous system between motor commands transmitted through ipsilateral pathways originating from one hemisphere, in conjunction with the predominant discharge through crossed cortico-spinal projections from the other hemisphere (Nass, 1985). Mirror movements are the consequence of simultaneous activation of crossed corticospinal pathways originating from both left and right motor cortices (Mayston *et al.*, 1999). As such, maturation of transcallosal inhibitory projections, a process by which each hemisphere suppresses the uncrossed descending pathways of the other hemisphere, may explain the age-dependent reduction of mirror activity in children without disabilities. A second mechanism that may underlie mirror activity is the bilateral activation of both hemispheres that occurs during unilateral tasks. Bilateral activation probably results from a lack of interhemispheric inhibition, which normally suppresses the motor cortex ipsilateral to the active hand (Ferbert *et al.*, 1992). Mayston *et al.* (1999) have recently suggested that this bilateral cortical activation is the main cause of mirror activity in healthy non-disabled children. As interhemispheric inhibition becomes more powerful with increasing age, cortical activity becomes more lateralised (Heinen *et al.*, 1998). It is therefore possible that ipsilateral corticospinal efferents are normally present but become more and more inhibited during the first ten years of development.

In the area of bimanual co-ordination, the maturation of the corpus callosum has also been linked with age-related changes in temporal and spatial co-ordination (Jeeves *et al.*, 1988; Njiokiktjien *et al.*, 1986). Njiokiktjien *et al.* (1986) showed that mirror-like supination/pronation movements are performed better than alternate movements in young children. Indeed, Fagard *et al.* (2001) did find that progress in interhemisperic communication was related to improvement in asymmetrical bimanual co-ordination. On the basis of these findings they conclude that better interhemispheric communication is one factor influencing the co-ordination of non-mirror movements. For, in order to perform a bimanual task with parallel movements, children must inhibit the tendency to make mirror movements. Resisting the attraction to in-phase patterns necessitates both hemispheres and thus interhemispheric connections. Conversely, the co-ordination of mirror-like bimanual movements may be controlled by a single hemisphere, by homologous motor neurons that are activated through noncortical descending pathways (Cohen, 1971).

Concurrent with an improvement in asymmetric bimanual co-ordination during the first ten years of life, an increase in stability of responding is observed (Fitzpatrick *et al.*, 1996; Robertson, 2001). Robertson (2001), using predictions from the dynamics systems theory with respect to intrinsic dynamics and variability of bimanual co-ordination modes, examined bimanual circle drawing at different developmental stages (4-, 6-, 8- and 10-year-old children). In the younger group more variability of responding and more transitions between in-phase and anti-phase were observed as compared to the older group, and to adults (e.g. Kelso, 1984). Thus, contrary to adults, children do not display preferred co-ordination modes and are more variable in responding. In sum, the results of these studies that are instigated from the dynamic systems approach showed that in-phase co-ordination patterns are most prominent in childhood and are enhanced with increasing age.

Hemiparetic cerebral palsy

Individuals with hemiparetic cerebral palsy suffer from a deviation in motor development as a consequence of lack of oxygen to the immature brain. Various definitions and classifications of cerebral palsy exist (e.g. Balf and Ingram, 1955; Minear, 1956; Kurland, 1957; and more recently Hagberg and Hagberg, 1993). Ingram has proposed a description of cerebral palsy that may be still be regarded as the standard definition:

> Cerebral palsy is an inclusive term used to describe a number of chronic non-progressive disorders of motor function, which occur in young children as a result of disease of the brain. Excluded by this definition are transient disorders of motor function, such as those that may occur in encephalitis or meningitis; disorders such as spina bifida, in which the disturbance of motor function is predominantly due to disease of the spinal cord; and degenerative conditions, including progressive demyelinations.
>
> (Ingram, 1996, p. 337)

Often, the cerebral damage also results in spasticity, a condition that can be described as a velocity-dependent increase in tonic reflexes, that results in an excessive and awkward activation of the muscles. Clinically, spasticity is associated with symptoms such as excessive co-activation of antagonistic muscles, hyperactive stretch reflexes, associated movements, stereotyped movement synergies and hypertonia (Shumway-Cook and Woollacott, 1995). In individuals with spastic hemiparesis resulting from cerebral palsy, the cerebral damage affects pre-dominantly one body side. As a consequence, problems are encountered with activities of daily living such as grasping objects. Obviously, these problems are enhanced when tasks have to be performed that necessitate both limbs.

One of the ubiquitous features of movement control in spastic hemiparesis is the general movement slowness at the impaired side (Steenbergen *et al.*, 1996). The difference in movement time between the impaired and unimpaired (or better, less impaired, see Baldissera *et al.*, 1994) hand is less for reaching than for grasping (Steenbergen *et al.*, 2000), primarily due to difficulties controlling the more distal hand and finger musculature of the impaired hand. The largest movement time differences between both hands occur in the so-called 'in contact phase'; that is, the phase demarcated by the first contact with the object and object lift (see also

Steenbergen *et al.*, 1998). In this phase, grip and lift forces are generated in order to hold and lift the object (cf. Johansson and Westling, 1984). Eliasson and co-workers (Eliasson *et al.*, 1991) have shown that precise force control is impaired in children with cerebral palsy. The parallel generation of grip and lift forces that is observed in control subjects when they grasp and lift objects (e.g. Johansson and Westling, 1988) is lacking in children with cerebral palsy. Rather, a positive increase in grip force is paralleled by a negative increase in load force in the first instance, resulting in a extended time spent in contact with the object before lifting it. Recently, it was shown that the between-hand difference in movement time virtually disappears in a hitting task (Van Thiel *et al.*, 2000). Children with hemiparetic cerebral palsy made hitting movements with a hand-held rod to stationary and moving targets that were presented on a screen in the fronto-parallel plane. Note that this task can primarily be performed by movements of the trunk, shoulder and elbow, without any involvement of distal finger movement.

Collectively, these studies suggest a proximal-to-distal increase in movement asymmetry between both body sides in spastic hemiparesis. Tasks involving distal musculature, such as grasping and to a lesser degree reaching, pose severe control problems for the impaired hand. There is neurophysiological evidence suggesting that the distal musculature is predominantly controlled from the contralateral hemisphere, whereas proximal (trunk) musculature is subserved on a bilateral basis (e.g. Brinkman and Kuypers, 1973; Wiesendanger *et al.*, 1994). As such, the distal hand and fingers may be exclusively controlled from the damaged hemisphere, while movements of the trunk may be controlled from the intact hemisphere on a bilateral basis. Given these neurophysiological findings of bilateral trunk innervation, it may be predicted that during upper limb movements, individuals with hemiparetic cerebral palsy show a preference for trunk involvement when moving with their impaired arm. This has indeed been repeatedly reported (e.g. Steenbergen *et al.*, 2000; Van Thiel and Steenbergen, 2001). However, there is a debate about the desirability of this increased trunk involvement. On the one hand it may reflect a disordered movement (re-)organisation (e.g. Archambault *et al.*, 1999), but on the other hand it may reflect adaptive movement control (Steenbergen *et al.*, 2000; Van Thiel and Steenbergen, 2001).

Other features of disordered upper limb control at the impaired side in spastic hemiparesis are segmentation and an increased variability of responding. Segmentation points to the phenomenon that during upper limb motion there is initially virtually no parallel shoulder and elbow involvement, but rather a large shoulder involvement followed by an increase in elbow involvement as the movement unfolds. Hence, there is a proximal-to-distal sequencing of the movement at the impaired side. This segmentation (or sequencing) was also found in a study with older hemiparetic stroke patients (Levin, 1996), and is also observed in the early phases of development (e.g. Berthier *et al.*, 1999). The other feature of movement control of the impaired arm that may hinder activities of daily living is an increased variability of responding both within and between individuals (e.g. Steenbergen *et al.*, 2000; Van Thiel *et al.*, 2000).

The above phenomena are related to the impaired hand when performing movements in isolation. Although performance of daily activities is hindered by these phenomena, in the majority of these cases the most obvious solution is that the unimpaired hand is used to perform the task. More serious problems occur when both hands are necessary to perform a task. Despite the fact that most daily manual activities require the co-operative interaction of both hands, remarkably little attention has been devoted to the study of bimanual co-ordination in individuals with hemiparetic cerebral palsy, let alone asymmetrical bimanual co-ordination.

As stated before, mirror movements are more pronounced after childhood hemiplegia (Woods and Teuber, 1978; Nass, 1985). Kutz-Buschbeck *et al.* (2000) showed that mirror activity was 15 times stronger in participants with cerebral palsy compared to a control group. However, there was no relationship between the amount of mirror activity and the degree of hemiplegia. The enhanced mirror activity in hemiparesis has been considered to reflect a compensatory reorganisation of the motor system after early unilateral brain injury (Woods and Teuber, 1978; Carr, 1996). The descending motor pathways may be reorganised such that cortico-spinal axons arising from the unimpaired hemisphere branch to innervate both left and right motor neuron pools simultaneously (Carr *et al.*, 1993). As a result, the unimpaired hemisphere participates in the voluntary control of both body sides, but at the expense of independent unilateral control (cf. Nirkko *et al.*, 1997). Netz (Netz *et al.*, 1997) examined the motor evoked responses of 15 patients with hemiparesis after ischaemic stroke and compared them to controls using focal transcranial magnetic stimulation of the unimpaired hemisphere. They found that responses to muscles ipsilateral to the stimulated hemisphere could be elicited at significantly lower thresholds in patients compared to controls (for similar results on ipsilateral responses to distal muscles, see Turton *et al.*, 1996). They concluded that after stroke, even the unaffected hemisphere is altered, including an unmasking of ipsilateral corticospinal projections.

Nass (1985) indicated that mirror movements in congenital hemiplegia are asymmetrical until age 10 (more pronounced in the unaffected hand), but are symmetrical after that age. A factor leading to more symmetrical mirror movements may be the maturation of transcallosal pathways that inhibit ipsilateral projections descending from the lesioned hemisphere. Kutz-Buscheck *et al.* (2000) further showed that strong mirror activity is associated with poor bimanual co-ordination. The negative influence of mirror movements on bimanual co-ordination is especially due to the symmetrical character of the mirror movements. It may therefore be hypothesised that at the behavioural level there exists an attraction to (egocentric) symmetrical movements involving homologous muscle groups, while asymmetrical movements are potentially more difficult to perform. We will next review behavioural data on bimanual co-ordination in children with hemiparetic cerebral palsy.

Recall the research of Kelso *et al.* (1979a), which showed high temporal invariance of movement responding despite asymmetries in task demands for both hands. Individuals with hemiparetic cerebral palsy have, what may be termed an 'unwanted movement asymmetry' as a consequence of cerebral damage predominantly to one hemisphere. Steenbergen *et al.* (1996) examined whether these asymmetries are decreased or eliminated when the two hands are required to perform functionally equivalent tasks. Children with hemiparetic cerebral palsy (n = 14) were asked to pick up a small ball (12 mm) and place it into a hole as quickly as possible. Uni- and bimanual movement conditions were tested, and equal and unequal hole sizes were used in the bimanual conditions. Reaction time and total movement time were recorded. The results in the unimanual conditions confirmed other findings in subjects with unilateral cerebral lesions (e.g. Brown *et al.*, 1989; Fisk and Goodale, 1988; Jeannerod, 1988; Trombly, 1992, 1993). Large differences between both hands were present for reaction time and total movement time. However, these asymmetries were diminished to a large extent (92 per cent) in the bimanual movement conditions, predominantly due to a unidirectional accommodation. The unimpaired hand adopted the time frame of the impaired hand and slowed down to the level of unimanual responding of the impaired hand. Mutual accommodation, i.e. the impaired hand speeding up and the unimpaired hand slowing down, was not observed (see also Steenbergen *et al.*, 2000). However, similar to the results of Kelso *et al.* (1979a), asymmetry of responding was reasserted when the difference in accuracy demands for both hands increased, especially in conditions where the impaired hand moved to the small hole and the unimpaired hand moved to the large hole.

Sugden and Utley (1995; Utley and Sugden, 1998), testing young children with hemiparetic cerebral palsy, also showed evidence for some form of co-operative action between both hands during bimanual reaching. Next to temporal coupling, they also studied postural coupling and spatial coupling to get a more complete picture of the coupling between both hands. Based on the assumption that moving at speed would reduce the attraction of the impaired hand to its preferred (impaired) state (cf. Walter *et al.*, 1993), Utley and Sugden (1998) stressed speed of responding. It was hypothesised that, during speeded bimanual responding, the unimpaired hand serves as a template for the impaired hand and, as such, the preferred postural state of the hemiparetic hand is broken down. Three different tasks were studied with increasing complexity, (1) reaching and touching, (2) reaching and grasping, (3) reaching, touching and grasping, under the assumption that discrete tasks of short duration would provide the system with little settling time, such that the preferred mode of responding at the impaired side was rarely attained. The results did indeed show that, in all three experiments, any form of coupling that was present was greatest during the first part of the movement. In the third task, the serial nature of the task reduced the benefits of moving at speed as the impaired hand had the time to adopt its preferred state, and the asymmetries between both hands consequently increased, or were re-established. Note that Sugden and Utley (1995; Utley and Sugden, 1998) were also among the first to examine the spatial interaction between both limbs. They showed that spatial trajectories were more similar during bimanual responding, despite a higher deviation in the *z*-direction (direction perpendicular to the tabletop) of the impaired side during unimanual responding. We (unpublished data) also noted a higher z-deviation at the impaired side during unimanual grasping, while trajectories of both hands were more similar in the bimanual conditions. This was mainly the result of an adaptation of the trajectory of the unimpaired hand. This hand increased its z-deviation in the bimanual movement conditions.

Whereas the analyses by Steenbergen *et al.* (1996), Sugden and Utley (1995) and Utley and Sugden (1998) were performed at the level of the kinematics of the end effector (i.e. the wrist), Steenbergen *et al.* (2000) showed coupling in interjoint co-ordination as well. Angular change of the impaired elbow was almost double that of the unimpaired elbow during unimanual responding. At the same time, when movements were made with the impaired hand in the unimanual conditions, displacement of the ipsilateral shoulder was more than twice that of the ipsilateral shoulder when movements were made with the unimpaired hand. In addition, contralateral shoulder displacement was virtually nil when reaching and grasping with unimpaired hand, but increased substantially when movements were made with the impaired hand. Thus, when the impaired side moved in the unimanual conditions, elbow extension is decreased and trunk involvement increased as compared to the unimpaired side. We also tested this movement reorganisation under bimanual responding. Again, movement reorganisation was such that even at this level the unimpaired side adapted its co-ordination to the impaired side. That is, elbow extension decreased to the level of the impaired side under unimanual responding, and displacement of both the ipsilateral and contralateral shoulders increased to the level of the ipsilateral shoulder involvement of the impaired side under unimanual responding. Hence, not only at the level of the kinematics of the end effector, but also with respect to elbow and shoulder (or trunk) involvement, a strong coupling of both body sides was present under bimanual responding. Again, the unimpaired side adapted to the impaired side. Or, to put it differently, the impaired side constrained the unimpaired side during bimanual movements (for similar results and reasoning, see Rice and Newell, 2001)

Taken collectively, the results on bimanual co-ordination in spastic hemiparesis suggest that at least in the temporal domain there is a tight coupling between both limbs, not only at the level of the end effector but also at the interjoint level. Additionally, the unimpaired side appears to be more flexible in altering its movement organisation among unimanual and bimanual responding. Note that in the studies discussed, only movement patterns that involved similar movements for both limbs were tested. That is, all experiments had tasks that are symmetrical from an egocentric frame of reference, hence involving homologous muscle groups. It is likely that the movement patterns observed in these tasks are naturally preferred by individuals with spastic hemiparesis because of the aforementioned increased occurrence of mirror movements in this group. As compared to these preferred (egocentric symmetrical) co-ordination modes, less compatible patterns with more diverging directional requirements have hardly been studied so far in spastic hemiparesis.

3. The role of allocentric and egocentric symmetry constraints on drawing semi-circles: preliminary results of a short-term learning experiment

In the remainder of this chapter we present some preliminary results of a study in which a semi-circle drawing task was employed to explore the effects of different symmetry constraints on the spatial characteristics of drawing traces of both hands in children with spastic hemiparesis. More specifically, the experiment that is described below is aimed at unraveling the influence of both the impaired hand on the unimpaired hand, and vice versa, when semi-circles are drawn that are either symmetrical from a egocentric frame of reference (involving homologous muscle groups) or symmetrical from an allocentric frame of reference (same direction in extrinsic [Euclidean] frame of reference). Subjects had to make drawing traces by one hand (baseline trials, $n = 3$) followed by the other hand (training trials, $n = 10$) and ending again with the 'starting' hand (test trials, $n = 5$) (see figure 10.2). We deliberately choose a unimanual learning task, as it was proven to be quite difficult for the subjects to perform a bimanual drawing task.

As stated before, Netz *et al.* (1997, but also Carr *et al.*, 1993; Turton *et al.*, 1996) showed that after hemiparesis the unimpaired hemisphere is reorganised such that it is involved in the control of both contralateral and ipsilateral movements. Or, as Netz *et al.* (1997) put it, there is an unmasking of ipsilateral corticospinal projections. From this it might be hypothesised that, in the present experiment, for the movement combination, unimpaired hand (intact hemisphere) – impaired hand (both hemispheres) – unimpaired hand (intact hemisphere), a template might be formed by the intact hemisphere after the first baseline trials. This template might also be used in the training trials with the impaired hand (control from the intact hemisphere) and again in the test trials with the unimpaired hand. Consequently, no 'conflict' would be present in the control of both limbs, as the template would be formed very early during practice. Conversely, for the combination impaired hand (both hemispheres) – unimpaired hand (intact hemisphere)– impaired hand (both hemispheres), the situation would be different. Here, in the baseline conditions, a template might be formed by the impaired hemisphere. However, in the training trials, a template for the unimpaired hand would be formed solely by the intact hemisphere and this template might 'conflict' with the one formed by the impaired hand in the baseline trials. Consequently, in the test trials with the impaired hand, the template formed by the intact hemisphere might also be used for the control of the impaired hand. Because this template would be different from the one in the baseline trials with the impaired hand, differences, or incongruencies between baseline and test trials for the impaired hand might be expected to be larger. Therefore we expected for the present experiment that any differences found between baseline and test trials would be largest for the conditions starting with the impaired hand. More speculative, as patterns that are symmetrical from an egocentric frame of reference are more easily performed, it might be expected that smaller transfer effects would be present from one hand to the other for these patterns compared to patterns that are symmetrical from an allocentric frame of reference.

Method and results

Seven children with hemiplegic cerebral palsy (mean age 16.9 years, standard deviation 1.1 years) participated in the experiment on a voluntary basis and gave signed consent prior to testing. Participants were pupils from the Werkenrode Institute where they received special education and adapted housing facilities. Clinical diagnosis of the group was based on neurological examinations, electro-encephalograms (EEGs), surgical records and CT scans performed at hospitals and rehabilitation centres throughout the Netherlands. One of the inclusion criteria for the experiment was that the participant had to be able to hold the pencil that was used for testing. In addition, they had to be able to sit independently, not show any hemineglect, and have the cognitive capacity to understand and perform the task. Although these selection criteria increased the homogeneity of the participant group, between-participant variability was still large (see below). Displayed in table 10.1 is additional participant information.

Participants were comfortably seated at a table. The task they had to perform consisted of drawing semi-circles with a pencil on a digitising tablet (Wacom Intuos™, spatial resolution of 100 lines/mm, accuracy < 0.25mm) that was placed directly in front of them on the table. The stem of the pencil was made thicker by covering it with foam (3 cm in diameter, 7 cm in length) so that grasping it was facilitated. Placed on the digitising tablet were two A4-sized papers on which two dots and one arrow were printed (see figure 10.1 for an example of one of the A4-sized papers).

At the start of a new trial, participants had to rest the pencil tip on the dot that was furthest away. Upon a start signal of the experimenter they had to draw a line from this dot to the dot that was closest to them by moving around the arrow that was halfway between the two dots (see figure 10.1 for exact measures). No speed demands were imposed. The only restriction was that they were not allowed to touch the arrow when drawing the semi-circle. The pencil did not leave a trace on the tablet, and drawing movements were virtually friction-free as transparent plastic was placed on top of the A4-sheets. Traces were sampled at 200 Hz.

Table 10.1 Participant information

Male/ female	Hemiparetic side	Age	IQ-score Verbal	Performal	Aetiology	Other
Male	Right	16.9	71	56	Cerebral palsy	epileptic, corrected vision
Male	Left	16.8	65	45	Cerebral palsy	epileptic
Male	Right	15.9	54	58	Cerebral palsy	epileptic, nystagmus
Male	Right	16.9	57	57	Cerebral palsy	epileptic
Male	Left	15.7	101	52	Cerebral palsy	corrected vision
Male	Right	19.5	89	48	Cerebral palsy	
Female	Left	16.9	76	96	Viral infection (Herpes encephalitis)	epileptic

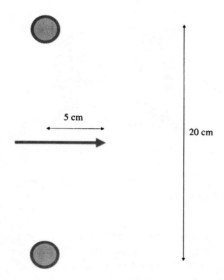

Figure 10.1 Example of one A4-sized paper. The two dots represent the start (top) and end (bottom) target. Drawing traces had to be made around the bold arrow

As noted earlier, a typical condition consisted of drawing three semi-circles with one hand (denoted *baseline* trials), followed by ten trials with the other hand (denoted *training* trials), and ending with five trials with the hand that was used for the baseline trials (denoted *test* trials), resulting in a total of eighteen trials per condition. Each participant was tested in eight unique conditions that constituted the manipulation of the following three variables: hand (unimpaired, impaired), symmetry (egocentric, allocentric) and arrow direction (left, right). This yielded a total of 144 traces to be made by each participant.

After the experiment, the X–Y position data of the drawing traces were analysed. First, the start and end of each individual trial were assessed by using custom-written semi-automatic segmentation routines. Following that, variables pertaining to the spatial characteristics of the drawing traces were calculated. For each variable, the average and standard deviation for the baseline, training and test conditions were calculated per participant. Here we will mainly focus on the spatial features of the traces by analysis of the following three variables: peak deviation in the x-direction (arrow direction, see figure 10.1), percentage y-distance travelled at peak x-deviation proportional to the total y-distance covered (as a measure of symmetry of the profiles), and total distance covered. As a control measure we also analysed movement time, as this variable is most commonly found to differentiate between the impaired and unimpaired side in spastic hemiparesis. Since we are mainly interested in the difference between the baseline and test trials, means and standard deviations were analyzed in a 2 (hand: unimpaired, impaired) × 2 (symmetry: allocentric, egocentric) × 2 (condition: baseline, test) repeated measures ANOVA design.

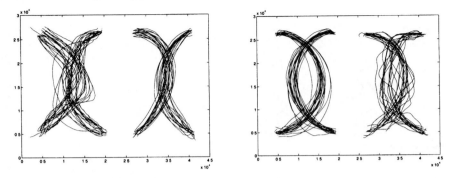

Figure 10.2 Two examples of the drawing traces made by a participant with left spastic hemiparesis (left) and right spastic hemiparesis (right)

Displayed in figure 10.2 are the drawing traces of two participants. It is clear from this figure that differences between participants were rather large. Therefore, 0.1 was chosen as significance level. In line with other studies, *movement time* of the impaired hand was significantly longer than that of the unimpaired hand, 646 ms versus 566 ms ($F[1,6] = 5.17, p = 0.063$). No further effects were found for this variable.

The hand × symmetry × trial interaction ($F[1,6] = 4.30, p = 0.083$) revealed that for the unimpaired hand no large difference existed for the peak deviation in the x-direction between the baseline and test conditions. For the impaired hand, however, baseline and test trials differed significantly. Moreover, the influence of the training trials was different for the allocentric and egocentric symmetrical patterns. For the allocentric symmetrical patterns, x-deviation increased from baseline to test trials, whereas this effect was opposite for the egocentric symmetrical patterns. In addition, we found a significant hand × symmetry interaction $F[1,6] = 4.50, p = 0.078$). Whereas, for the unimpaired hand, x-deviation was larger for the allocentric than for the egocentric symmetrical patterns (91.1 mm and 88.2 mm), this effect was opposite for the impaired hand. For this hand, x-deviation of the trajectories was smaller for the allocentric symmetrical patterns compared to the egocentric symmetrical patterns (90.3 mm and 93.9 mm). For the standard deviation we only found a main hand effect on peak x-deviation ($F[1,6] = 10.03, p = 0.019$). Standard deviation of the unimpaired hand (8.98 mm) was significantly smaller than that of the impaired hand (13.79 mm), suggesting a more stable performance of the unimpaired hand.

To obtain an impression of the symmetry of the semi-circles we looked at the *proportional y-distance covered at peak x-deviation as a function of total y-distance covered* (perfect symmetry would yield 50 per cent for this measure). The significant hand × symmetry × trial interaction ($F[1,6] = 5.93, p = 0.051$) showed that the largest difference between baseline and test trials was found for the impaired hand when allocentric symmetrical patterns were drawn (values of the baseline and test; 52.4 per cent versus 54.2 per cent). The semi-circles were more asymmetrical in the test trials. Additionally, we found a main hand effect ($F[1,6] = 5.34$, $p = 0.060$). Trajectories of the unimpaired hand were more positively skewed (48.8 per cent) as compared to the impaired hand (52.3 per cent). Finally, we found a significant hand × symmetry interaction ($F[1,6] = 5.81$, $p = 0.058$). With respect to the standard deviation of this measure we found main effects of hand ($F[1,6] = 14.14$, $p = 0.009$) and symmetry ($F[1,6] = 4.36$, $p = 0.082$). Again, standard deviation was larger for the impaired hand (9.7 per cent) compared to the unimpaired hand (5.1 per cent). Also, standard deviation was larger for the allocentric symmetrical patterns (7.8 per cent) compared to egocentric symmetrical patterns (6.9 per cent).

The only effect found for the *total distance covered* was a significant hand × symmetry × trial interaction ($F[1,6] = 5.38$, $p = 0.059$). For the allocentric symmetrical patterns, total distance covered was larger for the unimpaired hand compared to the impaired hand, but for both hands it did not differ between the baseline and test conditions. This differed from the egocentric symmetrical patterns. There was a differential effect of this constraint on both hands in the baseline and test trials. For the unimpaired hand, total distance increased from baseline to test trials with egocentric symmetrical patterns (282 mm to 287 mm), whereas for the impaired hand, total distance decreased from baseline to test trials for these patterns (288 mm 279 mm). As may be clear from the values, all these effects were rather small. For the standard deviation of this measure we only found a significant main effect of hand ($F[1,6] = 4.17$, $p = 0.087$). Again, the standard deviation for the impaired hand (22.8 mm) was larger compared to the unimpaired hand (13.9 mm).

Conclusion and discussion

One of the results that stands out is the large standard deviation at the impaired side for all spatial measures. This enlarged standard deviation was not affected by the training trials, pointing to a pathological constant at the impaired side. Although we have to be careful with drawing conclusions about this on the basis of the relatively small amount of learning trials in the present experiment, it is a finding that has been repeatedly reported in previous studies (e.g. Steenbergen *et al.*, 1996; 2000; Van Thiel *et al.*, 2000; Van Thiel and Steenbergen, 2001; Utley and Sugden, 1998). In addition, differences among both sides for the control measure, viz. movement time, were not very large. This may be ascribed to the relative proximal nature of the task. The task was predominantly carried out by shoulder and elbow movements, whereas the fingers were fixed on the pencil. Previous studies have shown a proximo-distal increase in movement asymmetry in spastic hemiparesis (e.g. Steenbergen *et al.*, 2000; Van Thiel and Steenbergen, 2001). For example, movement asymmetry was very small in a hitting task (Van Thiel and Steenbergen, 2001), a task in which, similar to the present study, an object (a rod) was held fixed in the hand.

The between-hand-transfer effects and the effects pertaining to the identity of the patterns were unequivocal. Based on findings that indicated a reorganisation of the intact hemisphere after hemiparesis (e.g. Netz *et al.*, 1997; Carr *et al.*, 1993; Turton *et al.*, 1996) we hypothesised that the largest differences between baseline and test conditions would be present in the conditions in which the impaired hand started to draw the semi-circles. For peak deviation in the *x*-direction and for the symmetry measure of the semi-circles, we did find a difference between baseline and test conditions when the impaired hand started. This difference was not found when the unimpaired hand started. Interestingly, peak *x*-deviation of the impaired hand in the test trials was virtually similar to peak *x*-deviation of the unimpaired hand (remember that this hand performed the training trials), for both allocentric and egocentric symmetrical patterns. Thus, there existed differential effects of the type of symmetry on the test trials of the impaired had, but at the same time these test trials resembled the training trials of the unimpaired hand. This finding in particular suggests that the template formed by the intact hemisphere in the training trials is indeed used for control in the test trials with the impaired hand. Still, this argument does not hold for the reverse order; that is, when conditions started with the unimpaired hand. With respect to the manipulation of symmetry of the patterns (either ego- or allocentric) the results were more diverse among the spatial variables measured. Owing to this, we are not able to draw any conclusions at this point. It is nonetheless promising for future studies to find that these manipulations were effective and as such represent an essential control dimension.

4. Clinical implications and further research

The central reorganisation of the hemispheres, in particular the intact hemisphere, has important implications for therapy as well. As was suggested by the results of the present experiment, training with the unimpaired hand may help to form a template that may be used in the control of the impaired hand as well (for a similar reasoning, see Utley and Sugden, 1998). Exercising the unimpaired limb may therefore have consequences for the central control of the impaired limb. Surely, for medical reasons, making movements with the impaired side (either actively or passively) will be of benefit, for contractures and other more peripheral disturbances need to be avoided. However, in the early stages of recovery, when movements are difficult to perform with the impaired side, training the unimpaired hand may help recovery of the impaired side as well. Therefore, both in experiments and in practice, transfer of training should be thoroughly investigated in future research. One way to test these suggestions further is to train very thoroughly the unimpaired hand on a novel task, a task for which, therefore, no existing template is expected to be present. Next, have the subjects perform the task with the impaired hand and look for signs of facilitation. If there is facilitation on this novel task, it may be assumed that control is predominantly left to the intact hemisphere. From a clinical point of view, facilitation of movement patterns for the impaired hand may be the ultimate goal. More theoretically, transfer effects may inform us about central reorganisation after early cerebral damage.

Acknowledgements

This research was conducted while the first author was supported by a grant awarded by The Netherlands Organization for Scientific Research (NWO) for the research project 'Adaptation in movement disorder'.

References

Archambault, P., Pigeon, P., Feldman, A.G. and Levin, M.F. (1999) Recruitment and sequencing of different degrees of freedom during pointing movements involving the trunk in healthy and hemiparetic subjects. *Experimental Brain Research*, 126, 55–67.

Baldissera, F., Cavallari, P. and Civaschi, P. (1982) Preferential coupling between voluntary movements of ipsilateral limbs. *Neuroscience Letters*, 34, 95–100.

Baldissera, F., Cavallari, P. and Tesio, L. (1994) Coordination of cyclic coupled movements of hand and foot in normal subjects and on the healthy side of hemiparetic patients. In S. Swinnen, H. Heuer, J. Massion and P. Casaer (eds), *Interlimb Coordination: Neural, Dynamical, and Cognitive Constraints* (pp. 229–42). San Diego: Academic Press.

Balf, C.L. and Ingram, T.T.S. (1955) Problems in the classification of cerebral palsy. *British Medical Journal*, 2, 163–6.

Berthier, N.E., Clifton, R.K., McCall, D.D. and Robin, D.J. (1999) Proximo-distal structure of early reaching in human infants. *Experimental Brain Research*, 127, 259–69.

Boessenkool, J.J., Nijhof E.J. and Erkelens, C.J. (1999) Variability and correlations in bimanual pointing movements. *Human Movement Science*, 18, 525–52.

Bogaerts, H. and Swinnen, S.P. (2001) Spatial interactions during bimanual coordination patterns: the effect of directional compatibility. *Motor Control*, 2, 183–99.

Brinkman, J. and Kuypers, H.G.J.M. (1973) Cerebral control of contralateral and ipsilateral arm, hand and finger movements in the split-brain rhesus monkey. *Brain*, 96, 653–74.

Brown, J.V., Schumacher, U., Rohlmann, A., Ettlinger, G., Schmidt, R.C. and Skreczek, W. (1989) Aimed movements to visual targets in hemiplegic and normal children: is the 'good' hand of children with infantile hemiplegia also normal? *Neuropsychologia*, 27, 283–302.

Carr, L.J. (1996) Development and reorganization of descending motor pathways in children with hemiplegic cerebral palsy. *Acta Pediatrica Supplement*, 416, 53–7.

Carr, L.J., Harrison, L.M., Evans, A.L. and Stephens, J.A. (1993) Patterns of central motor reorganization in hemiplegic cerebral palsy. *Brain*, 116, 1223–47.

Cohen, L. (1971) Synchronous bimanual movements performed by homologous and non-homologous muscles. *Perceptual and Motor Skills*, 32, 639–44.

Connolly, K. and Stratton, P. (1968) Developmental changes in associated movements. *Developmental Medicine and Child Neurology*, 33, 661–70.

Donchin, O., De Oliveira, S.C. and Vaadia, E. (1999) Who tells one hand what the other is doing: the neurophysiology of bimanual movements. *Neuron*, 23, 15–18.

Eliasson, A.C., Gordon, A.M. and Forssberg, H. (1991) Basic co-ordination of manipulative forces of children with cerebral palsy. *Developmental Medicine and Child Neurology*, 33, 661–70.

Fagard, J. (1987) Bimanual stereotypes: bimanual coordination in children as a function of movements and relative velocity. *Journal of Motor Behavior*, 19, 355–66.

Fagard, J., Hardy-Léger, I., Kervella, C. and Marks, A. (2001) Changes in interhemispheric transfer rate and the development of bimanual coordination during childhood. *Journal of Experimental Child Psychology*, 80, 1–22.

Fagard, J., Morioka, M. and Wolff, P.H. (1985) Early stages in the acquisition of a bimanual motor skill. *Neuropsychologia*, 23, 535–43.

Farber, D.A. and Knyazeva, M.G. (1991) Electrophysiological correlates of interhemispheric interaction in ontogenesis. In G. Ramaekers and C. Njiokiktjien (eds), *Pediatric Behavioral Neurology*, Vol. I. Amsterdam: Suyi Publications.

Ferbert, A., Priori, A., Rothwell, J.C., Day, B.L., Colebatch, J.G. and Marsden, C.D. (1992) Interhemispheric inhibition of the human motor cortex. *Journal of Physiology*, 453, 525–46.

Fisk, J.D. and Goodale, M.A. (1988) The effects of unilateral brain damage on visually guided reaching: hemispheric differences in the nature of the deficit. *Experimental Brain Research*, 72, 425–35.

Fitts, P.M. (1954) The information capacity of the human motor system in controlling the amplitude of the movement. *Journal of Experimental Psychology*, 47, 381–91.

Fitzpatrick, P., Schmidt, R.C. and Lockman, J.J. (1996) Dynamical patterns in the development of clapping. *Child Development*, 67, 2691–708.

Franz. E.A. and Ramachandran, V.S. (1998) Bimanual coupling in amputees with phantom limbs. *Nature Neuroscience*, 1, 443–4.

Franz, E.A., Zelaznik, H.N. and McGabe, G. (1991) Spatial topological constraints in a bimanual task. *Acta Psychologica*, 77, 137–51.

Franz, E.A., Eliassen, J., Ivry, R.B. and Gazzaniga, M. (1996) Dissociation of spatial and temporal coupling in the bimanual movements of callotosomy patients. *Psychological Science*, 7, 306–10.

Fowler, B., Duck, T., Mosher, M. and Mathieson, B. (1991) The coordination of bimanual aiming movements: evidence for progressive desynchronization. *Quarterly Journal of Experimental Psychology* [A], 43, 205–21.

Georgopoulos, A.P. (1991) Higher order motor control. *Annual Review of Neuroscience*, 14, 361–77.

Georgopoulos, A.P., Kettner, R.E. and Schwartz, A.B. (1988) Primate motor cortex and free arm movements to visual targets in three-dimensional space, II. Coding of the direction of movement by a neuronal population. *Journal of Neuroscience*, 8, 2928–37.

Georgopoulos, A.P., Taira, M. and Lukashin, A. (1993) Cognitive neurophysiology of the motor cortex. *Science*, 260, 47–52.

Goodman, D., Kobayashi, R.B. and Kelso, J.A.S. (1983) Maintenance of symmetry as a constraint in motor control. *Canadian Journal of Applied Sport Sciences*, 8, 238.

Hagberg, B. and Hagberg, G. (1993) The origins of cerebral palsy. In T.S. David (ed), *Recent Advances in Pediatrics* (pp. 67–83). Churchill: Livingstone.

Heinen, F., Glocker, F.X., Fietzek, U., Meyer, B.U., Lücking, C.H. and Korinthenberg, R. (1998) Absence of transcallosal inhibition following focal magnetic stimulation in preschool children. *Annals of Neurology*, 43, 608–12.

Ingram, T.T.S. (1966) The neurology of cerebral palsy. *Archives of Disabled Childhood*, 41, 337–57.

Jeannerod, M. (1988) *The Neural and Behavioral Organization of Goal directed Movements*. New York: Oxford University Press.

Jeeves, M.A., Silver, P.H. and Milne, A.B. (1988) Role of the corpus callosum in the development of a bimanual motor skill. *Developmental Neuropsychology*, 4, 305–23.

Johansson, R.S. and Westling, G. (1984) Roles of glabrous skin receptors and sensorimotor memory in automatic control of precision grip when lifting rougher or more slippery objects. *Experimental Brain Research*, 56, 550–64.

Johansson, R.S. and Westling, G. (1988) Coordinated isometric muscle command adequately and erronously programmed for the weight during lifting tasks with precision grip. *Experimental Brain Research*, 71, 59–71.

Kelso, J.A.S. (1984) Phase transitions and critical behavior in bimanual coordination. *American Journal of Physiology: Regulatory Integrative Comparative Physiology*, 15, R1000–4.

Kelso, J.A.S., Putnam, C.A. and Goodman, D. (1983) On the space–time structure of human interlimb coordination. *Quarterly Journal of Experimental Psychology* [A], 35, 347–75.

Kelso, J.A.S., Southard, D.L. and Goodman, D. (1979a) On the coordination of bimanual movements. *Journal of Experimental Psychology: Human Perception and Performance*, 5, 229–38.

Kelso, J.A.S., Southard, D.L. and Goodman, D. (1979b) On the nature of human interlimb coordination. *Science*, 203, 1029–31.

Kurland, L.T. (1957) Definitions of cerebral palsy and their role in epidemiologic research. *Neurology*, 7, 641–54.

Kutz-Buschbeck, J.P., Sundholm, L.K., Eliasson, A.C. and Forssberg, H. (2000) Quantitative assessment of mirror movements in children and adolescents with hemiplegic cerebral palsy. *Developmental Medicine and Child Neurology*, 42, 728–36.

Lazarus, J.A. and Todor, J.L. (1987) Age differences in the magnitude of associated movement. *Developmental Medicine and Child Neurology*, 29, 726–33.

Levin, M.F. (1996) Interjoint coordination during pointing movements is disrupted in spastic hemiparesis. *Brain*, 199, 281–93.

Marteniuk, R.G., MacKenzie, C.L. and Baba, D.M. (1984) Bimanual movement control: information processing and interaction effects. *Quarterly Journal of Experimental Psychology* [A], 36, 335–65.

Mayston, M.J., Harrison, L.M. and Stephens, J.A. (1999) A neurophysiological study of mirror movements in adults and children. *Annals of Neurology*, 45, 583–94.

Minear, W.L. (1956) A classification of cerebral palsy. *Pediatrics*, 18, 841–52.

Nass, R. (1985) Mirror movement asymmetries in congenital hemiplegia: the inhibition hypothesis revisited. *Neurology*, 35, 1059–62.

Nirkko, A.C., Rösler, K.M., Ozboda, C., Heid, O., Schroth, G. and Hess, C.W. (1997) Human cortical plasticity: functional recovery with mirror movements. *Neurology*, 48, 1090–3.

Njiokiktjien, C., Driessen, M. and Habraken, L. (1986) Development of supination-pronation movements in normal children. *Human Neurobiology*, 5, 199–203.

Netz, J., Lammers, T. and Hömberg, V. (1997) Reorganization of motor output in the non-affected hemisphere after stroke. *Brain*, 120, 1579–86.

Rice, M.S. and Newell, K.M. (2001) Interlimb coupling and left hemiplegia because of right cerebral vascular accident. *Occupational Therapy Journal of Research*, 21, 12–28.

Robertson, S.D. (2001) Development of bimanual skill: the search for stable patterns of coordination. *Journal of Motor Behavior*, 33, 114–26.

Shumway-Cook, A. and Woollacott, M.H. (1995) *Motor Control: Theory and Practical Implications*. Baltimore: Williams and Wilkins.

Steenbergen, B., Hulstijn, W., De Vries, A. and Berger, M. (1996) Bimanual movement coordination in spastic hemiparesis. *Experimental Brain Research*, 110, 91–8.

Steenbergen, B., Hulstijn, W., Lemmens, I.H.L. and Meulenbroek, R.G.J. (1998) The timing of prehension movements in subjects with cerebral palsy. *Developmental Medicine and Child Neurology*, 40, 108–14.

Steenbergen, B., Van Thiel, E., Hulstijn, W. and Meulenbroek, R.G.J. (2000) The coordination of reaching and grasping in spastic hemiparesis. *Human Movement Science*, 19, 75–105.

Sugden, D.A. and Utley, A. (1995) Inter-limb coupling in children with hemiplegic cerebral palsy. *Developmental Medicine and Child Neurology*, 37, 293–309.

Swinnen, S.P., Jardin, K., Meulenbroek, R.G.J., Dounskaia, N. and Hofkens-Van Den Brandt, M. (1997) Egocentric and allocentric constraints in the expression of patterns of interlimb coordination. *Journal of Cognitive Neuroscience*, 9, 348–77.

Swinnen, S.P., Jardin, K., Verschueren, S., Meulenbroek, R.G.J., Franz, E.A., Dounskaia, N. and Walter, C.B. (1998) Exploring interlimb constraints during bimanual graphic performance: effects of muscle grouping and direction. *Behavioral Brain Research*, 90, 79–87.

Trombly, C.A. (1992) Deficits of reaching in subjects with left hemiparesis: a pilot study. *American Journal of Occupational Therapy*, 46, 887–97.

Trombly, C.A. (1993) Observations of improvement of reaching in five subjects with left hemiparesis. *Journal of Neurology, Neurosurgery and Psychiatry*, 56, 40–5.

Turton, A., Wroe, S., Trepte, N., Fraser, C. and Lemon, R.B. (1996) Contralateral and ipsilateral EMG responses to transcranial magnetic stimulation during recovery of arm and hand function after stroke. *Electroencephalography and Clinical Neurophysiology*, 85, 273–9.

Utley, A. and Sugden, D.A. (1998) Interlimb coupling in children with hemiplegic cerebral palsy during reaching and grasping at speed. *Developmental Medicine and Child Neurology*, 40, 396–404.

Van Thiel, E. and Steenbergen, B. (2001) Shoulder and hand displacements during hitting, reaching, and grasping movements in hemiparetic cerebral palsy. *Motor Control*, 2, 166–82.

Van Thiel, E., Meulenbroek, R.G.J., Hulstijn, W. and Steenbergen, B. (2000) Kinematics of fast hemiparetic aiming movements towards stationary and moving targets. *Experimental Brain Research*, 132, 230–42.

Walter, C.B., Swinnen, S.P. and Franz, E.A. (1993) Stability of symmetric and asymmetric discrete bimanual actions. In K.M. Newell and D.M. Corcos (eds), *Variability and Motor Control* (pp. 359–81). Champagne IL: Human Kinetics.

Wiesendanger, M., Wicki, U. and Rouiller, E. (1994) Are there unifying structures in the brain responsible for interlimb coordination? In: S. Swinnen, H. Heuer, J. Massion and P. Casaer (eds), *Interlimb Coordination: Neural, Dynamical, and Cognitive Constraints* (pp. 179–207). San Diego: Academic Press.

Woods, B.T. and Teuber, T.L. (1978) Mirror movements after childhood hemiplegia. *Neurology*, 28, 1152–8.

11 Locomotion in children with cerebral palsy

Early predictive factors for ambulation and gait analysis

Annick Ledebt

1. Introduction

The aim of this chapter is to present two aspects of ambulatory problems in children with spastic cerebral palsy (CP). The first aspect concerns the identification of criteria for long-term prognosis with respect to walking in the young child with cerebral palsy. The second aspect concerns gait analysis and the difficulty in identifying the primary causes of gait abnormalities in children with CP who can walk.

Cerebral palsy is a condition caused by non-progressive brain damage that usually occurs before, during or shortly after birth. The effect on the body can result in progressive deformities and disabilities that develop in a variety of different forms and degrees of severity depending upon the location and the extent of the damage. Despite the variety of the consequences there are certain common features including:

- Abnormal muscle tone (e.g. dystonia and spasticity). Spasticity refers to increased tone or tension in a muscle whereas dystonia corresponds to sustained involuntary muscle contractions and spasms. Spastic cerebral palsy occurs with varying degrees of spasticity and is the most frequent form of CP. In spastic CP, the tone imbalance between agonist and antagonist muscle groups can lead to contractures of the shortened muscles;
- Deficient recruitment of motor units (paretic component);
- Unselective muscle control (e.g. co-activation);
- Changes in the properties of the muscles (non-neural component), like the transformation of motor units that takes place following a supraspinal lesion (Dietz and Berger, 1995).

Three main subgroups of patients can be distinguished according to the body part affected by the symptoms: involvement of either half of the body (left or right side) (hemiplegia), predominant involvement of the lower limbs (diplegia), or involvement of all four limbs (quadriplegia).

CP is generally recognised in the early years but the diagnosis is rarely given before the age of three years, as developmental delay becomes apparent. Although recent brain imaging techniques can help identify some brain abnormalities, the disorder is most often seen in its symptoms. Usually, at the moment CP is diagnosed, the child is not yet able to walk but the question whether s/he will achieve walking rapidly arises (da Paz Junior *et al.*, 1994). Predictive factors that can help clinicians to evaluate the possibilities of a child will be discussed in the first part of this chapter.

For the children with CP who acquire walking, the main motor impairments are balance, co-ordination problems (upper and lower limbs), and deviations from normal walking. Gait abnormalities that occur are a combination of primary consequences imposed by the brain damage, and of secondary deviations, which result from adaptations to circumvent the primary deficits (Gage and Koop, 1995). Although the number of gait abnormalities present varies between individuals, three main common gait abnormalities can be distinguished:

1   Limited range of motion of joints: especially critical in the sagittal plane, since walking mainly occurs in this plane. The limitation of joint motion during walking can be due to muscle contracture, and/or co-spasticity or co-contraction of agonists and antagonists.
2   Rotational deformities of bone: in the lower limbs, bone torsion causes malalignments of the joints that will impair the moments and powers the muscles can generate. Bone deformities are mainly due to the influence of spastic muscles that do not develop normal rotational pull.
3   Apparent weakness (low joint power) which can arise directly from the central lesion, or peripherally from changes of the muscle properties and/or a too short lever arm upon which a muscle works.

At the behavioural level, gait abnormalities in children with spastic CP manifest themselves through a common gait pattern that may include flexion, adduction and internal rotation of the hips, flexion at the knees (known as crouched gait), equinus and external/internal rotation of the ankle and feet (Gage and Ounpuu, 1991). This pattern often occurs together with toe walking, often called gait equinus, an obligate toe-strike maintained throughout stance in the gait cycle, for one or both legs, which results in a poor base of support in stance and instability during this phase. The second part of this chapter will show how gait analysis can offer a new perspective to understand and treat toe walking in children with spastic CP.

2. Walking prognosis in cerebral palsy

Several retrospective and prospective studies have examined different factors that might predict locomotor outcome at an early age. The type of CP gives a rough estimation of future walking possibilities, though a change in diagnosis can occur between the clinical type diagnosed early during infancy and later during childhood (Watt *et al.*, 1989). One of the general results is that hemiplegic and ataxic infants have a very good potential for walking, whereas infants with hypotonic CP have almost no likelihood of walking (Molnar and Gordon, 1976; Watt *et al.*, 1989). With all the other clinical types of CP (i.e. spastic diplegia and quadriplegia, spastic-athetoid, and athetoid) there are variable probabilities that walking will be possible. Different predictors have been proposed for these last diagnostic categories.

The first proposed predictors were the persistence or absence of primary reflexes (Bleck, 1975; Molnar and Gordon, 1976; Watt *et al.*, 1989). In the study of Molnar and Gordon (1976), almost all infants who showed the persistence of six primitive motor reactions (i.e. Moro, asymmetrical and symmetrical tonic neck, tonic labyrinthine reflexes, and supporting reaction and predominant extensor pattern of the legs in vertical suspension) at 18 months never became ambulatory. Persistence was not a reliable sign before 12 months, since they occasionally observed it in infants of this age who later reached walking. This was confirmed by Trahan and Marcoux (1994) who showed that the association between the inability to walk (with or without aid) at 6 years and the presence of primary automatisms was stronger in children evaluated after 12 months of age than in those evaluated earlier. Watt *et al.* (1989) found the same kind of results with a different age limit. In fact, they showed that the persistence of four of the reflexes at 24 months was significantly associated with non-ambulatory status at 8 years, whereas the absence of reflexes did not guarantee later walking. But, as Badell-Ribera (1985) noticed, the degree of persistence is difficult to quantify because it is subject to modifications in the infant's state, and the subjective appreciation of examiners, who have different skills and methods of assessment and handling of the infants. The investigation of postural and motor abilities proposed to avoid these problems. Assessments of different motor milestones, especially during the first two years after birth, were made according to either behavioural categories defined by each research or standardised categories (e.g. Gross Motor Function Classification System, Bayley test). The use of motor milestones as serial screening tests was shown to be a quite reliable predictor of CP in very preterm infants by as early as 9 months (Allen and Alexander, 1997). Delays in motor milestone attainment were also used to predict later locomotor status of infants already diagnosed as having CP.

In general, different studies agree that the rate of attainment of motor milestones is related to later ambulatory status and, particularly, that the age at which sitting without support is achieved is predictive for walking, but that none of them predict the age at which walking will be reached. In the studies that defined walking as the ability to locomote without assistive devices, the capacity to sit by 2 years (Fedrizzi *et al.*, 2000; Molnar and Gordon, 1976), or at the latest at 2½ years (Badell-Ribera, 1985) was predictive for later independent walking. This was also true for studies that did not make the distinction between walking with and without aids (crutches or walkers) in groups of children with all types of CP (Watt *et al.*, 1989), and for di- and quadriplegia (da Paz Junior *et al.*, 1994). Complementary to these results, Trahan and Marcoux (1994) found that the inability to sit after the age of 12 months increased the probability of non-ambulatory status at 6 years.

Contrary to sitting, there is no agreement on crawling ability as a predictive factor. Badell-Ribera (1985) found that all community ambulators at the age of 6 years or more had the capacity to crawl by 2½ years. However, the result of a multivariate analysis showed that the acquisition of crawling was not related to the ability to walk at the age of 6 years (Trahan and Marcoux, 1994). This apparent contradiction could be explained by different clinical categories of CP included in the studies, combined with the different definitions of the ambulatory status. For example, Badell-Ribera studied children with diplegia, whereas Trahan and Marcoux analysed the data from children with diplegia and quadriplegia. It is, then, possible that the non-predictive value of crawling in the Trahan and Marcoux study is due to the fact that they studied the children with quadriplegia who could crawl but who were less likely to walk than those with diplegia. Furthermore, the first author defined ambulation as walking without aid, though the second authors defined it as the capacity to walk without or with aid. So the predictive value could be restricted to the ability to walk without aid. In children with spastic quadriplegia,[1] the non-ambulatory status at the age of 4 years seems to diminish the chance to acquire independent walking afterwards (Barnhart and Liemohn, 1995).

Recently, Wood and Rosenbaum (2000) proposed that the Gross Motor Function Classification System (GMFCS) applied to clinical notes might be used as a prognostic tool. This stratification system has already been used for objective classification of the patterns of motor disability in children with CP according to four age ranges 1 to 2, 2 to 4, 4 to 6, and 6 to 12 years, and five levels of gross motor function (Palisano *et al.*, 1997). Wood and Rosenbaum (2000) showed that this system also has a predictive validity for the ultimate gross motor function with some reasonable degree of confidence. This is based on the fact that, in general, a child stays at the same level of the GMFCS from age 1 to 2 years to age 6 to 12 years. The likelihood of a child walking at age 6 to 12 years can be calculated by knowing the child's GMFCS level and the age at which s/he was assessed.

Drawing a clear conclusion from the nine studies that looked for early predictive signs is rather difficult because of the different clinical groups and the different definitions of walking (see table 11.1). Indeed, in some studies a child can be qualified as a walker if s/he is able to walk 15 metres without falling and eventually with crutches (Bleck, 1975) or walkers (Barnhart and Liemohn, 1995; Trahan and Marcoux, 1994; Watt *et al.*, 1989), whereas other studies distinguish different levels in the capacity to walk (Badell-Ribera, 1985; Fedrizzi *et al.*, 2000; Wood and Rosenbaum, 2000). It seems important to make the distinction between a household ambulator with low endurance (limited to short indoors distances), a household ambulator with high endurance, a community ambulator (without crutches but eventually with braces) whose endurance is functional for walking outdoors, and those who are able to walk on uneven surfaces and inclines. Only one study took this distinction into account for the calculation of predictive milestones for three outcome groups, i.e. walking without aid, walking with aid, and no walking at 3 to 5 years of age (Fedrizzi *et al.*, 2000).

Despite these two problems, it seems that the most reliable predictor for, at the least, aided locomotion (with crutches and walkers), and at the best, independent walking, is the ability to sit without support by the age of 2 years (see also positive factors in table 11.1). The first detectable signs that might predict low probability of achieving walking (see factors related to negative outcome in table 11.1) are abnormal tonic and postural primary reactions after 12 months of age, and the

Table 11.1 Early predictive factors for locomotor outcome in children with CP according to nine studies

Authors	n	Clinical type	Type of study	Definition of walking	Positive factors	Factors related to negative outcome
Bleck (1975)	73	all types of CP	prospective	with AND without aid (crutches)	—	two or more abnormal postural and tonic activities at about 12 months (best predictor out of 5 = extensor thrust)
Molnar and Gordon (1976)	233	all types of CP	prospective	without aid	sitting by 2 years	– di-, quadriplegia, athetose – persistent primary reflexes at 18 months
Badell-Ribera (1985)	50	diplegia	prospective	without aid	sitting and crawling at the latest at 2½ years	—
Watt et al. (1989)	74	all types of CP	prospective	with AND without aid	sitting by 2 years	– persistent primary reflexes at 24 months
Da Paz et al. (1994)	272	di- tri- and quadriplegia	retrospective	with AND without aid	– head balance by 9 months – sitting by 2 years	– no head balance by 20 months – no sitting before 36 months
Trahan and Marcoux (1994)	264	di- and quadriplegia	retrospective	with AND without aid	—	– persistent primary reflexes after 12 months – incapacity to sit after 12 months
Barnhart and Liemohn (1995)	19	quadriplegia	retrospective	with AND without aid	—	remote prospect of walking when non-ambulatory status at 4 years
Fedrizzi et al. (2000)	31	di- and triplegia	prospective	with OR without aid	– weight on hands while prone and roll from supine to prone at 18 months – sitting by 2 years	four or less gross motor skills (from an 18-item protocol) acquired at the age of 2 years
Wood and Rosenbaum (2000)	85	all types of CP	retrospective	with OR without aid	I and II GMFCS's levels at age 1 to 2 years	IV and V GMFCS's levels at age 1 to 2 years. (mixed outcomes for level III)

Notes:
NB: (—) information not given by the authors. Definition of walking: 'AND' stands for studies that do not distinguish walking with and without assistive devices for calculating the predictors, whereas 'OR' concerns studies that do make the distinction

inability to sit before (at the latest) 36 months. The combination of these two signs is certainly a strong sign of negative outcome with respect to walking with or without support.

Though delays of early motor development and the abnormal persistence of infantile automatism are good predictors of future walking ability, it seems that associated handicaps, especially mental retardation and epilepsy (seizures), also affect the possibility to walk (Fedrizzi *et al.*, 2000; Molnar and Gordon, 1976; Trahan and Marcoux, 1994). For example, in the study of Molnar and Gordon (1976), 81 per cent of the children with CP (hemiplegic and ataxic patients excluded) who reached locomotion between 5 and 7 years were retarded. In a population of patients with spastic diplegia or triplegia, Fedrizzi *et al.* (2000) observed that 73 per cent of the children who could not walk at all by the age of 8 years had abnormal general quotients on the Griffiths mental development scale, compared to 16 per cent for those who could walk independently. The possible explanation for this association is that mental retardation and epilepsy could be indicators of more severe neurological lesion.

3. Gait analysis: identification of primary and secondary gait deviations

It has been proposed that gait analysis can help clinicians in making therapeutic decisions (Morton, 1999). Therefore, the analysis has to focus on the movement itself, instead of a global outcome measure like gait velocity. Gait velocity is, on average, reduced in children with CP (Norlin and Odenrick, 1986) and is strongly correlated with gross motor functions (Damiano and Abel, 1996) and the severity of the disability (Drouin *et al.*, 1996). However, reduced velocity is only a sign that one has problems walking and is the end result of multiple factors, as is the case for the elderly or adults with different type of injuries (Brandstater *et al.*, 1983). When considered alone, velocity does not give any valuable information about the reasons of the problems in walking. Gait analysis based on three-dimensional movement analyses (kinematics), ground reactive forces (kinetics) and electrical muscle activity (surface EMG) provides documentation of aspects which are difficult to visualise, which might give insights about the cause of gait abnormalities (Gage and Ounpuu, 1991). Sophisticated gait analysis allows observation in a more detailed and precise way but it is still subject to the interpretation of the researchers and/or clinicians who have to collate an impressive amount of data. Nevertheless, gait analysis has been found to give decisive information for surgical decision-making compared to clinical assessment and video recording alone (DeLuca, Davis, Ounpuu, Rose and Sirkin, 1997). The study of DeLuca *et al.* (1997), which involved 91 children with CP, showed that 47 of the recommendations changed when new information from the gait analysis was given to experienced clinicians, including changes in planned surgery and the cancellation of interventions. Though more studies comparing surgical interventions based upon gait analysis with those on clinical assessment alone are needed, it seems now quite clear that gait analysis is useful as a means both to evaluate complex gait abnormalities and to assess the effects of intervention (Morton, 1999).

As soon as treatment is envisaged, it is crucial to disentangle the primary causes of gait deviation from the compensations. To have an effect, surgical intervention has to address the primary causes, which will as a consequence eliminate the coping responses, whereas treating the compensation will increase the problems that the patient has to face (Gage, 1993). The importance of making the distinction between primary and secondary gait abnormalities was recently demonstrated in studies on toe walking, one of the most common gait deviations in children with CP. Two main explanations of toe walking are available, which result in two different treatments that have opposite physiological effects on the muscle (Lin and Brown, 1992).

The classical explanation of toe walking considers that ankle plantar flexors are abnormally shortened with a high tonic activity due to contracture of the triceps surae and/or excessive strong contraction of the ankle plantarflexors (Winters *et al.*, 1987). The usual proposed treatment is to reach normal muscle length either with the help of drugs that reduce muscle tone (Boyd *et al.*, 2000; Koman *et al.*, 2000) or with surgery that, for example, lengthens the Achilles tendon (Kling *et al.*, 1985). These types of intervention further weaken the already weak spastic muscles. Successful outcomes are not systematic, and additional treatments through casts or orthotic devices are often required (Sala *et al.*, 1997).

Another point of view considers toe walking more as compensation for weak plantar flexors rather than directly due to overactivity in those muscles (Davids *et al.*, 1999; Kerrigan *et al.*, 2000). Toe walking is then viewed as an adaptive response to weak calf muscles. A first indication that toe walking is not necessarily a consequence of too short plantar flexors stems from the study of Lin and Brown (1992) that analysed the relation between the characteristics of the ankle joint and muscles and gait equinus in 24 children with hemiplegia. The authors did not find any fixed equinus among the children (all joints could be passively dorsiflexed) though nine children showed gait equinus on their affected side. Furthermore, a comparison between the groups with and without gait equinus showed no significant differences in leg length, ankle-joint range of motion or toe dexterity, or any difference in muscle tone at rest in the affected limbs. Passive equinus (ankle compliance when passively dorsiflexed) was observed in 16 children but did not systematically imply gait equinus. The lack of a clear correlation between dorsiflexor weakness and gait equinus showed that toe walking is more complex than a simple, central, paralytic foot-drop.

Moreover, a biomechanical analysis of toe walking showed that it offers certain compensatory advantages insofar as it can require less peak strength about the ankle and knee than normal heel–toe walking, and could thus be a solution to cope with both weak calf muscles and the requirements of walking (Kerrigan *et al.*, 2000). According to these results, Kerrigan *et al.* (2000) suggested that the adapted treatment is to strengthen the plantar flexors instead of to weaken them (i.e. lengthening or neurectomies). The study of Carmick (1995) gives an argument in favour of the hypothesis that strengthening the calf muscles can decrease the equinovarus posture of the foot and lead to plantigrade walk in toe walkers. In her study, three children with CP who had equinus walk received neuromuscular electrical stimulation (NMES) on the calf muscle during walking to strengthen it. After NMES the toe walkers became plantigrade without increasing the spasticity (Carmick, 1995).

Patterns of muscle activity, in combination with joint moment and power, are commonly used descriptors to check the eventual source of gait deviations in children with CP. However, gait analysis has to take other issues into account; for example, the fact that some of the abnormal co-activities in the leg muscles may be due to biomechanical constraints of the gait pattern as opposed to being a direct consequence of loss of selective control of those muscles. In fact, constant rectus femoris activity through the entire gait cycle is often considered to be an indicator for surgical transfer of the distal end of the rectus femoris to the sartorius (Miller *et al.*, 1997). In this way, the action of the muscle as a hip flexor is preserved, while converting its action as a knee extensor to that of a knee flexor. But taken alone this indicator may mask the fact that the overactivity of the rectus femoris together with activity of other postural muscles at the knee and ankle level achieves dynamic stability during stance. This was verified with the comparison of dynamic EMG between voluntary (able-bodied children) and obligatory toe walkers, i.e. children with CP (Davids *et al.*, 1999). The results of Davids *et al.* (1999) showed that the rectus femoris activity during the swing phase, and the co-activation of agonist and antagonist muscle groups at the ankle and the knee during midstance, were present in both voluntary and obligatory toe walkers, and probably used to enhance stability on the toes. The loss of selective muscle control observed in children with CP during toe walking could thus result from postural requirements rather than an abnormal distribution of common synaptic drives arising from abnormally branched inputs. In fact, it seems that abnormal patterns of muscle contraction and the widespread distribution of reflex responses observed in the lower limbs of children with CP cannot be attributed to abnormal branching to the motor-neurone pools innervating lower limbs (Gibbs *et al.*, 1999).

4. Conclusion

The present chapter presented two fields of research concerning locomotion in children with CP: the prognostic value of early signs for future locomotor outcome and the explanatory value of gait analysis for understanding gait abnormalities. Studies on the detection of predictive signs for later walking appeared to be difficult to compare because of crucial methodological differences, especially in terms of walking definitions and the population studied. Nevertheless, statistical analyses have isolated positive (in favour of later walking) and negative factors that can be detected during the first 3 years of life.

Recent studies based on gait analysis showed that kinematic, kinetic and EMG data have to be carefully interpreted before being used for treatment recommendation. For example, the phenomenon of co-activation of agonist and antagonist muscles, a frequent characteristic in spastic CP, is probably not due to abnormal branching of inputs to motor neurones (Gibbs *et al.*, 1999). In the case of toe walking, the fact that co-activation seems to be linked to the modification of the movement itself should be taken into account when surgical muscle transfers are proposed.

The results of several studies have converged to give an alternative explanation for another typical feature of spastic gait. In fact, the restricted range of motion at a joint during walking (e.g. gait equinus, and internally leg-rotated walk) can be the result of either strong and shortened spastic agonist (classical interpretation) or weak agonists (plantar flexors in the case of toe walking). The later explanation thus suggests that toe walking is a compensation for weak calf muscles and that an attempt should be made to strengthen rather than weaken these muscles.

Generally, however, studies investigating the possible causes and treatments for toe walking have never addressed the issue of balance, though they have implicitly agreed that heel–toe walking provides a greater base of support and, as a consequence, a better balance. Of note is the fact that while treatments are aimed to modify a deviant range of motion and moments in order to normalise them, such treatments may indeed improve some local characteristics but without improving the general gait efficiency. As Kerrigan *et al.* (2000) noticed, there is no support for the proposition that toe walking predisposes to more falls than heel–toe walking, and that treatments that weaken the ankle plantar flexors and/or lengthen the Achilles tendon to achieve heel–toe walking improve balance. Rather, these treatments could impair the important postural role that the plantar flexors play in keeping upright equilibrium. Studies on gait equinus should concentrate not only on localised consequences of treatments (e.g. the increase of heel strike and range of motion of the ankle) but also on the global level of balance and the related risk of falls.

Note

1   Retrospective study on 19 children who received physical therapy through childhood but no other type of treatment (e.g. surgery, medicine).

References

Allen, M.C. and Alexander, G.R. (1997) Using motor milestones as a multistep process to screen preterm infants for cerebral palsy. *Developmental Medicine and Child Neurology*, 39, 12–16.

Badell-Ribera, A. (1985) Cerebral palsy: postural-locomotor prognosis in spastic diplegia. *Archives of Physical Medicine and Rehabilitation*, 66, 614–19.

Barnhart, R.C. and Liemohn, W.P. (1995) Ambulatory status of children with cerebral palsy: a retrospective study. *Perceptual and Motor Skills*, 81, 571–4.

Bleck, E.E. (1975) Locomotor prognosis in cerebral palsy. *Developmental Medicine and Child Neurology*, 17, 18–25.

Boyd, R.N., Pliatsios, V., Starr, R., Wolfe, R. and Graham, H.K. (2000) Biomechanical transformation of the gastroc-soleus muscle with botulinum toxin A in children with cerebral palsy. *Developmental Medicine and Child Neurology*, 42, 32–41.

Brandstater, M.E., de Bruin, H., Gowland, C. and Clark, B.M. (1983) Hemiplegic gait: analysis of temporal variables. *Archives of Physical Medicine and Rehabilitation*, 64, 583–7.

Carmick, J. (1995) Managing equinus in children with cerebral palsy: electrical stimulation to strengthen the triceps surae muscle. *Developmental Medicine and Child Neurology*, 37, 965–75.

da Paz Junior, A.C., Burnett, S.M. and Braga, L.W. (1994) Walking prognosis in cerebral palsy: a 22-year retrospective analysis. *Developmental Medicine and Child Neurology*, 36, 130–4.

Damiano, D.L. and Abel, M.F. (1996) Relation of gait analysis to gross motor function in cerebral palsy. *Developmental Medicine and Child Neurology*, 38, 389–96.

Davids, J.R., Foti, T., Dabelstein, J. and Bagley, A. (1999) Voluntary (normal) versus obligatory (cerebral palsy) toe-walking in children: a kinematic, kinetic, and electromyographic analysis. *Journal of Pediatric Orthopedics*, 19, 461–9.

DeLuca, P.A., Davis, R.B., Ounpuu, S., Rose, S. and Sirkin, R. (1997) Alterations in surgical decision making in patients with cerebral palsy based on three-dimensional gait analysis. *Journal of Pediatric Orthopedics*, 17, 608–14.

Dietz, V. and Berger, W. (1995) Cerebral palsy and muscle transformation. *Developmental Medicine and Child Neurology*, 37, 180–4.

Drouin, L.M., Malouin, F., Richards, C.L. and Marcoux, S. (1996) Correlation between the gross motor function measure scores and gait spatiotemporal measures in children with neurological impairments. *Developmental Medicine and Child Neurology*, 38, 1007–19.

Fedrizzi, E., Facchin, P., Marzaroli, M., Pagliano, E., Botteon, G., Percivalle, L. and Fazzi, E. (2000) Predictors of independent walking in children with spastic diplegia. *Journal of Child Neurology*, 15, 228–34.

Gage, J.R. (1993) Gait analysis: an essential tool in the treatment of cerebral palsy. *Clinical Orthopaedics*, 126, 126–34.

Gage, J.R. and Koop, S.E. (1995) Clinical gait analysis: application to management of cerebral palsy. In P. Allard, I.A.F. Stokes and J.-P. Blanchi (eds), *Three-dimensional Analysis of Human Movement* (pp. 349–62). Champaign, IL: Human Kinetics.

Gage, J.R. and Ounpuu, S. (1991) Surgical intervention in the correction of primary and secondary gait abnormalities. In A.E. Patla (ed.), *Adaptability of Human Gait* (pp. 359–85). Amsterdam: Elsevier Science Publishers.

Gibbs, J., Harrison, L.M., Stephens, J.A. and Evans, A.L. (1999) Does abnormal branching of inputs to motor neurones explain abnormal muscle cocontraction in cerebral palsy? *Developmental Medicine and Child Neurology*, 41, 465–72.

Kerrigan, D.C., Riley, P.O., Rogan, S. and Burke, D.T. (2000) Compensatory advantages of toe walking. *Archives of Physical Medicine and Rehabilitation*, 81, 38–44.

Kling, T.F., Kaufer, H. and Hensinger, R.N. (1985) Split posterior tibial-tendon transfers in children with cerebral spastic paralysis and equinovarus deformity. *Journal of Bone and Joint Surgery*, 67, 186–94.

Koman, L.A., Mooney, J.F., Smith, B.P., Walker, F. and Leon, J.M. (2000) Botulinum toxin type A neuromuscular blockade in the treatment of lower extremity spasticity in cerebral palsy: a randomized, double-blind, placebo-controlled trial. BOTOX Study Group. *Journal of Pediatric Orthopedics*, 20, 108–15.

Lin, J.P. and Brown, J.K. (1992) Peripheral and central mechanisms of hindfoot equinus in childhood hemiplegia. *Developmental Medicine and Child Neurology*, 34, 949–65.

Miller, F., Cardoso Dias, R., Lipton, G.E., Albarracin, J.P., Dabney, K.W. and Castagno, P. (1997) The effect of rectus EMG patterns on the outcome of rectus femoris transfers. *Journal of Pediatric Orthopedics*, 17, 603–7.

Molnar, G.E. and Gordon, S.U. (1976) Cerebral palsy: predictive value of selected clinical signs for early prognostication of motor function. *Archives of Physical Medicine and Rehabilitation*, 57, 153–8.

Morton, R. (1999) New surgical interventions for cerebral palsy and the place of gait analysis. *Developmental Medicine and Child Neurology*, 41, 424–8.

Norlin, R. and Odenrick, P. (1986) Development of gait in spastic children with cerebral palsy. *Journal of Pediatric Orthopedics*, 6, 674–80.

Palisano, R., Rosenbaum, P., Walter, S., Russell, D., Wood, E. and Galuppi, B. (1997) Development and reliability of a system to classify gross motor function in children with cerebral palsy. *Developmental Medicine and Child Neurology*, 39, 214–23.

Sala, D.A., Grant, A.D. and Kummer, F.J. (1997) Equinus deformity in cerebral palsy: recurrence after tendo Achillis lengthening. *Developmental Medicine and Child Neurology*, 39, 45–8.

Trahan, J. and Marcoux, S. (1994) Factors associated with the inability of children with cerebral palsy to walk at six years: a retrospective study [see comments]. *Developmental Medicine and Child Neurology*, 36, 787–95.

Watt, J.M., Robertson, C.M. and Grace, M.G. (1989) Early prognosis for ambulation of neonatal intensive care survivors with cerebral palsy. *Developmental Medicine and Child Neurology*, 31, 766–73.

Winters, T.F., Gage, J.R. and Hicks, R. (1987) Gait patterns in spastic hemiplegia in children and young adults. *Journal of Bone and Joint Surgery*, 69, 437–41.

Wood, E. and Rosenbaum, P. (2000) The gross motor function classification system for cerebral palsy: a study of reliability and stability over time. *Developmental Medicine and Child Neurology*, 42, 292–6.

Part III
Sport

12 Catching action development

Geert Savelsbergh, Karl Rosengren,
John van der Kamp and
Martine Verheul

1. Introduction

Catching skills are an essential part of many diverse sports. For instance, baseball, football, rugby, basketball, and team handball all involve the interception of a ball. In all these circumstances, players demonstrate highly skilled co-ordinated behaviour. To reach such high levels of performance and flexibility often takes years of development, learning and practice. An important characteristic of skilled performance is precise tuning of the action to the continuously changing circumstances of the environment. Perception is indispensable in this respect, because successful catching demands conformity to highly constrained spatial and timing requirements. In order to make a successful catch, the catcher not only has to time her/his catch accurately but she/he also has to orient and locate the hand at a precise location at a precise time. In addition, the catcher needs to anticipate the exact moment the ball will hit the hand in order to close the fingers around the ball. A classic high-speed film analysis of Alderson, Scully and Scully (1974) in the early 1970s of the last century showed that when the ball approaches with a velocity of 10 m/s, the catcher has only a time-window of 60 ms in order to avoid timing errors in grasping. In most sport situations the approach velocity of the ball reaches a higher value, e.g. 160–190 km/hour a for tennis serve, 80–90 km/hour for a cricket ball (Land and McLeod, 2000) and 140–160 km/hour for baseball pitch (Bahill and LaRitz, 1984).

Describing the development of catching

The skill of catching develops gradually throughout childhood. Wickstrom (1983) gives a particularly detailed description of the development of catching, from its early onset to the various applications in sporting situations. Catching, defined as the stopping and controlling of an aerial ball or object by the use of hand(s) and/or other parts of the body, develops from the age of 3. Perceptual–motor skills that underlie catching can already be seen in infancy, such as stopping a ball that rolls towards a sitting child or chasing and stopping a bouncing ball. Like many other skills, the development of catching follows a proximal–distal pattern. This means that the skill involves large trunk and arm movements in the early stage and more refined hand and finger movements at later stages. Initially, catching involves 'trapping', meaning that the ball is stopped between the trunk and arms. This type of catching often coincides with a 'fear reaction' in children, where a child may turn his/her head to the side and slightly bend his/her trunk backwards. Experience with various ball sizes, including smaller balls, encourages the child to increase the contribution of the hands and progress from a trapping style of catching to a more mature technique. As the child acquires more advanced catching skills, he/she starts to lower his/her arms, with the elbows flexed and pointing downwards, and position the palms and fingers in anticipation of a two-handed catch. In a successful catch, the hands make contact with the ball simultaneously. The mature form of catching, observed in late childhood, is characterised by correctly positioning the hand(s) with regard to the trajectory of the object and by successfully grasping the object. The latter phase involves 'giving way' with the object, increasing the time to perform the actual grasping motion and the distance over which to exert force to stop the ball. Various sporting situations require specialised catching actions, but these basic characteristics remain observable in all of these situations. For a detailed account of catching in basketball, football and baseball, see Wickstrom (1983).

The goal of this chapter is to elaborate upon the role of visual information in the co-ordination and control of the development of catching.[1] Section 2 focuses on the theoretical perspective; that is, the role of constraints in the learning and development of complex motor skills. Section 3 discusses the role of informational constraints in the control of simple one-handed catching in adults and children. The chapter concludes with a model with respect to different stages in learning and development in information–movement couplings.

2. The theoretical perspective

In the first two years an infant has already acquired a variety of different goal-directed motor behaviours, such as reaching, grasping, sitting, crawling and walking. These so-called motor milestones have been well known since the work of Gesell (1929), McGraw (1945) and Shirley (1933). The description of these milestones was based in part on the assumption that motor development was a rather rigid and gradual unfolding of postures and movements that was mainly attributed to the general process of maturation of the central nervous system. From a neural-maturation perspective, the development of movement co-ordination is regarded as a gradual unfolding of predetermined patterns (from cephalo-to-caudal and central-to-distal sequences) in the central nervous system and an increasing cortical control over lower reflexes. In contrast, the theoretical paradigm for this chapter is based on the work of Bernstein (1967), Gibson (1979), Newell (1986) and Kugler *et al.* (1982). From this perspective, development of movement co-ordination is brought about by changes in the constraints imposed upon the organism–environment system. Particular constraints may act, at certain developmental times, as rate-limiting factors in the emergence of new behaviours, in the mastering of new actions, or even in the sustaining of highly skilled actions. For instance, rapid changes in the physiology of an adult can be quite disruptive for motor functioning. Van der Kamp *et al.* (1996), report that, shortly after winning the world title in gymnastics in 1987, Aurelia Dobre was plagued by growth spurts. As a result, she failed to maintain her high level of performance, and she abruptly disappeared from the international competition. In this case, a change in an organismic constraint disrupted the acquired movement organisation. A central aim of the constraint-led perspective is, by identifying the environmental and organism constraints and their relative contributions, to develop accurate explanations for changes in an observed behaviour. In this manner, the constraint perspective moves well beyond the descriptive accounts that have dominated the field of motor development.

Constraints in movement organisation

To shed light on the role of constraints in catching movement organisation, different kinds of categorisations have been proposed. Among the best known are Newell's (1986) distinction between organismic, environmental, and task constraints, in which constraints are ordered with respect to their origin. For instance, the action pattern that emerges when children have to grasp (task constraint) can be understood by the relation between organismic and environmental constraints. A good example of this relation was demonstrated by Van der Kamp *et al.* (1998), who showed that the ratio between object size (environmental constraint) and hand size (organismic constraint) determined when children shifted from a one-handed to a two-handed grasping pattern.

Another classic example which illustrates how muscle strength can be a constraint, is provided by research of Thelen and her colleagues with respect to the development of leg movements (Thelen *et al.*, 1984). These researchers found that in 8-week-old infants held upright, the stepping movements observed at a younger age disappeared. However, when the infants were lying supine, they performed kicking movements that were kinematically similar to the earlier observed stepping movements. Moreover, when the same infants were held upright in water, the stepping pattern re-emerged. If the disappearance was due to cortical inhibition, as the traditional explanation would have it, why would the cortex inhibit movements in the upright posture but not in the supine posture? Thelen explained this disappearance of new-born stepping movements as a consequence of the disproportionate growth of leg muscles and fat tissues. Specifically, during this period of development infants acquire fat at a greater rate than muscle mass, which leads to relatively less muscle force. Thus, the occurrence of stepping movements (task) is a consequence of the interaction between organismic constraints (body proportions) and environmental constraints (orientation to the gravity vector), and not uniquely determined by neuro-maturational constraints. Similar observations have been made with respect to infant reaching by Savelsbergh and Van der Kamp (1994).

In a more recent experiment, conducted by Van Hof *et al.* (2002), it was shown that the development of midline crossings during reaching is not exclusively dependent on the maturation of hemispheric connections, but depends also on their interaction with particular environmental constraints. Previously, it was held that the development of midline crossing is uniquely determined by maturation of the hemispheric specialisation (Provine and Westerman, 1979) or the maturation of spinal tracts (Morange and Bloch, 1996). Van Hof *et al.* observed infants longitudinally at 12, 18 and 26 weeks of age while reaching for two balls (3 and 8 cm in diameter) at three positions (ipsilateral, midline and contralateral). With age, the infants increasingly adapted the number of hands used to the size of the object. The number of reaches crossing the body midline also increased with age. Furthermore, the majority of the midline crossings were part of two-handed reaches for the large ball and occurred at or after onset of bimanual reaching. Together, these results strongly suggest that the development of crossing the body midline emerges in the context of bimanual reaching. It is concluded that the need to grasp a large ball positioned contralaterally with two hands induces midline crossing. Hence, the development of midline crossings is not exclusively dependent on organismic constraints (e.g. the maturation of hemispheric connections).

To summarise, there is now clear empirical evidence that constraints act as rate-limiting factors on the emergence of new motor abilities. A rather small change in one of the constraints (e.g. fat/muscle ratio change, or change in object size) can lead to changes the observed co-ordination pattern.

Visual information as a constraint

Information can guide the grasping pattern and it is in this sense that information may act as a constraint. Informational constraints, in a Gibsonian sense, serve to tune parameters to tailor the movement to the changing conditions of the local environment. How should we consider this tuning? Gibson's (1979) theory of direct perception placed an emphasis on the nature of information for action. By stressing the circularity between perception and action, Gibson refuted traditional theories of perception that considered perception as consisting of passively sensed retinal images, which through inference and recourse to memory are built into meaningful representations of the world. In contrast, Gibson argued that information for perception and action is provided by the change or persistence of optical patterns in the environment. The specific visual patterns in the environment are determined both by the movements of the observers and by events in the environment. Gibson's ideas have resulted in a research strategy of identifying visual information (optic variables) that uniquely specify events, examining the subject's sensitivity to such variables, and demonstrating that the identified information source is actually used in controlling action. In the next section we will discuss the latter position in the context of catching.

3. Informational constraints on catching

In catching, both spatial and temporal requirements have to be met in order for a successful catch to be accomplished. Alderson *et al.* (1974) discerned different phases in the performance of a simple one-handed catch: a gross spatial orientation phase, a fine orientation phase, and a grasp and hold phase. To ensure catching success, the hand first has to be roughly positioned at the interception point, followed by spatial adjustments of the hand such that the ball makes contact with the hand in the metacarpal region. Eventually the grasp needs to be initiated and completed within a restricted time-window, depending on the speed of the approaching ball, thus requiring precise timing. In addition to these arm and hand movements, it is sometimes also necessary to move the whole body to the future landing position of a ball, as is the case for an outfielder in baseball.

Information for spatial predictions

Chapman (1968) proposed that in order to intercept a baseball, the catcher has to run in such a way that he or she is zeroing out vertical optical acceleration. This hypothesis was empirically tested and supported by several researchers (for instance, Babler and Dannemiller, 1993; McBeath, Shaffer and Kaiser, 1995; McLeod and Dienes, 1993; Michaels and Oudejans, 1992). When a ball is travelling in the sagittal plane heading for the catcher's eye, the optical height of the ball on the image plane rises linearly during the ball's approach. Thus, when running for the ball, the only thing the catcher has to do is to keep the optical velocity constant. This strategy always brings the catcher at the interception point without the need to know the landing position in advance. Oudejans and Michaels have shown that all the catcher needs to do to get to the right place at the right time, is to zero out the ball's vertical optical acceleration (Oudejans, 1996; Michaels and Oudejans, 1992). This strategy of zeroing out vertical optical acceleration, however, breaks down a few hundred milliseconds before completion of the catch; that is, during the orientation and grasping phase.

To predict the future passing distance of a ball, information about the current distance of the ball is also required. Peper *et al.* (1994) derived an alternative, where future passing distance, in units of ball size, is specified by the ratio of the velocity of sideward displacement of the centre of expansion and the rate of expansion of the object image. Although the perception of future passing distance appears to be in units of ball size, it is also affected by the angle of approach of the ball, eventually leading the authors to propose a catching strategy in which the sideward arm movement is regulated by continuously gearing the movement velocity of the arm to the optically (i.e. ball) and kinesthetically (i.e. hand) specified required velocity. Such information 'does not specify when to be where, but how to be at the right place in the right time, regardless of where this might be' (Peper *et al.*, 1994, p. 610).

More recently, Montagne and co-workers (1999) put the model to the test in a catching experiment (Montagne *et al.*, 1999). Their findings show that catchers do indeed use a prospective control strategy. That is, the catchers maintained a relation beween ball approach and hand movements that ensured the attainment of success. This result provides an indication of the tight coupling between information and movement.

In summary, experimental studies and theoretical considerations show that the necessary spatio-temporal information for successful catching is available in the environment. In the remainder of this section, the potential optical information sources constraining the timing of catching behaviour will be evaluated.

Information for timing

To time the grasping phase in catching, the catcher has to know how long it takes for the ball to reach the hand. The time to contact of a ball heading for the catcher is determined by its distance from the catcher divided by its speed of approach. Lee and Young (1985) called this the tau-margin, after the optic variable tau that specifies time to contact. The optical variable tau is defined as the inverse of the rate of dilation of the retinal image of an approaching object (Lee, 1976). Provided that the relative velocity between the ball and the catcher is constant, tau specifies the actual time remaining before the ball hits the eye. Therefore, if subjects behave in accordance with a tau-margin strategy, they are expected to initiate their actions at a constant time before contact, independent of object velocity. Is tau actually used to time the grasping phase in catching?

Savelsbergh *et al.* (1992) had subjects catch balls projected from a distance of 6m and approaching with different speeds (11.9, 13.9, and 16.2 m/s). For each catch, the tau-margin at the moment of initiation of the grasp was determined. It was found that the onset of muscular activity in the hand and forearm was geared to a constant tau-margin rather than to the speed of the ball, thereby providing evidence for the use of tau in controlling interceptive timing. Moreover, Lee *et al.* (1983) showed that even with non-constant, accelerative approaches, as in the case of attempting to punch a falling ball, subjects guided their actions to the optical variable tau rather than to the actual time to contact.

However, both these and other studies mainly show that the subjects' actions are consistent with a tau-strategy; whether tau was actually used was not put to the test. More direct evidence for the use of tau was provided in the 'deflating ball experiment' of Savelsbergh *et al.* (1991; see also Savelsbergh *et al.*, 1993). In this study, subjects were required to catch a luminous ball attached to a pendulum in a totally dark room. Three balls with different diameters were used. Two of them had a constant size of 5.5 cm or 7.5 cm, while the third one changed its size during flight from 7.5 cm to 5.5 cm. In comparison to the constant balls, the deflating ball specified a longer time to contact, thereby allowing for a direct test of the role of tau in one-handed catching. Examining the timing of the grasp, Savelsbergh *et al.* (1991) found that the moment of maximal closing velocity occurred later for the deflating ball (see figure 12.1), strongly suggesting the use of tau in timing the grasp.

As recently put forward by Michaels and Beek (1995) and Wann (1996), how-ever, the timing differences between the constant and the deflating balls as reported by Savelsbergh *et al.* (1991) are smaller than would be predicted from a uniquely tau based-strategy. This is particularly true in case of the binocular viewing condition (Tresilian, 1994; Savelsbergh, 1995). Thus, although the deflating ball

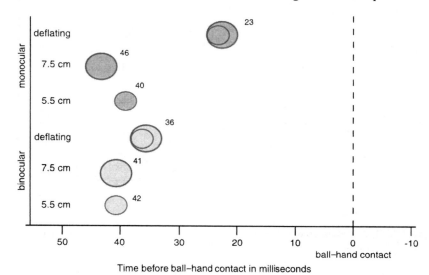

Figure 12.1 The timing of the catch in the deflating ball experiment under monocular and binocular viewing (Savelsbergh *et al.*, 1991). Illustrated is the moment of maximal closing velocity of the hand.

experiment shows the use of tau, it also suggests it is not used exclusively, but rather that informational constraints originating from binocular vision are involved as well. Supporting evidence in this respect comes from Judge and Bradford (1988) who had subjects catch balls while wearing a telestereoscope, which increased the effective inter-ocular separation by displacing the line of sight of each eye laterally. As a consequence, disparity increases and objects will be perceived closer to the observer (see figure 12.2).

In this study, balls were thrown to the subject from a distance of 3m and an average velocity of about 4.9 m/s. Wearing the telestereoscope exerted a powerful influence on the catching behaviour of the subjects. The findings showed that subjects closed their hands earlier when wearing the telestereoscope. However, it remains unclear from this investigation whether this early closing of the hand was due to temporal or spatial errors.

The findings are somewhat ambiguous with respect to the information sources controlling interceptive timing. A few studies suggest that, depending on the circumstances, different information sources (e.g. tau or binocular information sources) constrain the temporal characteristics of the catch. At present, the precise contribution of other information sources is still an empirically open question. Therefore, to examine the range of the contribution of tau (i.e. the inverse of the rate of dilation), not only should the alter-tau alter-action hypothesis (Michaels and Beek, 1995) be examined, but so also should the not-alter-tau not-alter-action hypothesis.

This was the goal set by Van der Kamp *et al.* (1997). Subjects were required to catch randomly presented luminous balls of different sizes under both monocular

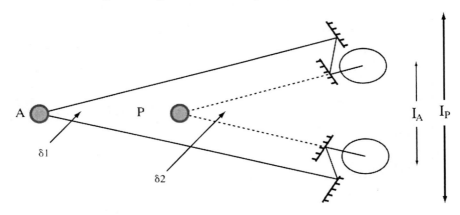

Figure 12.2 The telestereoscope. By means of four small mirrors the effective interocular distance is increased.

and binocular viewing conditions in a totally dark room. The balls were transported by a specially devised Ball Transport Apparatus (BallTrAp) and approached the subjects with a constant deceleration (average velocity 1.5 m/s). The balls were transported into the hand in a spatially fixed trajectory such that only temporal judgements were necessary. After contacting the hand, the ball immediately returned to its starting position giving rise to a time window of ±350 ms. Kinematics of the temporal characteristics of the grasp phase in the binocular viewing condition showed no differences for the moment of onset of the grasp, the moment of maximal aperture of the hand, or the moment of completion of the catch (see figure 12.3). In other words, subjects behaved in accordance with a constant time-to-contact or tau-margin strategy. In contrast, in the monocular condition subjects opened and closed their hand earlier, and also at different times before contact for the different ball sizes.

In sum, although a constant time-to-contact strategy seemed to be used in the binocular condition, in the monocular condition this strategy was lost. In other words, depending on the circumstances, different informational sources constrain the temporal characteristics of the grasp phase in catching. It would be illogical to argue from these results that tau (i.e. the inverse of the relative rate of dilation) was used in the binocular condition only. Clearly, it is a binocular information source which results in a constant time-to-contact strategy. Hence, the conclusion from previous studies (e.g. Lee *et al.*, 1983; Savelsbergh *et al.*, 1992) that (monocular) tau controlled the timing of the act might have been premature, because the subjects in these studies had binocular information sources available. The finding in the Van der Kamp *et al.* (1997) study, that in the monocular condition larger balls resulted in an earlier grasp, even questions the use of tau when only monocular information sources are available. That is not to say that tau is not used at all (see for instance Savelsbergh *et al.*, 1991), but that tau does not exclusively control the timing of the grasp phase in catching.

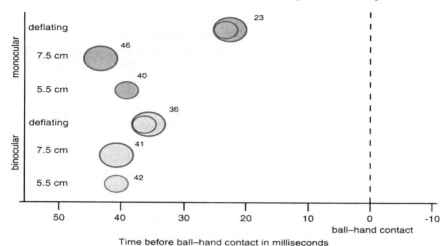

Time before ball–hand contact in milliseconds

Figure 12.3 The timing of the catch for balls of different diameters under monocular and binocular viewing (Van der Kamp *et al.*, 1997). Illustrated are, from left to right, the moment of onset of the catch, the moment of maximal hand aperture, and the moment of completion of the catch.

What binocular information sources might be involved? Heuer (1993) argued that

> any variable p that is accessible to the visual system and that satisfies the condition $\tau(t) = p(t)/p'(t) = -D(t)/D'(t)$ is suited. This equation will be satisfied by all proximal variables that are proportional to the reciprocal distance of an object. Among them are accommodation of the lens, the angle of convergence, and the sum of the angle of convergence and the retinal disparity.
>
> (Heuer, 1993, p. 550)

Following Heuer's proposal, Laurent *et al.* (1996) demonstrated mathematically that for head-on approaches, the tau-function of vergence (i.e. the angle subtended by the ball and the points of observation divided by its change) can indeed provide information about time to contact. Interestingly, the predictions based on this information source are in close alignment with those of tau as defined by Lee (1976). For instance, in case of a constant velocity approach, a constant time-to-contact strategy is expected to occur.

Bennett and his colleagues have examined whether the timing of one-handed catching is consistent with a binocular tau-function strategy. Participants in this study wore a telestereoscope to increase the effective interocular separation (figure 12.2), under binocular and monocular viewing (Bennett *et al.*, 1999). The data showed that under binocular viewing, the opening and closing of the hand during the grasp occurred earlier. No effects were found of wearing the telestereoscope under monocular viewing. These findings suggest that binocular information is important in the timing of the grasp. The timing results are also not consistent with the use of the binocular tau-function as proposed by Laurent *et al.* (1996).

Wann (1996), in reviewing the existing evidence of tau, argues that subjects actually use a relative-distance strategy during catching. That is, movements are initiated at the moment that the distance from the object to the observer divided by the initial distance between object and observer (zeta) reaches a particular value. Wann demonstrated that the use of zeta might provide a better explanation of the subjects' behaviour in the punching ball experiment (see Lee *et al.*, 1983) than tau. Note that for different velocities, subjects are not expected to behave in accordance with a constant time-to-contact strategy. Hence, the actual contribution of the tau-function of vergence and zeta in controlling the timing of the catch might be discerned by using different velocity profiles for the approaching ball.

The zeta-strategy holds that movements are initiated when the distance from the object to the observer divided by the initial distance between object and observer reaches a critical value. In contrast to the generalised tau-hypothesis from Bootsma and Tresilian, which predicts a constant time-to-contact strategy for constant approach velocities, the zeta-hypothesis predicts that in case of lower velocities the catch will be initiated earlier. To test this, Van der Kamp (1999) had subjects catch balls approaching at different constant velocities (i.e. 0.5, 1.0, 1.5, 2.0 and 2.5 m/s). In agreement with the zeta-hypothesis, catchers initiated the grasp earlier, the slower the approach. However, calculations indicate that the differences between the velocity conditions are not in agreement with a relative-distance strategy. In contrast, a strategy based on the relative rate of constriction of the gap between the moving ball and the hand seem to fit the observed temporal grasping patterns best.

To summarise, these results do not lend support for the strong version of direct perception theory. Indeed, these results suggest that a one-to-one mapping between information and action seems difficult to support. The presence of multiple information sources guiding the timing of the grasp in catching suggests a many (or few)-to-one mapping as proposed by directed perception theory (Cutting, 1986; Laurent *et al.*, 1996). Consequently, the catcher (or any other observer) has to deal with more perceptual degrees of freedom and, depending on the task circumstances, has to select the most appropriate information source available. These findings suggest that an appropriate research strategy is first to identify the different information sources contributing to guiding an action and then to explore the particular selection mechanisms involved in the emergence of skilled action (Laurent *et al.*, 1996).

4. Constraints and the development of catching

As shown by Von Hofsten (1983), catching starts to develop quite early in life, even in infancy. Nevertheless, considerable changes in catching ability can be found until about 12 years of age. Alderson (1974) observed that, at least from 7 to 12 years of age, the ability to locate the hand in the correct position seems to be an important factor in determining catching performance. Fischman *et al.* (1992) examined the influence of age, gender and ball location (e.g. approach of the ball above the head, out to the side, at waist height or shoulder height). They showed that catching performance between 5 to 12 years improved with age, with boys generally performing better than girls did. By 5 years of age children were found to have begun to exhibit the rudiments of skill in one-handed catching. However, at this age, children's performance (in terms of successful catches) was only slightly better than chance. By the age of 12, children had essentially mastered the skill of catching.

Ball location appears to be an important task constraint in catching performance, although the effect of ball location appears similar across age and gender. Tosses that were farthest from the trunk region (e.g. above the head and out to the side) were much more definitive in forcing the use of an appropriate hand orientation than tosses that were closer to the body (e.g. shoulder height). Thus, the location of the ball approach constrains the child's selection of an appropriate hand–arm orientation. In addition, Fischman and co-workers found that some young children selected a correct hand orientation but were not able to catch the ball successfully. In contrast, some older children selected an inappropriate hand orientation but were able to catch the ball successfully. Specifically, for 11- and 12-year-old boys, a combined total of 34 inappropriate hand orientations were observed for a toss at the waist, yet 33 of these (97 per cent) resulted in successful catches. These findings were similar to ones obtained by Strohmeyer and co-workers (Strohmeyer *et al.*, 1991), who suggest that some of the older subjects may have 'played' with the way they responded when tosses were to less challenging locations. As children become more skillful, they have more freedom to experiment with their responses. From a constraint-led perspective, one could argue that these findings indicate a freeing of the degrees of freedom as children explore the task. Before explaining this issue further a short intermezzo is necessary to explain the degrees of freedom concept.

Degrees of freedom and constraints

An important characteristic of successful performance is that the movements of all the components (e.g. muscles, tendons, joints etc.) of the motor apparatus of the human body have to be controlled. Bernstein (1967) realised that the non-linear nature of the interactions among these different components of the human body makes separate regulation impossible. Bernstein inferred that to be able to control all these components, or degrees of freedom, these movements have to be co-ordinated. Co-ordination, therefore, is the process of mastering the redundant degrees of freedom into a controllable system (Bernstein, 1967, p.127). Several researchers (e.g. Vereijken *et al.*, 1992; Steenbergen *et al.*, 1995) have provided evidence for three stages in learning with respect to Bernstein's degrees of freedom, namely *freezing*, *freeing* and *exploiting* the degrees for freedom. Vereijken *et al.* (1992) provide a nice example of this concept in a study that examined learning to ski on a ski-simulator. Skiing on a simulator involves standing on a platform attached to a spring and moving the platform to the side in a ski-like fashion. Vereijken *et al.* (1992) found that, at the beginning of practice, novices tried to apply force to the platform at a biomechanically inefficient moment. When using this strategy one does not benefit from available elastic forces stored in the stretched springs. With experience, subjects learned to exploit the characteristics of the apparatus, postponing their application of force until after the platform had passed the centre of the apparatus and started to slow down. With this strategy, subjects made use of the elastic forces that gave them a 'free ride' back to the centre of the apparatus and beyond, allowing them to reduce their active muscle forces.

The catching findings of Strohmeyer *et al.* (1991) and Fischman *et al.* (1992), indicate that as children become more skilful, they experiment more freely with their responses. In Bernstein's terms this exploration can be described as a shift from freezing to freeing of the degrees of freedom. Another example of this concept stems from a paper published in 1937, where Wellman identified three levels of development in two-handed catching (Wellman, 1937). At the age of 3½ years children hold their arms stiff and straight at the elbows, in front of their body (freezing of degrees of freedom). At 4 years of age the children open their hands to receive the object even though the arms remain stiff. By 5 years of age, children assume a more relaxed position, with arms bent at the elbow and hands ready to receive the ball (freeing of degrees of freedom).

In order to examine the impact of postural constraints on catching, Davids and his colleagues ball (Davids *et al.*, 2000) had good and poor catchers (10-year-olds) perform a one-handed catching action in both a seated and standing condition. In the standing position the act of raising the arm to align the hand with the flight path of the approaching ball is constrained by the upright posture, which also influences the perception of spatio-temporal information about the coupling of the hand and ball (Davids *et al.*, 2000). The findings show that poor catchers performed better in the seated condition than while standing. This result suggests that for the poor catchers reducing the degrees of freedom (freezing) served to improve performance. For good catchers the opposite result was obtained, with the best catching performance occurring during the standing condition. These results suggest that reducing the degrees of freedom available (freezing) to be exploited in the seated condition places the good catchers at a disadvantage. The standing position provides the good catchers with additional degrees of freedom that they are able to exploit in order to make corrections at the last instance prior to grasping the ball.

Visual information and the development of catching

With respect to learning and development, one might ask whether subjects become attentive or sensitive to different or additional visual information sources or whether the selection mechanisms themselves change. Some insight into this issue can be gained from a study conducted by Bennett and colleagues (Bennett *et al.*, 1999a). These researchers examined one-handed catching under various informational constraints in 9- to 10-year-old children. One group of children practised under restricted visual conditions; that is, neither the hand nor the ball was visible for the last 150 ms of the ball flight. After this practice the children performed the catching task with full visual information. A separate group of children caught first in the full vision condition, followed by the restricted visual condition. The visually restricted group showed a greater increase in catching performance than the full vision practice group. The authors suggest that the children under the restricted vision conditions were forced to seek additional information. In other words, by varying the visual informational constraints, they were encouraged to pay attention to different or additional information for catching.

Van der Kamp *et al.* (1996) investigated a similar question; namely, whether children are attentive to the same information sources during the development of the timing of catching. That is to say, do the same information sources constrain the timing of the grasp in catching over the course of childhood? If it is indeed, at least partly, the temporal accuracy that develops in one-handed catching during childhood, is this due to improvements in timing the grasp, and what is the role of informational constraints? In other words, do children become sensitive or attentive to different information sources during the acquisition of simple one-handed catching? A preliminary answer might be found in a study of Isaac (1983), in which 5- to 12-year-old children were required to time the closure of their hand. To this end, children were provided with a row of lights that were illuminated successively, simulating two different approach velocities (about 2.2 and 4.4 m/s). At the moment the light reached the target, the children had to close their hand around a ball. The two approach velocities led to differences in timing, although among 11- and 12-year-olds these differences disappeared. Isaac argued that because completion of the grasp in all conditions occurred within a very restricted time range, from about 30 ms before until 50 ms after the target light lit up, this result cannot explain the increment in catching performance with age. After all, the amount of variability was such that it did not fall outside the time-window for a successful one-handed catch. However, the presence of velocity effects, except for the older children, suggests that younger children, in contrast to adults, did not use a constant time-to-contact or tau-margin strategy. But, because the available information from a row of lights is vastly different from the information generated by an approaching ball, it might be that Isaac's (1983) findings can not be generalised to actual catching. Nevertheless, the results suggest a change in information sources used to control the timing of the grasp.

Van der Kamp *et al.* (1996) investigated the timing of the grasp in one-handed catching in 4- to 11-years-olds. One of the purposes of the study was to examine whether catching performance was hampered by the inability of the children to time their catch accurately. These investigators also wanted to determine whether, throughout childhood, there is a change in the information sources contributing to the control of the temporal properties of hand closure. The experimental setting was similar to that of Van der Kamp *et al.* (1997) described above. Children were required to catch three different sized balls (between 3 and 7 cm, depending on hand size) under both binocular and monocular viewing conditions. Both the younger (4 to 7 years) and the older (8 to 11 years) children performed well; on average only about 4 out of 30 balls were missed.

Kinematic analyses did not show any significant differences in timing between the younger and older children, although there was a tendency for the younger children to initiate their grasp somewhat earlier.

As figure 12.4 illustrates, children from both age groups behaved in accordance with a constant time-to-contact or tau-margin strategy when provided with binocular vision. In contrast, in the monocular viewing condition, the grasp was initiated and completed later for the smaller balls; that is to say, a constant time to contact was not present. Note that these findings were similar to those found in adults (Van der Kamp *et al.*, 1996). Thus, dependent on the circumstances (task constraints), children as well as adults use different information sources, and this leads to small differences in the timing of the catch. (Although small, the differences between monocular and binocular viewing conditions are meaningful in the sense that the number of caught balls is less when monocular viewing is used.)

From early on in childhood, children seem to be attentive to the same informational constraints as adults when timing the grasp phase in simple one-handed catching. That is, early in childhood the control of the temporal characteristics of the grasp is similar to that in adults. As a default argument, what is learned in the development of catching during childhood is not so much control over the grasp and hold phase, but control over the gross and fine orientation phase, that is to say, over the spatial (and temporal?) positioning of the hand in the flight trajectory of the ball.

Recently, Savelsbergh and Van der Kamp (2000) defended the thesis that information and movement are tightly coupled. As a result of this tight coupling,

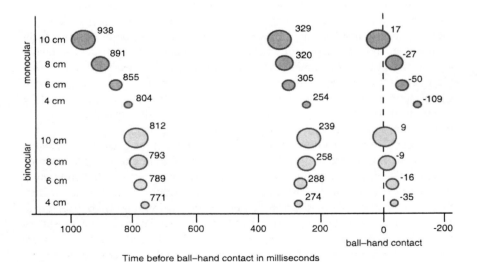

Figure 12.4 The timing of the catch for balls of different diameters under monocular and binocular viewing in children from 4 to 11 years of age. Illustrated are, from left to right, the moment of onset of the catch, the moment of maximal hand aperture, and the moment of completion of the catch.

they argue that specificity of training is required in order to get meaningful learning effects. These authors illustrated this thesis by elaborating upon the role of informational constraints in the control and learning of one-handed catching. They proposed the existence of different phases in the learning of information–movement coupling in order to explain the sometimes contradictory experimental findings with respect to adults' catching performance. The next section discusses the relevance of the model for the development of catching.

5. Stages in the coupling of information and movement

Savelsbergh and Van der Kamp (2000) consider the learning (and development) of information–movement coupling to be analogous to the learning sequence of freezing, freeing and exploiting the degrees of freedom as proposed by Bernstein. The basic idea is that depending on the specific constraints, i.e. the available visual information, multiple information sources are involved. That is to say, different types of visual information at different times (in development) may be used to perform the required job successfully. The idea is that, as Bernstein has described degrees of freedom with respect to the motor system (Bernstein, 1967), the concept of degrees of freedom can also be used with respect to the visual system. We refer to this concept as 'perceptual degrees of freedom', suggesting that multiple sources of information are available for controlling the same task. During learning and development, analogous to the movement degrees of freedom, perceptual degrees of freedom show the same sequence of freezing, freeing and exploiting. More specifically, the couplings of information and movement take place following this sequence. First, the learning and developmental process starts with the emergence and strengthening of a coupling between information and movement (the freezing; figure 12.5a). That is, within a certain set of constraints, a particular coupling between information and movement emerges, which fits the task requirements. With repetition the strength of this (successful) coupling increases. In other words, the movement gets tuned to information. As such, it enhances the probability that this coupling re-occurs under a similar set of constraints. This eventually results in a freezing out of other potential couplings, and an increasing stability of the pattern. However, when in this early phase of learning and development the particular set or interaction of constraints changes, the coupling will be disturbed and the action will break down. An alternative coupling between information and movement may not be available or may be too weak to lead to successful performance. More practice will then be required to strengthen the alternative coupling between information and movement that is specific to the new set of constraints. This brings us to the next stage.

The second stage involves freeing different information–movement couplings (figure 12.5b). Practice and experience under different sets of constraints will eventually lead to a whole repertoire of possible information–movement couplings for a certain task. Hence, if certain constraints change, the actor will be able to realise another available coupling, without the need to learn it from scratch. Moreover, in contrast to the early stage of learning, such a change of constraints

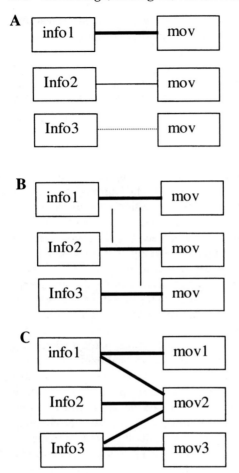

Figure 12.5 Stages of learning: (A) the strengthening: the coupling between information (info1) and movement (mov) gets stronger during practice, but not for info2 and mov etc.; (B) freeing: one can jump from one strong coupling to another, and (C), exploiting: information (info1) can be used for different actions (mov1 and mov2) and different perceptual information (info2 and info3) for the same movement (mov2) (Adapted from Savelsbergh and Van der Kamp, 2000).

will not lead to a complete breakdown of the action. Skilled performance, from our perspective, can be characterised by the ability to exploit different information–movement couplings (figure 12.5c). Because the child has a whole repertoire of information–movement couplings, it is possible for him/her to exploit the information that is available under a different set of constraints. That is to say, information (e.g. about time to contact) may be tuned to one movement (e.g. catching), but it may also be exploited for another movement (e.g. avoidance behaviour). Moreover, when the required information is absent, the child may use different information (e.g. monocular or binocular tau; see section 3 of this chapter) for the same movement (e.g. punching a ball).

From this perspective, the development of catching can be understood as a constraint-led approach in which the child will go through the three stages (freezing, freeing, exploiting) every time a new coupling of information and movement emerges as a result of changing constraints.

6. Conclusions and practical applications

Research into human movement has been heavily inspired by the work of two seminal workers, the Russian physiologist Bernstein and the American psychologist Gibson. Combining the ideas of Bernstein and Gibson, the ecological approach to perception and action searches for 'constraints on action' that reduce the total number of degrees of freedom. The identification of these constraints is a fruitful avenue for investigating the motor performance, learning, and development of goal-directed actions like catching. As reflected in this chapter, considerable progress has been made on how informational constraints tune skilled movements to the environment. In contrast, studies examining the development of visual and haptical control of movements seem to be rather sparse (but see Adolph *et al.*, 1993; Gibson, 1969). However, with respect to children it is still to be determined what visual information is important for catching, and how exactly visual information controls the development of catching. For instance, the large changes in the visual system during the first year of life, such as the emergence of binocular vision, the increase in acuity, and the growth of the visual field (Van Hof-Van Duin, 1989), suggest that informational constraints must have an important role in the development of action. This conclusion was also reached in a study by Van der Meer *et al.* (1995), who showed that in healthy infants from 6 to 12 months, the timing of catching laterally moving objects changes from a distance-to-contact to a time-to-contact strategy, suggesting a change in the information sources used to control action. It is realistic to assume that such changes occur during development all the time. The model suggested by Savelsbergh and Van der Kamp (2000) is a first attempt to explore and eventually understand the role of informational constraints in development and learning. The model can act as a framework to understand why information and movement are coupled under certain sets of constraints. What does this model imply for teachers and coaches?

First, visual information also 'tells' how and when to move for instance, in the case of a child heading a ball after a corner kick in soccer, the child must move at a precise time to successfully score a goal (Savelsbergh and Van der Kamp, 2001). To be successful in catching a fly ball in baseball, an outfielder must be at the right time at the right spot. Again, accurate perception is indispensable. Visual information about the ball flight trajectory 'tells' the child or the outfielder how and when to run. When a fielder tracks the ball, a moving image of the ball will form on the individual's retina. Research shows (see section 3; e.g. Oudejans, 1996) that the child should run such that he/she cancels out the acceleration of the ball's image on the retina. If s/he manages this, s/he is sure to intercept the ball.

Hence, visual information specifies how to move, or to put it differently, information and movement are tightly coupled.

Second, the inseparability of perception and movement implies that specificity of practice is very important (Savelsbergh and Van der Kamp, 2001). That is to say, what should be learned during practice is to couple information and movement. For instance, training should match the game situation as closely as possible. The visual information available during training should correspond with the information during the match. In the case of teaching a child to head a ball, the training should involve running and jumping for the ball. Training involving just a few jumps from a standing position or tossing a ball to a stationary player is not likely going to enable the child to get his/her head to right place at the right time during the actual match. The key point here is that the set of constraints should be the same in the training and game situations. If they are not the same, then children may use different information to perform the task in the training and game situation and thus not be able to perform successfully during a game. During practice sessions, a teacher or coach should create an environment (a set of constraints) in which a specific coupling of information and movement is facilitated. In other words, a teacher has to create a training environment whereby the child is 'forced' to tune to a specific information–movement coupling. We call such an environment a facilitative environment (see Buekers, 2000).

Third, because information and movements are tightly coupled, changes in the information that is available will lead to changes in action and overall performance. At the same time, changes in action lead to perceptual changes. This means for a coach or teacher that s/he may be able to change movements by giving a type of instruction that makes children attune to specific perceptual information.

Fourth, the learning sequence is of great importance. From the present perspective, the processes of learning and development serve to establish and further refine information–movement couplings. We have argued that the learning process of coupling information to movement consists of a sequence of mutually overlapping phases; that is, freezing, freeing and exploiting perceptual information. Consider a youngster learning to contact and catch a ball. The approaching ball provides a huge amount of visual information sources that can be used: information that 'tells' the time until the ball reaches the hand, the speed and direction of the ball's approach, the distance between ball and hand etc. The youngster faces the problem of finding out what information results in optimal performance; that is, positioning the hand correctly and absorbing the impact of the ball. Early in learning, the youngster selects one of multiple information sources that will do the job. At this stage the choice is likely not to lead to optimal performance. For example, distance information can be used to position the hand more or less correctly. Practice under a similar set of circumstances will refine or increase the strength of the coupling between distance information and positioning the hand. However, for accurate ball control, distance information alone leads to errors. Under slightly different conditions (e.g. high ball speed) the coupling gets disrupted, leading to failure to control the ball (the hand is positioned late or the ball bounces from the hand).

After reaching a certain degree of stability in performance, the second learning phase starts where alternative information–movement couplings are explored (freeing). Practice will unavoidably take place under different circumstances at this phase. The child at this phase is forced to explore other sources of visual information as a means to control the ball: distance information alone appears insufficient. Eventually, this leads to a whole repertoire of information–movement couplings for the task of contacting and controlling a ball. As a result, the performance of the youngster becomes much more flexible, and s/he learns to adapt to changing conditions, i.e. tunes in to different couplings, without starting from scratch each time. The child is on his or her way to become a skilled performer.

Skilled performance is characterised by the ability not only to use different information couplings, but to exploit them as well. Since the youngster now has a whole repertoire available, he or she may use them for tasks other than controlling the ball. That is, information (e.g. about ball approach) may get coupled not only to the original movement (e.g. contacting and controlling a ball) but also to other movements in different conditions (e.g. hitting or heading). In short, the original information-movement coupling forms the foundation for new couplings to emerge.

In conclusion, particularly during the early phase of learning, specificity of practice is implied. In the first instance, information gets coupled to movement only under similar conditions. Hence, specificity of practice is needed. During latter phases, however, practice should take place under more variable conditions such that a repertoire of couplings can be formed and further exploited. What does this mean for the organisation of practice?

First, as said before, the coach or teacher should create a certain set of conditions that pushes the player to become attuned to a specific information–movement coupling. Instead of forcing the player, the coach needs to create a facilitative environment (Buekers, 2000). Second, the specificity of practice should dominate the early, but *not* the later, phases of learning. At these later phases, the child should build on the established couplings to exploit other information–movement couplings under different conditions.

In general, many coaches, trainers and teachers already use different types of environmental facilitators (e.g. piles, or other players). However, these 'environmental facilitators' should always be similar to circumstances in game situations, as otherwise the relevant information–movement coupling will not be established.

Acknowledgement

This chapter was written while the third author was supported by the Foundation for Behavioural Sciences (grant number 490-00-243), which is funded by the Netherlands Organisation for Scientific Research (NWO).

Note

1 The chapter is based on two published papers, namely Van der Kamp, Vereijken and Savelsbergh (1996) and Savelsbergh and Van der Kamp (2000).

References

Adolph, K.E., Eppler, M.A. and Gibson, E.J. (1993) Development of perception of affordances. In C. Rovee-Collier and L.P. Lipsitt (eds), *Advances in Infancy Research*, 8 (pp. 51–89). Norwood, NJ: Ablex.

Alderson, G.J.K. (1974) The development of motion prediction ability in the context of sport skills. Unpublished PhD thesis, Department of Physical Education, University of Leeds.

Alderson, G.J.K., Sully, D.J. and Sully, H.G. (1974) An operational analysis of a one-handed catching task using high speed photography. *Journal of Motor Behaviour*, 6, 217–26.

Bahill, A.T. and LaRitz, T (1984) Why can't batters keep their eyes on the ball. *American Scientist*, 72, 249–53.

Babler, T.G. and Dannemiller, J.L. (1993) Role of image acceleration in judging landing location of free-falling projectiles. *Journal of Experimental Psychology: Human Perception and Performance*, 19, 15–31.

Bernstein, N.A. (1967) *The Co-ordination and Regulation of Movements*. Oxford: Pergamon Press.

Bennett, S.J., Button, C., Kingsbury, D. and Davids, K. (1999a) Manipulating visual informational constraints during pratice enhances the acquisition of catching skill in children. *Research Quarterly for Exercise and Sport*, 70, 220–32.

Bennett, S.J., Van der Kamp, J., Savelsbergh, G.J.P. and Davids, K. (1999) Timing a one-handed catch: I. Effects of telestereoscopic viewing. *Experimental Brain Research*, 129, 362–8.

Buekers, M. (2000) Can we be so specific to claim that specificity is the solution for learning sport skills? *International Journal of Sport Psychology*, 31, 485–9.

Chapman, S. (1968) Catching a base-ball. American *Journal of Physics*, 36, 868–70.

Cutting, J.E. (1986) *Perception with an Eye for Motion*. Cambridge, MA: The MIT Press.

Davids, K., Bennett, S.J., Kingsbury, D., Jolley, L. and Brain, T. (2000) Effects of postural constraints on children's catching behavior. *Research Quarterly for Exercise and Sport*, 71, 69–73.

Fischman, M.G., Moore, J. and Steele, K. (1992) Children's one-handed catching as a function of age, gender, and ball location. *Research Quarterly for Exercise and Sport*, 63, 349–55.

Gesell, A. (1929) Maturation and infants behavior pattern. *Psychological Review*, 36, 307–19.

Gibson, E.J. (1969) *Principles of Perceptual Learning and Development*. Englewood Cliffs, NJ: Prentice-Hall.

Gibson, J.J. (1979) *The Ecological Approach to Visual Perception*. Boston: Houghton Mifflin.

Heuer, H. (1993) Estimates of time to contact based on changing size and changing target vergence. *Perception*, 22, 549–63.

Isaac, L.D. (1983) Coincidence-anticipation in simple catching. *Journal of Human Movement Studies*, 9, 194–201.

Judge, S.J. and Bradford, C.M. (1988) Adaptation to telestereoscopic viewing measured by one-handed ball-catching performance. *Perception*, 17, 783–802.

Kugler, P.N., Kelso, J.A.S. and Turvey, M.T. (1982) On the control and coordination of naturally developing systems. In J.A.S. Kelso and J.E. Clark (eds), *The Development of Movement control and Coordination* (pp. 5–78). New York: John Wiley and Sons.

Land, M.F. and McLeod, P. (2000) From eye movements to actions: How batsmen hit the ball. *Nature Neuroscience*, 3, 1340–5.

Laurent, M., Montagne, G. and Durey, A. (1996) Binocular invariants in interceptive tasks: a directed perception approach. *Perception*, 25, 1437–50

Lee, D.N. (1976) A theory of visual control of braking based on information about time-to-collision. *Perception*, 5, 437–59.

Lee, D.N. and Young, D.S. (1985) Visual timing in interceptive actions. In D.J. Ingle, M. Jeannerod and D.N. Lee (eds), *Brain Mechanisms and Spatial Vision* (pp. 1–30). Dordrecht: Martinus Nijhoff.

Lee, D.N., Young, D.S., Reddish, D.E., Lough, S. and Clayton, T.M.H. (1983) Visual timing in hitting an accelerating ball. *Quarterly Journal of Experimental Psychology*, 35a, 333–46.

McBeath, M.K., Shaffer, D.M. and Kaiser, M.K. (1995) How baseball outfielders determine where to run catch fly balls. *Science*, 268, 569–73.

McGraw, M.B. (1945) *The Neuromuscular Maturation of the Human Infant*. New York: Columbia University Press.

McLeod, P. and Dienes, Z. (1993) Running to catch the ball. *Nature*, 362, 23.

Michaels, C.F. and Beek, P.J. (1995) The state of ecological psychology. *Ecological Psychology*, 7, 259–78.

Michaels, C.F. and Oudejans, R.R.D. (1992) The optics and actions of catching fly balls: Zeroing out optical acceleration. *Ecological Psychology*, 4, 199–222

Montagne, G., Laurent, M., Durey, A. and Bootsma, R. (1999) Movement reversals in ball catching. *Experimental Brain Research*, 129, 87–92.

Morange, F. and Bloch, H. (1996) Laterlization of the approach movement and the prehension movement in infants from 4 to 7 months. *Early Development and Parenting*, 5, 81–92.

Newell, K.M. (1986) Constraints on the development of coordination. In M. Wade and H.T.A. Whiting (eds), *Motor Development in Children: Aspects of Coordination and Control* (pp. 341–60). Dordrecht: Martinus Nijhoff.

Oudejans, R.D.D. (1996) *The Optics and Actions of Catching Fly Balls*. PhD thesis. Enschede: PrintPartners Ipskamp.

Peper, L., Bootsma, R.J., Mestre, D. and Bakker, F.C. (1994) Catching balls: how to get the hand to the right place at the right time. *Journal of Experimental Psychology: Human Perception and Performance*, 20, 591–612.

Provine, R.R. and Westerman, J.A. (1979) Crossing the midline: Limits of early eye-hand behavior. *Child Development*, 50, 437–41.

Savelsbergh, G.J.P. (1995) Catching 'Grasping tau': Comments on J.R. Tresilian (1994) *Human Movement Science*, 14, 125–7.

Savelsbergh, G.J.P. and Van der Kamp, J. (1994) The effect of body orientation to gravity on early infant reaching. *Journal of Experimental Child Psychology*, 58, 510–28.

Savelsbergh, G.J.P. and Van der Kamp, J. (2000) Information in learning to co-ordinate and control movements: Is there a need for specificity of practice? *International Journal of Sport Psychology*, 31, 467–84.

Savelsbergh, G.J.P. and Van der Kamp, J. (2001) Training must be as specific as possible, but not always! *Insight*, 4, 48–9.

Savelsbergh, G.J.P., Whiting, H.T.A. and Bootsma, R.J. (1991) 'Grasping' Tau. *Journal of Experimental Psychology: Human Perception and Performance*, 19, 315–22.

Savelsbergh, G.J.P., Whiting, H.T.A., Burden, A.M. and Bartlett, R.M. (1992) The role of predictive visual temporal information in the coordination of muscle activity in catching. *Experimental Brain Research*, 89, 223–8.

212 *Savelsbergh, Rosengren, van der Kamp and Verheul*

Savelsbergh, G.J.P., Whiting, H.T.A., Pijpers, J.R. and van Santvoord, A.M.M. (1993) The visual guidance of catching. *Experimental Brain Research*, 93, 146–56.

Shirley, M.M. (1933/1976) *The First Two Years: A Study of Twenty-five Babies: I Postural and Locomotor Development*. Minneapolis: University of Minnesota Press.

Steenbergen, B., Marteniuk, R.G. and Kalbfleisch, L.E. (1995) Achieving coordination in prehension: Joint freezing and postural contributions. *Journal of Motor Behavior*, 27, 333–48.

Strohmeyer, H.S., Williams, K. and Schaub-George, D. (1991) Developmental sequences for catching a small ball; A prelongitudinal screening. *Research Quarterly for Exercise and Sport*, 62, 257–66.

Thelen, E. Fischer, D.M. and Ridley-Johnson, R. (1984) The relationship between physical growth and newborn reflex. *Infant Behavior and Development*, 7, 479–93.

Tresilian, J.R. (1994) Perceptual and motor processes in interceptive timing. *Human Movement Sciences*, 13, 335–73.

Van Hof-Van Duin, J.J. (1989) The development and study of visual acuity. *Developmental Medicine and Child Neurology*, 31, 543–52.

Van der Kamp, J. (1999) *The Information-based Regulation of Interceptive Actions*. PhD thesis. Nieuwegein: Digital Printing Partners Utrecht.

Van der Kamp, J., Savelsbergh, G.J.P. and Davis, W.E. (1998) Body-scaled ratio as control parameter for prehension of 5–9 year old children. *Developmental Psychobiology*, 33, 351–61.

Van der Kamp, J., Savelsbergh, G.J.P. and Smeets, J.B. (1997) Multiple information sources in interceptive timing. *Human Movement Science*, 16, 787–822.

Van der Kamp, J., Vereijken, B. and Savelsbergh, G.J.P. (1996) Physical and informational constraints in the coordination and control of human movement. *Corpus, Psyche et Societas*, 3, 102–18.

Van der Meer, A.L.H., Van der Weel, F.R., Lee, D.N., Laing, I.A. and Lin, J.P. (1995) Development of prospective control of catching moving objects in preterm at-risk infants. *Developmental Medicine and Child Neurology*, 37, 145–58.

Van Hof, P., Van der Kamp, J. and Savelsbergh, G.J.P. (2002) The relation of unimanual and bimanual reaching to crossing the midline *Child Development*, 73, 1353–62.

Vereijken, B., Whiting, H.T.A. and Beek, W.J. (1992) A dynamical systems approach towards skill acquisition. *Quarterly Journal of Experimental Psychology*, 45A, 323–44.

Von Hofsten, C. (1983) Catching skills in infancy. *Journal of Experimental Psychology: Human Perception and Performance*, 9, 75–85.

Wann, J. (1996) Anticipating arrival: is the Tau margin a specious theory? *Journal of Experimental Psychology: Human Perception and Performance*, 22, 1031–48.

Wellman, B.L. (1937) Motor achievements of preschool children. *Childhood Education*, 13, 311–16.

Wickstrom, R.L. (1983) *Fundamental Motor Patterns*. Philadelphia: Lea Febiger.

13 Degrees of freedom, movement co-ordination and interceptive action of children with and without cerebral palsy

Annieck Ricken, Geert Savelsbergh and Simon J. Bennett

1. Introduction

Many activities combine walking with the interception of a target (e.g. reaching/ hitting a tennis ball). Successful performance of these tasks requires a fine-tuned organisation of the motor control system. For children with cerebral palsy (CP) who have motor disorders caused by damage to the brain, this requires a specific type of movement co-ordination. In this chapter a model is described (see figure 13.1), which is inspired by theories and ideas falling under the rubric of ecological psychology, that is used to understand and describe the organisation of movement co-ordination of children with spastic hemiplegia CP during interceptive actions. The model is derived from concepts and theories of Newell (1986), Gibson (1979) and Bernstein (1967) (for a discussion see chapter 12). It shows us how movement co-ordination emerges from the control of the multiple degrees of freedom (DF) of the biomechanical movement system (joints, muscles and nerves) and the perceptual system and, more importantly, the interaction between them in the form of information–movement couplings.

According to the ecological approach, the interaction between information and movement depends on the constraints that are imposed by the environment, the task and the organism. Movement creates information, which in its turn is used to control movement. Using the model depicted in figure 13.1, this chapter describes how the movement co-ordination of children with and without CP in interceptive action tasks is organised. It provides insight into how children with CP are able to

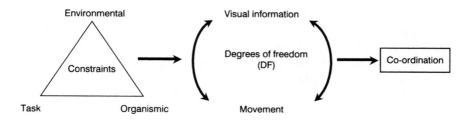

Figure 13.1 Theoretical model of movement co-ordination (see text for explanation)

adapt to their changed constraints (motor disorders) and when and how they are organizing the movement co-ordination in interceptive action. This knowledge may be used to inform rehabilitation procedures and the teaching of sports to children with CP.

2. Theoretical model for describing movement co-ordination

According to Bernstein (1967), movement co-ordination involves the free(z)ing of the redundant degrees of freedom (DF) of joints, muscles, nerves and cells. By freezing the redundant DF, limb and joint movements become temporarily coupled and a co-ordination emerges that satisfies the task goal. However, early in practice this co-ordination is often not optimal in terms of energy efficiency (Sparrow and Irizarry-Lopez, 1987) or performance outcome (Vereijken, 1991; Vereijken *et al.*, 1992). As skill acquisition progresses, the DF are gradually released and a more appropriate co-ordination emerges that takes advantage of passive and elastic forces such as gravity and stored mechanical energy. According to this perspective, the process of free(z)ing DF, and the resulting co-ordination, self-organise under constraints. For example, when a full cup has to be picked up (i.e. task constraint), the DF in the shoulder and elbow joints are tightly coupled to act as a single unit (i.e. frozen), while the DF of the trunk are released in order to achieve smooth movement of the distal end of the effector, and hence not spill the cup's contents (Steenbergen *et al.*, 1995). With an empty or half empty cup the task constraints are altered (i.e. less necessity for smooth movement) and a different co-ordination between the DF emerges.

While different definitions of the constraints on the process of co-ordination have been reported (see Van der Kamp *et al.*, 1996) the idea that they act to constrain the redundant DF is a common theme. According to Newell (1986), there are three categories of constraints; environmental, task and organismic, which form the boundaries that limit the subsequent co-ordination. Environmental constraints are defined as constraints that are external to the organism. Newell distinguishes *general* environmental constraints, which are not manipulated by the experimenter and are relatively time-independent (e.g. natural light, gravity), and *task-specific* environmental constraints, which can be manipulated by changing the environment in which the activity takes place. Task constraints are imposed by the goal, rules and implements or machines used. Intercepting a ball during walking is a task constraint on movement co-ordination, as the resulting co-ordination of the upper limb in relation to the ball will be limited by the act of walking. Organismic constraints are functional constraints of the body (e.g. mechanical, physiological, cognitive and anatomical). During development, organismic constraints can change very quickly and therefore they may be associated with large-scale changes in co-ordination (Thelen and Fisher, 1982).

The self-organisation of co-ordination under constraints is a dynamical process that is dependent on the perception of information related to key properties (e.g. time to contact) of the relationship between the performer (e.g. haptic information from muscles and joints) and the environment (e.g. visual information from an approaching ball). A change in constraints that is not perceived will not 'inform' the performer that a change in co-ordination is necessary. Clearly then, the nature of the surrounding constraints determines the perceptual information available. For example, a moving ball will provide additional sources of information about the spatial and temporal properties of the performer–environment relationship compared to a stationary ball (e.g. relative rate of expansion). When developing perceptual–motor skills, the performer explores their environment to obtain information about how to co-ordinate their movements. Consequently, there is a continuous information–movement coupling between the performer and their environment (Gibson, 1979). Information that becomes available about an event, an object or the layout of the environment affords a particular action. Upon the performance of this action, information is made available that is used to further explore the environment. The development of perceptual–motor skills and information–movement couplings, may therefore be influenced by the surrounding constraints (see Ulrich, 1989 for a discussion of how locomotion is influenced by constraints imposed by the environment).

3. CP as an organismic constraint on movement co-ordination

Cerebral palsy (CP) is an 'umbrella term' used to cover a group of non-progressive disorders of motor function, which often differ between individuals. Such disorders are a result of a lesion to the immature brain (Ingram, 1966; Hagberg and Hagberg, 1993) and occur before, during or after birth. The location of the lesion determines the resulting symptoms. CP can be divided in several subgroups based on the affected limb or limbs: hemiplegia, diplegia and quadriplegia. CP can also be described on the level of motor functioning: spastic, athetoid and ataxic. These terms are usually combined in the literature. Also, their motor disorders may engender visual–spatial deficits (Abercrombie, 1964).

In children with spastic hemiplegic CP, the spasticity in the legs and/or arms acts as an organismic constraint on movement co-ordination. The spastic arm muscles and the rigid elbow and wrist joints constrain the available DF to act as a single unit. Consequently, DF in other joints and muscles will be released to find an optimal movement co-ordination (see Archaumbault *et al.*, 1999; Steenbergen *et al.*, 2000). The organismic constraints in CP children are substantially different from those in healthy children, and therefore result in quite different motor development and movement co-ordination. In addition, the exploration of the environment and the resulting information–movement couplings will be different in children with CP compared to healthy children, due to the movement disorders (e.g. spasticity, athetoid and ataxia). The influence of spastic hemiplegic CP as an organismic constraint on co-ordination in interceptive action will be discussed in the following sections.

4. Interceptive action in children with CP

Recently, some research has been done on co-ordination of the upper limbs in interceptive action tasks (e.g. reaching and grasping) in adults with hemiplegic

CP (Van Thiel, 2001; Steenbergen, 2000; Roby-Brami *et al.*, 1997) (see chapter 10). These studies showed that adults with CP co-ordinate an interceptive action differently, by free(z)ing DF in other joints and performing more segmented movements. Hence, they exemplify an adaptive movement strategy to the constraints imposed by CP. Although there has been little research on interceptive action in children with CP, this section will explain the different aspects in the co-ordination of interceptive action in children with CP.

Perception–action coupling and cerebral palsy

Recently, a unified approach to perception and action has been adopted in studying the perception–action coupling of adults or children with CP or spastic hemiparesis caused by stroke (Lough, 1985; Howard and Henderson, 1989; Lee *et al.*, 1990; Van der Weel *et al.*, 1991, 1996; Savelsbergh *et al.*, 1998; Steenbergen *et al.*, 1998; Van Thiel *et al.*, 2000). Results from these studies showed that adults and children with CP use different strategies in co-ordinating interceptive actions compared to those without.

Katz *et al.* (1998) showed that children with left hemiplegia (right hemisphere damage) might have relatively greater attentional and perceptual problems than children with right hemiplegia (left hemisphere damage). However, this does not clearly indicate a left unilateral neglect. Children with right hemiplegia also have attentional and perceptual problems relative to controls, particularly on complex tasks. The left hemisphere plays a role in the organisation and execution of voluntary movement, while it is well known that the right hemisphere plays a role in spatial processing.

Howard and Henderson (1989) examined the perceptual judgement of door apertures in relation to body size of children with and without CP. Children had to judge whether or not they could walk through the opening. Their findings showed that children with CP were less accurate in this task than the control group. This significant difference in judgements could be due to lack of motor experience with the task at hand. A more recent study by Savelsbergh *et al.* (1998) examined judgements of, in comparison to actual walking through, door apertures by children with and without CP. With respect to judgements, differences were found between 5- to 7-year-old CP children in comparison to children without CP. The young children with CP were less accurate in their judgements. However, no differences were found when the actual task was carried out, with children with CP performing as accurately as the controls. This indicates that experience of coupling movement with the relevant information (e.g. door width) is of great importance.

Affordances and cerebral palsy

Perceiving affordances play an important role in guiding an action. It tells us whether an organism is able to perceive what is within reach, what is graspable and what locomotor pathways are available. The use of this kind of information relates to a higher level of decision-making and is dependent on knowledge of our body and the world of objects, and more importantly the relationship between the them. All optical variables contain (i.e. afford) important body- or action-scaled information about distance, size and velocity, as well as about time. The perception of affordances is based on intrinsic optical information and the relationship between environmental properties and properties of the observer's own action system (Warren, 1984). Therefore, what is afforded depends on the action capabilities of the individual (Konczak *et al.*, 1992). For example, a 5-year-old child perceives the environment in relation to its own action capabilities and will respond to this in a different way from a 10-year-old child. The same applies for a child with CP, who perceives objects in the environment in relation to their action capabilities. Anthropometrics and biomechanical constraints, such as force generation and flexibility of movements, which are different in children with and without CP, define the action capabilities. This is also called body-scaled or action-scaled information. In a study by Van der Meer (1997) children with CP had to pass under a barrier of various heights. It was found that children with CP scale perceptual information in terms of their body characteristics and action capabilities, and therefore they were able to perceive the affordance of the barrier. Försstrom and Von Hofsten (1982) studied children with neurological problems who had to perform a task that required the interception of a small object on the end of a moving rod. Results suggested that the disabled children took into account a projected movement delay in intercepting the object, thus demonstrating body/action scaling in relation to the perceptual information.

Constraints, degrees of freedom and cerebral palsy

The co-ordination of interceptive action depends on the constraints that are imposed. Considering spastic hemiplegic CP children, the limbs of one side of the body show muscular co-contraction. The spasticity in the arm does not enable it to stretch fully, and this organismic constraint therefore results in a modified way of co-ordinating arm movements such as reaching for a ball. As we know from Newell's model and theory, the system is able to adapt to constraints and searches for solutions to the problem of co-ordinating movements. According to Bernstein's theory, redundant degrees of freedom are recruited and used to solve the co-ordination problem. In the case of children with CP reaching for a ball with the spastic arm, this may result in compensation from the trunk while reaching for a ball. In the next section the compensating strategies in interceptive action tasks will be further explained with reference to previous research in individuals with CP performing interceptive actions.

Interceptive action and cerebral palsy

The interceptive action of reaching and grasping involves moving the upper limb segments away from the body towards the object. It involves the co-ordination of the many degrees of freedom of the shoulder, elbow, wrist and trunk, such that they move fluently and efficiently (i.e. sequencing of body segments). This is achieved by free(z)ing the DF in the body. Steenbergen *et al.* (2000) studied the kinematics of upper limbs, the joint and trunk involvement and the interlimb coupling in unimanual and bimanual reaching and grasping in young adults with spastic hemiplegic CP. These individuals are characterised as having spasticity in the muscles on one side of the body. Results of the study showed that angular change in the elbow and shoulder joints of the CP participants on the impaired side was reduced, while trunk involvement was increased when reaching for an object. Further, individuals with CP showed more segmented movements.

Van Thiel and Steenbergen (2001) studied shoulder and hand displacements during hitting, reaching and grasping in hemiparetic CP. It was found that there was more shoulder displacement, due to trunk translation and rotation. This may reflect an adaptive strategy which people with CP use, as they actively avoid extreme joint angles because of the increased stretch reflexes that occur near the end of joint excursion during reaching. This results in a decrease in functional angular changes in the elbow and shoulder, which results in the impaired limb being less involved in daily activities, which in turn promotes the occurrence of muscle contracture. To summarise, people with CP have less DF available in the impaired arm to co-ordinate movements. To complete a task successfully, they will therefore recruit DF in other parts of the body, as indicated by more trunk movement or shoulder rotation during the interceptive action task. Although other DF in the body are used, the movement is often co-ordinated optimally, in terms of total movement costs, and functionally, in terms of end-posture comfort within their action capabilities (Steenbergen, 2000). For example, picking up a cup always occurs with a specific posture of hand, arm and trunk (functionally) through which the total energy movement cost is kept low (optimally). The redundancy of the DF of the movement system allows adaptive movement behaviour when constraints change. The trunk involvement may be considered as an efficient adaptation to the altered constraints. It is a successful, adaptive reaction to reduced joint mobility in the affected arm of people with spastic hemiplegic CP. It is adaptive because participants are capable of flexibly recruiting and sequencing the various DF of their impaired side required for successful task completion, albeit in different magnitudes and sequenced differently.

Similar results have been reported by Archaumbault *et al.* (1999), Cirstea and Levin (2000) and Roby-Brami *et al.* (1997). They studied adults with hemiparesis, due to cerebrovascular lesions, performing reaching/pointing and grasping tasks. Movements of the hemiparetic participants were more segmented and slower compared to healthy adults. They concluded that in people with hemiparesis, the recruiting and sequencing of degrees of freedom might be impaired or that new DF were recruited that were typically not used by a healthy population. These studies showed that adults with CP or hemiplegia co-ordinate an interceptive action differently compared to healthy participants, because of free(z)ing DF in other parts of the body and by showing more segmented movements.

It is expected that the above findings hold true for children with CP (6–12 years). However, there has been little research on the organisation of movement co-ordination of children with CP to substantiate this claim. Utley and Sugden

(1998) studied the interlimb coupling during unimanual and bimanual reaching and grasping in children with CP. They showed that these children coupled their hands temporally. This coupling reduced some of the movement difficulties that are often seen in children with CP. Van der Weel *et al.* (1991) studied the movement co-ordination of children with CP when performing abstract (non-functional) and concrete (functional) tasks. The children with CP found non-functional tasks, such as extending the arm as much as possible, more difficult than functional tasks, such as reaching to grasp an object. The above studies of the interceptive action in children with CP show that they are able to make more co-ordinated interceptive actions when the interceptive action is performed under a different set of constraints.

Although there has been some studies of relatively simple tasks, there has been no work studying movement co-ordination of children with CP in more complex tasks, such as performing an interception with the upper limb while walking towards a target. This is a task that can be seen in most sport activities, which requires a complex co-ordination between upper and lower limbs in relation to an external target. A recent study by Ricken *et al.* (2002) has examined movement co-ordination during interceptive action and locomotion in healthy children (for a study with healthy adults see Marteniuk *et al.*, 2000, and Marteniuk and Bertram, 2001). The authors looked at the displacement of the hand relative to a fixed, world-centered frame of reference (e.g. a table in a room) and relative to a body-centered frame of reference (the trunk). The latter method of analysis effectively eliminates the movement of the trunk (including any contribution from gait) from the movement of the hand. Therefore, it allows the movement of the hand to be viewed independently from the movement of the rest of the body. The results showed that participants reached with a skewed bell-shaped trajectory of the wrist in both standing and walking conditions when analysed from a world-centred frame of reference. However, when the trajectory of the hand was analysed relative to the subject's trunk, a body-centered frame of reference, a far more complicated pattern was observed in the walking condition than when compared to the standing condition. There was no longer a skewed, bell-shaped trajectory, and in fact the net displacement of the hand was backward towards the trunk in the walking condition (see figure 13.2).

The results showed that locomotion influences the degree of trunk contribution, with more flexion and rotation being exhibited. The combination of an interception with the hand while walking towards the target required a re-organisation of the redundant DF. The movements of the hand in the walking condition reflect a compensation for the trunk's forward displacement during locomotion. Apparently the arm and body-movements of healthy children are acting in co-operation to produce smooth bell-shape trajectories when it involves complex, combined locomotion and interceptive action tasks.

To our knowledge no research has been conducted on interceptive action during locomotion in children with CP. Ongoing research expects to find that the trajectory of the hand will not be as smooth and bell-shaped as that of a healthy child, due to the problems in locomotion and the problems in controlling the spastic muscles of the arm. When analysing the co-ordination from a body-centered point of view, it

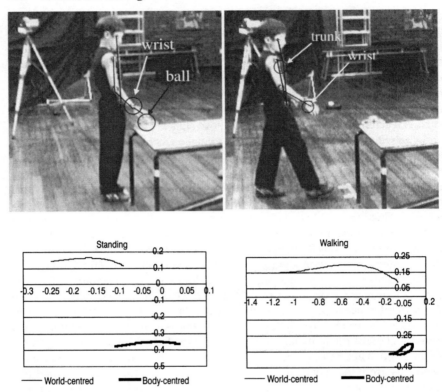

Figure 13.2 Interception of a stationary ball, analysed from a world (A) – and body (B) centered frame of reference in a standing (C) and a walking (D) condition

is expected that the results will demonstrate more trunk involvement. This will evidence how the two systems act in co-operation in children with CP who have altered DF in the arm due to its spasticity. Studying the way in which children with CP use the DF available to them will give us more insight into the organisation of movement co-ordination in different task conditions, and this might be useful in an early stage of development and also useful for teachers/trainers of physical education/sport.

5. Practical implications

Performing a sport requires controlling not only the degrees of freedom of the joints, muscles and nerves, but also the degrees of freedom of the information–movement couplings. Ball sports require a complex combination of picking up visual information and anticipating where to move, and finally co-ordinating the motor action in order to be in the right position at the right time to make a successful interception. Children with CP have difficulty performing these actions, but are still able to perform all kinds of sports in a very professional way (for example the paralympics).

Sport activities require a specific movement co-ordination and perception–action coupling to perform the tasks correctly. Children with CP, as well as healthy children, are able to perceive the necessary information sources in sport activities and couple these to their movement. Although it is unknown if they use the same information sources as healthy children to support action, it can still be reasoned that in learning sports, where interceptive action is involved, children with CP are freeing and freezing out certain information–movement couplings to perform the interceptive action correctly. Smyth *et al.* (2001) recently showed that children with movement disorders use less visual information that is available to them compared to children without movement disorders (see also chapter 8). In catching a ball with one hand, a child with spastic hemiplegic CP will find and use the information source that results in optimal control of the non-impaired or impaired hand. This is positioning the hand correctly at the right time by freeing or freezing certain DF in joints and muscles, and absorbing the impact of the ball to keep it in the hand. Following practice under similar circumstances, t!.e strength of the information–movement coupling will be refined or increased (Savelsbergh and Van der Kamp, 2000). Practice must therefore take place under different circumstances, where alternative information–movement couplings can be explored for perfect control of interceptive action. Eventually, this leads to a whole repertoire of information–movement couplings for action. As a result, the performance of the child becomes more flexible and the child learns to adapt to changing conditions, i.e. tunes into different couplings.

Other means of improving practice, and hence learning, in children with CP are also required. Essentially, these should involve the task being performed to be simplified during practice (Brown, 1987). This may involve reducing the confusion of visual information, thereby simplifying the decision-making process, or reducing the available DF in the body by simplifying the task (sitting instead of standing, or standing in stead of walking). It may also involve the use of alternative materials to simplify the motor actions. Large balls are easier to handle than small ones and are easier to see. Catching a small ball requires very accurate visual tracking ability and fine manipulation, and also the placement of the hands is necessary with only a small margin of error between success and failure. Teachers or coaches should organise problem-solving situations which allow the children to experiment and discover individual patterns of movement (such as additional use of degrees of freedom in for example trunk, shoulder etc.) that are efficient in producing reasonable accuracy. This approach should lead to the children learning to discover their action capabilities in a variety of situations and should also lead to their discovering fundamental principles about the information–movement coupling. It is also necessary to decide if supplementary information must be provided to perform a task successfully, as stated in previous section.

Research has to be conducted to find out what are the best methods of teaching children with CP during sport activities to develop information–movement couplings and to adapt to their altered constraints. Physiotherapy should therefore not only concentrate on promoting movement patterns, which may or may not transfer to perceptuo-motor activities of daily life, but should also concentrate on allowing the children discover the information–movement couplings within their own action capabilities.

References

Abercrombie, M.L.J. (1964) *Perceptual and Visuomotor Disorders in Cerebral Palsy. A Survey of Literature.* London: Spastics Society Med. Educ. and Information Unit.

Archambault, P., Pigeon, P. and Feldman, A.G. (1999) Recruitment and sequencing of different degrees of freedom during pointing movements involving the trunk in healthy and hemiparetic subjects. *Experimental Brain Research,* 126, 55–67.

Bernstein, N.A. (1967) *The Co-ordination and Regulation of Movements.* London: Pergamon Press.

Brown, A. (1987) *Active Games for Children with Movement Problems.* London: Harper and Row.

Carnahan, H., McFadyen, B.J., Cockell, D.L. and Halverson, A.H. (1996) The combined control of locomotion and prehension. *Neuroscience Research Communications,* 19, 91–100.

Cirstea, M.C. and Levin, M.F. (2000), Compensatory strategies for reaching in stroke. Brain, 123, 940–953.

Försstrom, A. and Von Hofsten, C. (1982) Visually directed reaching of children with motor impairments. *Developmental Medicine and Child Neurology,* 24, 653–61.

Gibson, J.J. (1979) *The Ecological Approach to Visual Perception.* Boston: Houghton Mifflin.

Hagberg, B. and Hagberg, G. (1993) The origins of cerebral palsy. In: T.S. David (ed.), *Recent Advances in Paediatrics,* pp. 67–83. Churchill Livingstone.

Howard, E.M. and Henderson, S.E. (1989) Perceptual problems in cerebral palsied children: a real-world example. *Human Movement Science,* 8, 141–60.

Ingram, T.T.S. (1966) The neurology of cerebral palsy. *Archives of Disease in Childhood,* 41, 337–57.

Katz, N., Cermak, S., Shamir, Y., (1998) Unilateral neglect in children with hemiplegic cerebral palsy. *Perceptual and Motor Skills,* 86, 539–50.

Konczak, J., Meeuwsen, H.J. and Cress, M.E. (1992) Changing affordances in stair climbing: the perception of maximum climb-ability in young and older adults. *Journal of Experimental Psychology: Human Perception and Performance,* 18, 691–7.

Lee, D.N., Daniel, B.M. and Turnbull, J. (1990) Basic perceptuo–motor dysfunctions in cerebral palsy. In M. Jeannerod (ed.), *Attention and Performance XIII Motor Representation and Control* (pp. 583–603), Hilsdale, NY: Erlbaum, Associates.

Lough, S. (1985) Visuo–motor control following stroke: a motor skills perspective. PhD thesis, Edinburgh University.

Marteniuk, R.G. and Bertram, C.P. (2001) Contributions of gait and trunk movements to prehension from world- and body-centered co-ordinates. *Motor Control,* 2, 151–65.

Marteniuk, R.G., Ivens, C.J. and Bertram, C.P. (2000) Evidence of motor equivalence in a pointing task involving locomotion. *Motor Control,* 4, 165–84.

Newell, K.M. (1986) Constraints on the development of co-ordination. In M. Wade and H.T.A. Whiting (eds), *Motor Development in Children: Aspects of Co-ordination and Control* (pp. 341–60). Dordrecht: Martinus Nijhof.

Ricken, A.X.C., Savelsbergh, G.J.P. and Bennett, S.J. (2002) Co-ordination of interceptive action during locomotion of children. In C. Craig, L. Fernandez and R.J. Bootsma (eds), *Proceedings of 7th European Workshop on Ecological Psychology*, pp. 47–8. Bendor Island, France.

Roby-Brami, A., Fuchs, S., Mokhtari, M. and Bussel, B. (1997) Reaching and grasping strategies in hemiparetic patients. *Motor Control*, 1, 72–91.

Savelsbergh, G.J.P. and Van der Kamp, J. (2000) Information in learning to co-ordinate and control movements: Is there a need for specificity of practice? *International Journal of Sport Psychology*, 31, 467–84.

Savelsbergh, G.J.P., Douwes Dekker, L., Vermeer, A. and Hopkins, B. (1998) Locomoting through apertures of different width: a study of children with CP. *Pediatric Rehabilitation*, 2, 5–13.

Smyth, M.M., Anderson, H.I. and Churchill, A. (2001) Visual information and the control of reaching in children: a comparison between children with and without developmental co-ordination disorder. *Journal of Motor Behaviour*, 33, 306–20.

Sparrow, W.A., Irizarry-Lopez, V.M. (1987) Mechanical efficiency and metabolic cost as measures of learning a novel gross motor skill. Journal of *Motor Behavior*, 19, 240–64.

Steenbergen, B. (2000) The Planning and Co-ordination of Prehension Movements in Spastic Hemiparesis. Nijmegen: Universal Press Veenendaal.

Steenbergen, B., Marteniuk, R.G. and Kalbfleisch, L.E. (1995) Achieving co-ordination in prehension: joint freezing and postural contributions. *Journal of Motor Behavior*, 27, 333–48.

Steenbergen, B., Hulstijn, W., Lemmens, I.H.L. and Meulenbroek, R.G.J. (1998) The timing of prehensile movements in subjects with CP. *Developmental Medicine and Child Neurology*, 40, 108–14.

Steenbergen, B., Van Thiel, E., Hulstijn, W. and Meulenbroek, R.G.J. (2000) The coordination of reaching and grasping in spastic hemiparesis. *Human Movement Science*, 19, 75–105.

Thelen, E. and Fisher, D.M. (1982) Newborn stepping: an explanation for a 'disappearing' reflex. *Developmental Psychology*, 18, 760–75.

Ulrich, B.D. (1989) Development of Stepping Patterns in Human Infants: A Dynamical Systems Perspective. *Journal of Motor Behavior*, 21, no. 4, 392–408.

Utley, A. and Sugden, D. (1998) Interlimb coupling in children with hemiplegic cerebral palsy during reaching and grasping at speed. *Developmental Medicine and Child Neurology*, 40, 396–404.

Van der Kamp, J., Vereijken, B. and Savelsbergh, G.J.P. (1996) Physical and informational constraints in the coordination and control of human movement. *Corpus, Psyche et Societas*, 3, 102–18.

Van der Meer, A.L.H. (1997) Visual guidance of passing under a barrier. *Early Developmental Parenting*, 6, 149–57.

Van der Weel, F.R., Van der Meer, A. and Lee, D.N. (1991) Effect of task on movement control in cerebral palsy: implications for assessment and therapy. *Developmental Medicine and Child Neurology*, 33, 419–26.

Van der Weel, F.R., Van der Meer, A. and Lee, D.N. (1996), Measuring dysfunction of basic movement control in cerebral palsy. *Human Movement Science*, 15, 253–83.

Van Thiel, E. (2001) *(Dis)ordered Motor Control: Characterizing Arm Movements in Hemiparetic Cerebral Palsy*. Nijmegen: Universal Press Veendaal.

Van Thiel, E. and Steenbergen, B. (2001) Shoulder and hand displacements during hitting, reaching and grasping movements in hemiparetic cerebral palsy. *Motor Control*, 2, 166–82.

Van Thiel, E., Meulenbroek, R.G.J., Hulstijn, W. and Steenbergen, B. (2000) Kinematics of fast hemiparetic aiming movements toward stationary and moving targets. *Experimental Brain Research*, 132, 230–42.

Vereijken, B. (1991) The dynamics of skill acquisition. Unpublished doctoral dissertation, Free University, Amsterdam.

Vereijken, B., Van Emmerik, R.E.A., Whiting, H.T.A. and Newell, K.M. (1992) Free(z)ing degrees of freedom in skill acquisition. *Journal of Motor Behavior*, 24, 133–42.

Warren, W.H., Jr. (1984) Perceiving affordances: Visual guidance of stair climbing. *Journal of Experimental Psychology: Human Perception and Performance*, 13, 371–83.

14 The development of throwing behaviour

Allen W. Burton and
Richard W. Rodgerson

1. Introduction

The onset of locomotion around 6 to 8 months opens for infants a new world to be explored by direct manipulation. This event profoundly affects an infant's perceptual, social, and cognitive development (Bertenthal *et al.*, 1984). Bipedal locomotion, emerging at an average age of about 12 to 13 months, changes a child's visual perspective, enhances mobility, and frees the hands to continue to explore and interact with the environment. Two other developmental skills allow children to interact with the environment without direct touch or manipulation: language (verbal and nonverbal) and throwing. Verbal language and throwing begin to be used in a functional manner at about the same age that walking appears (Halverson, 1940; Lenneberg, 1967), and both offer children opportunities to extend their sphere of influence beyond the boundaries of the body.

In most motor development textbooks, information on throwing – as well as other object-control skills such as catching, striking, kicking, and dribbling – is limited to tasks using balls. Indeed, most research on the development of throwing involves the throwing of balls, or perhaps bean bags, but many objects other than balls are thrown by children and adults. Accordingly, we assume a broad definition of throwing, as articulated by Halverson (1940): 'Throwing is long-distance placement of objects' (p. 84). Also, we want to emphasise along with Halverson that throwing 'projects the hand through the intervening space toward the spot by means of the object' (p. 84).

This broad definition of throwing fits well with Newell's (1986) model of constraints on motor development. From an ecological perspective, Newell argues that an optimal pattern of co-ordination and control for any activity is determined by three categories of constraints: performer, environment, and task. The performer category addresses who is the performer and the unique set of personal attributes that may affect movement co-ordination for that person. The environment category considers where and with what the person is performing, and the task category considers why a person is performing. In this model, Newell acknowledges that different people may throw a wide variety of objects, in a wide variety of settings, for a wide variety of reasons. The final question, how the person performs a skill, is a consequence of the three factors, depicted by Newell as a triangle of constraints.

In this chapter, we want to provide a broad perspective of the development of throwing behaviour in children from 4 to 12 years of age. We begin by considering why humans throw, exploring the connections between anatomical evolution, hunting, throwing, and sport and games. Then research on changes in throwing outcomes across the elementary-school years is presented, followed by a section on research related to changes in throwing form. We end the paper by discussing some ideas for future investigation.

2. Why do humans throw?

Humans throw because their anatomy and physiology has been shaped over time to allow them to throw; in other words, they throw because they can. Throwing is deeply implicated in the phylogenetic history of humans. Indeed, throwing is sometimes referred to as a phylogenetic skill (Gallahue and Ozmun, 1998). An organism must have a hand to be able to throw, and primates, unlike other mammals, have hands that are able to grasp and manipulate objects with some sophistication (Fragaszy, 1998). Researchers have reported aimed throwing in nonhuman primate species, such as capuchin monkeys (Westergaard and Suomi, 1994) and Japanese macaques (Tokida *et al.*, 1994). For example, Tokida *et al.* wrote that one female macaque developed an underhand throwing technique to free apples from a pipe. Jane Goodall (1986) observed many instances of hurling and throwing in her Gombe troop of chimpanzees. She commented that

> In addition to the generalized hurling of objects during displays, chimpanzees throw stones, rocks, or sticks at definite objectives such as conspecifics, baboons, humans, or a variety of other species. Aimed throwing may be overhand or underhand: larger missiles are more often thrown underhand, and sometimes launched with both hands.
>
> (Goodall, 1986 p. 550)

Goodall further noted that chimpanzees have good aim, but that their throws often fall short of the target, and that males are more likely to throw than females.

The achievement of bipedal locomotion frees the hands of an infant to manipulate objects and throw; in a similar manner, the phylogenetic milestone of bipedal locomotion acted as a launching pad for the reorganisation of hominid bones, muscles, and neurons, shaping the capacity to throw. Morphological changes associated with the emergence of Homo habilis between 1.6 and 2.0 million years ago included evolved changes to the hand and thumb leading to increased dexterity and a more powerful grip (Trinkaus, 1986). Considerable paleoanthropological evidence suggests that hunting and the concomitant sexual division of labour was a major selective agent in human evolution (Tooby and DeVore, 1987). The specific skill of throwing allowed hunters to capture prey beyond the reach of their limbs and provided a distinct survival advantage.

Fossil evidence suggests differences between Neanderthal and early modern humans in scapular glenoid physiology. These differences, associated with an increase in the potential range of motion of the human arm, have been linked to throwing and projectile use in early modern humans (Churchill and Trinkaus, 1990). Marzke, Longhill, and Rasmussen (1988) posited a connection between gluteus maximus muscle function in the origin of bipedal locomotion and trunk rotation required to throw and club with force. Wilson (1998) summarised the fossil and archeological evidence association with the evolutionary history of the human hand and concluded,

> The ownership of the old arm, mounted on a new pelvis, aided by a highly advanced visual system and bipedality, and stimulated by the reality of having no real alternative to living on the savannah, meant that ballistics would become the inaugural centerpiece of a new hominid survival strategy.
>
> (Wilson, 1998, p. 76)

However, the performer constraint explanation that humans throw because they can is not adequate in Newell's (1986) scheme, nor is congruent with the fundamentals of evolution. Newell argues that the task and environment must be considered in explaining the development of co-ordination, and evolutionary theory dictates that anatomical and physiological changes must be driven by survival advantage. So, humans threw in our evolutionary past because elusive prey offered nourishing and tasty moving targets in the environment, and throwing provided an effective means of accomplishing the task of hunting and, ultimately, surviving. In modern societies, throwing is no longer used much for hunting and surviving, although it is used in many functional activities, such as getting a piece of trash into a garbage bin, quickly relaying a tool or toy to another person, or scaring off a nearby animal. Nevertheless, the throwing tasks of hunting and survival are still reflected in the games and sports throughout history.

The play of young animals has been theorised to fit them for the tasks of later life (Groos, 1911) and the psychological appeal of the games and sports children and adults play has been suggested to be directly homologous with our ancestral past (Tiger, 1984). Most games and sports involve running (chasing and escaping), aiming and throwing (hunting), or wrestling and fighting (male dominance activities). Throwing games, in particular, are an important part of play for children around the world. Eibl-Eibesfeldt (1989), for example, describes make-believe arrow wars among the Eipo of New Guinea, where boys throw spear-like hardened grasses at one another. Eibl-Eibesfeldt also describes the 'melon ball dance' in which women and girls from the Kalahari Bushmen tribe in South Africa dance and rhythmically clap as they gently toss a melon from dancer to dancer. A study by the National Federation of State High School Associations (1997) listed the most popular interscholastic sports in the US for boys and girls separately and revealed that three of the top four for the boys (football, basketball, and baseball) and two of the top four for the girls (basketball and softball) contained some element of throwing.

Competitive throwing games also have an ancient lineage. Gardiner (1930), in his book *Athletics of the Ancient World*, described many forms of competitive throwing games. The javelin competition in the Olympic Games was derived from a common weapon of war and hunting for the Greeks. He added that the Greek word 'diskos' meant 'a thing for throwing', and that early discus and shot-put competitions involved throwing stones for distance. Competitive throwing games, including team games, were so important in ancient Sparta that males in their first year of manhood were called 'ball players'.

In explaining why humans throw, we have emphasised the links between a wide variety of games and sports and throwing, between throwing and hunting, and ultimately between hunting and evolved anatomy and physiology. Some scholars who study throwing and targeting behaviour have used the throwing–hunting–evolution connection as a theoretical foundation. For instance, Calvin (1982, 1994) speculated that the very narrow 'launch window' involved in accurate throwing and the related central processing requirements led to a phylogenetic expansion of neuronal circuits and that this expansion also allowed language to emerge. Kolakowski and Malina (1974) connected throwing with special abilities associated with hunting, such as navigational skills and spatial perception. Later, Jardine and Martin (1983) examined this same connection with respect to sex differences in throwing and spatial abilities.

The centrality of the task in Newell's (1986) model leads us to organise the measurement of throwing behaviour in developmental research according to a functional sequence. In hunting, its corollaries in modern games and sports, and other tasks, the primary goal is accuracy. An object thrown very fast at an animal is useless unless the animal is struck; a fast throw in baseball, basketball, or football is useless unless it reaches its intended target. Indeed, velocity needs to be adjusted according to the size and motion of the target (Indermill and Husak, 1984). Throwing form, then, must accommodate the accuracy and velocity requirements of the task. This is consistent with Oslin and Mitchell's (1998) 'form-follows-function' concept and Burton and Miller's (1998) three-step, top-down assessment sequence. In their sequenced strategy for assessing movement proficiency, Burton and Miller begin with functional movement outcomes (related to the task and the environment), move on next to movement patterns or form, and finally examine movement skill foundation (related to performer attributes). In the next section, we address the research on changes in throwing outcomes across the elementary-school years, followed by a section in which we consider the research related to changes in throwing form.

3. Changes in throwing outcomes across childhood

Accuracy, the most important outcome measure in throwing, has not been given much attention in the developmental literature, and most studies that have examined age-related changes in accuracy have some significant limitations. Further, a variety of measures have been used to quantify throwing accuracy, such as radial error or peculiar scoring systems based on a series of concentric target rings, so comparisons across studies are difficult.

Hoffman, Imwold, and Koller (1983) investigated the accuracy of first-, third- and fifth-grade boys and girls throwing small balls at a target only 1.6m away. This study was unique because four task conditions were presented to all participants: (a) person and target stationary (I); (b) person stationary, target moving (II); (c) person moving, target stationary (III); and (d) person and target moving (IV). Hoffman *et al.* found that the older children were significantly more accurate than the younger, the boys were significantly more accurate than the girls, and the difference between the boys and girls was greatest on Tasks II and IV, 'suggesting that gender-related performance differences were amplified as the complexity of the task was increased' (p. 39). The application of this research to most sport contexts was limited by the very short distance thrown, but it was impressive that age and sex differences still were revealed.

Rippee *et al.* (1991) conducted an ambitious study in which they examined throwing accuracy, velocity, distance, and form of first- and fourth-grade boys and girls. For the accuracy task, the children threw a baseball at a 48-inch-diameter target. The first graders threw from 10 and 15 feet, whereas the fourth graders threw from 20 and 25 feet. The scoring system showed that the fourth graders threw significantly more accurately than the first graders, and that the boys threw significantly more accurately than the girls. The attempt to account for differences in body sizes between the age groups by adjusting the throwing distances was commendable, but the fourth graders were not 67 per cent (25/15 = 1.67) to 100 per cent (20/10 = 200 per cent) taller than the first graders. Despite the relative disadvantage of the older children, they still threw significantly more accurately.

In a recent study, Burton *et al.* (2000) investigated age-related changes in both throwing accuracy and velocity. They had second-grade, fourth-grade, sixth-grade, and young adult males and females throw a baseball or softball at three distances: two, four, and six times the individual's height. Thus, both ball size and throwing distance were scaled to each individual's hand size and height. Another unique feature of this study was that the participants were encouraged to throw accurately rather than hard or fast by giving them a small amount of money for every throw going through the 12-inch-diameter target hole. The results showed that, at the two longer distances, mean radial error (the distance of a throw from the centre of the target hole) was significantly lower for sixth graders and adults than second graders, and significantly lower for males than females at the two longer distances. The actual number of 'hits' or throws through the target hole was significantly higher for males and older participants, regardless of the distance.

The combined results of three studies (Burton *et al.*, 2000; Halverson *et al.*, 1982; Sakurai and Miyashita, 1983) reveal a consistent, linear increase in maximum throwing velocity from kindergarten to seventh grade (5 to 12 years) for both boys and girls, and an increasing advantage of boys over girls with advancing age (see figure 14.1). The tasks were very similar in the three studies: Halverson *et al.*, in a longitudinal design, had their participants throw a tennis ball 'hard' through a 'velocimeter' placed 3 feet in front of them; Rippee *et al.* had their participants throw a baseball 'as hard as possible' a distance of 25 feet; and Burton *et al.* had their participants, at the end of their accuracy trials, throw a baseball or softball

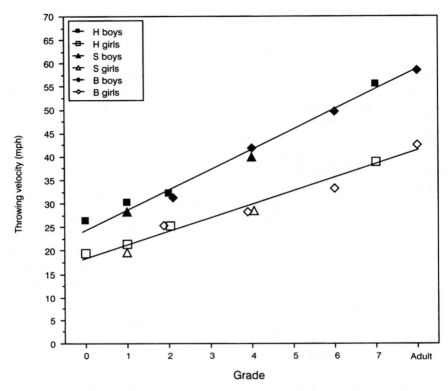

Figure 14.1 Mean throwing velocity for boys and girls by grade. Data from Halverson *et al.* (1982) [H], Sakurai and Miyashita (1983) [S], and Burton *et al.* (2000) [B].

'as fast as possible' a distance equivalent to six times their height. Halverson *et al.* did not examine the statistical significance of the age and sex effects, but both Rippee *et al.* and Burton *et al.* reported significant age and sex effects, as well as a significant age × sex interaction. Two of the co-authors in the Halverson *et al.* group recently replicated the throwing velocity aspects of original study only with seventh graders to determine if Title IX, federal legislation in the US to equalise sport opportunities for males and females, had any effect on sex differences in throwing velocity (Pulito *et al.*, 2000). They found no significant cohort effects nor any difference in the velocity gap between boys and girls, as also shown by Burton *et al.*'s data (see figure 14.1).

The best study of changes in maximum throwing distance across age was presented by Keogh (1969) in a technical report. Using a longitudinal design, he tested two cohorts of boys and girls over a period of four years at six-month intervals – one beginning at 6 years and the other at 8 years. The two cohorts followed a similar developmental path, with ball-throwing distance steadily increasing with age and boys throwing further than girls at all ages (see figure 14.2). In Rippee *et al'*.s (1991) throwing study, first- and fourth-grade boys and girls threw a softball

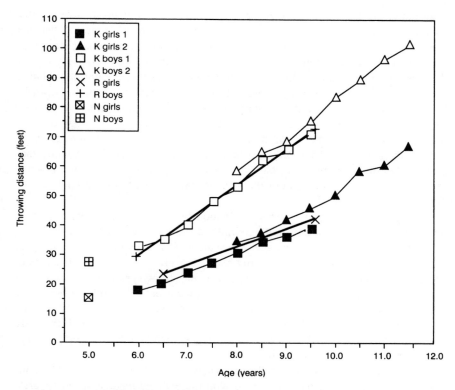

Figure 14.2 Mean throwing distance for boys and girls by age. Data from two longitudinal cohorts [1, 2] in Keogh (1969) [K], Rippee *et al.* (1991) [R], and Nelson *et al.* (1986) [N].

for maximum distance, and showed results very similar to Keogh's (see figure 14.2). They also reported statistically significant age and sex effects, and a significant age × sex interaction. The progression of throwing distance was extended down to 5-year-old boys and girls by Nelson *et al.* (1986), who reported a significant sex effect favouring boys and distances congruent with the developmental trends in Figure 2. This pattern of change for boys and girls matches the pattern found for changes in throwing velocity (compare figures 14.1 and 14.2), leading Rippee *et al.* to comment that distance and velocity 'are so highly correlated ($r = 0.90$) that for all practical purposes the two variables are the same' (p. 184).

Accuracy and velocity or distance are usually studied separately. Although an accurate throw requires a certain minimum velocity or distance, a fast or hard throw does not require a certain minimum accuracy. Thus, asking children to throw fast or hard without regard for accuracy, as done in most experiments, may not be very functional. Burton *et al.* (2000) perhaps were the first to examine the velocity of throws when the primary goal was accuracy. Because they measured maximum velocity after the accuracy trials were completed, Burton and colleagues could calculate the percentage of each individual's maximum velocity that was used in the accuracy trials. They found that percent maximum velocity did not significantly vary between males and females, but significantly interacted with age and distance such that the age effect was significant only at the two *shorter* distances. More specifically, at two and four times their height, the adults threw relatively slower than second, fourth, and sixth graders, but at six times their height, the relative velocities of the four age groups were not significantly different, ranging from 75 to 83 per cent of maximum velocity. Thus, despite significant age and sex differences at the longest distance for absolute velocity, the strategy used to maximise accuracy was essentially the same. The 75–83 per cent strategy at the longest distance was consistent with Indermill and Husak's (1984) finding that young adult males threw tennis balls at an archery target 12m away significantly more accurately at 75 per cent of their maximum velocity than at 50 per cent or 100 per cent.

The research on changes across childhood in throwing outcomes related to accuracy, maximum velocity, and maximum distance shows a consistent pattern of improvement with increasing age, boys performing better than girls at all ages, with the gap between them expanding over time. Burton *et al.* (2000) attribute these age-related changes in throwing performance to two primary factors: (a) the accumulation of practice and experience throwing balls and other objects for accuracy at a variety of distances, and (b) the continuing myelination of the cortico-spinal tract, which is 'the chief route through which the brain commands the body to perform voluntary movements, especially any kind of fine, fast, or highly skilled movement' (Eliot, 1999, p. 273).

Throwing differences between the sexes may well reflect the division of labour and intrasexual competition associated with the evolved history of our species. After studying sex differences in throwing performance for the past 15 years, Thomas (2000) offers three reasons why he believes that these differences reflect more than greater amounts of practice and opportunity for boys than girls: '(a) differences are three times as large as other motor performance tasks at ages 3–4 years; (b) biological variables are related to gender differences; and (c) differences are resistant to training' (p. 3). Thomas argues that throwing performances differences between males and females may be a remnant of an evolutionary adaptation. Phylogenetic adaptation has also been proposed by others to account for these robust findings (Geary, 1998; Jardine and Martin, 1983; Wilson 1998).

4. Changes in throwing form across childhood

The linkage between throwing performance and throwing form is eloquently stated by Hicks (1931): 'It is impossible to say that any one style of throwing is always best, for good throwing is throwing that produces good results' (p. 52). According to Davis and Burton (1991) in their ecological task analysis, the great variation in movement form across performers, environments, and tasks offers insight into how individuals perceive these three factors. Research conducted before Newell's (1986) landmark paper on constraints focused almost exclusively on variations in throwing form related to age and sex factors, holding the task (maximum force or velocity only) and environment constant. These investigations by Wild at the University of Wisconsin in the 1930s, Seefeldt and colleagues at Michigan State University in the 1960s, 1970s, and 1980s, and Roberton and colleagues at the University of Wisconsin in the 1970s and 1980s laid the foundation for under-standing developmental changes in throwing behaviour, but the manipulation of environmental and task factors is needed to completely understand this process.

Wild (1938) was one of the first researchers to study developmental changes in the form used to throw a ball overhand with force. After filming and analysing the throws of 2- to 12-year-old boys and girls, she described four stages of overhand throwing patterns: (a) directional movement of the upper body only; (b) horizontal turning of the trunk, but no step; (c) a shift in body weight with ipsilateral step; and (d) trunk rotation, arm adduction, and contralateral step. Earlier in the decade, Hicks (1931) observed 3- to 6-year-old boys and girls throw tennis balls at a moving target 5 feet away. He reported that 88 per cent of the throws performed overhand, 8 per cent underhand, and 4 per cent 'tossed', but found few differences in form by age or sex. When throwing overhand, most children used the arm and shoulder only, with no step, as in Wild's first stage.

In 1968, Seefeldt and his associates began a longitudinal study of fundamental movement skills that still continues today. From this extensive set of data, five stages of overhand throwing patterns were described (Seefeldt and Haubenstricker, 1974–6, as cited in Payne and Isaacs, 1999): stage 1 – feet usually stationary; little or no trunk rotation; force coming from hip flexion, shoulder protraction, and elbow extension; stage 2 – hips, spine, and shoulders rotating as one unit; either ipsilateral or contralateral step; arm brought forward in transverse plane, resembling a 'sling' rather than a throw; stage 3 – ipsilateral arm–leg action; little or no rotation of spine and hips in preparation for throw; ball placed above the shoulder by a vertical and posterior motion of the arm; stage 4 – contralateral arm–leg action; motion of the trunk and arm closely resembling stages 1 and 3; stage 5 – throwing hand moves in a downward arc and then backward as the contralateral leg moves forward; this action rotates the spine and hip into position for forceful derotation.

About 10 years after Seefeldt began his longitudinal study, Roberton (1977) serendipitously conceived a different approach to examine the development of overhand throwing patterns. She found that two sets of body component levels – one for arm action and the other for pelvic–spinal action – appeared to occur at different rates. Then, in a follow-up longitudinal study expanded to include three body components (humerus, forearm, and pelvis–spine), Roberton (1978) reported that from kindergarten to the second grade, 6 per cent of the participants progressed in all three components, 20 per cent in two, 39 per cent in only one, and 35 per cent showed no change or regressed in at least one. She concluded that 'the issue of "stages", then, must be confined to the ordering within the components rather than to the total body configuration, although the latter has been a traditional practice in motor development' (Roberton, 1978, p. 174). In a later account of this longitudinal study, Halverson *et al.* (1982) reported that boys were about one level advanced compared to girls – even as early as kindergarten, and first and second grades – in the humerus and forearm components. However, sex differences favouring the boys did not appear in the trunk (pelvis–spine) component until the seventh grade. Later, Roberton (1984) modified her developmental sequences of overhand throwing patterns for force to include five components (see figure 14.3).

Roberton's new component approach posed a challenge to the total-body-configuration approach used by Wild (1938) and Seefeldt and Haubenstricker (1974–6, as cited in Payne and Isaacs, 1999), in which each stage included a description of all relevant body components. Branta *et al.* (1984) admitted that they do not believe that 'all of the subroutines within a stage develop as an indivisible unit, or in lock-step fashion', but maintained that there is 'sufficient cohesion among certain characteristics of a pattern to define those as stages of development' (p. 470). Further, they argued that the total-body-configuration approach is the simplest way to describe a specific developmental task, like throwing overarm for force (Seefeldt and Haubenstricker, 1982).

Trunk component
1. no trunk action or forward–backward movements
2. upper trunk rotation or total trunk 'block' rotation
3. differentiated rotation

Backswing component
1. no backswing
2. elbow and some shoulder flexion (in front of head)
3. circular, upward backswing (behind head)
4. circular, downward backswing

Humerus component during forward swing
1. humerus oblique
2. humerus parallel, in front of shoulder at front-facing
3. humerus parallel, even or behind shoulders at front-facing ('lag')

Forearm component during forward swing
1. no forearm lag (ball and forearm move forward together)
2. forearm lag before front-facing
3. forearm lag delayed until after front-facing

Feet component
1. no step
2. homolateral or ipsilateral step
3. contralateral, short step
4. contralateral, long step

Figure 14.3 Levels of five components for the overhand throw for force (adapted from Roberton, 1984)

In 1993, Roberton and Langendorfer offered a rapprochement between the body-component and total-body-configuration views (Roberton and Langendorfer, 1993). They reanalysed throwing data from their original eight-year longitudinal study, involving only three body components with three levels for each component, and found only 11 of the 27 possible combinations of levels (3 humerus × 3 forearm × 3 trunk). Roberton and Langendorfer explained that the total-body-configuration approach focuses on the most frequently observed combinations, referring to them as 'strong attractor states'. However, they pointed out that less common transition combinations and combinations used in unique situations are not accounted for in this approach. In a more recent study, Langendorfer and Roberton (2000) examined the 'constellations of developmental levels' that occur with the highest level trunk pattern, differentiated rotation (see figure 14.3). They reported that on 89 per cent of the trials that involved differentiated rotation, circular-downward-backward backswing and humerus lag also were observed, and argued that 'intra-organismic constraints' are operating as the overarm throw develops. Thus, the total-body-configuration approach may be simpler and easier to use, which should be attractive to most practitioners, but the body-component approach accounts for more unique combinations of patterns, which should be important to researchers and practitioners who work with children with movement deficits.

Biomechanical analyses, in contrast to the qualitative analyses from the total-body-configuration or body-component views, offer more detailed information about changes in children's throwing patterns, but they are rarely reported in the published literature. Moreover, these biomechanical descriptions are difficult for practitioners to apply. Sakurai and Miyashita (1983) examined the throwing patterns of 3- to 9-year-old Japanese boys and girls using Wild's (1938) qualitative total-body-configuration system and a quantitative biomechanical analysis. Their biomechanical analysis showed that boys had a significant advantage over girls in elbow and wrist velocity as early as five years, and the ratio of initial ball velocity to wrist velocity at time of ball release ('snap' ratio) was significantly higher in boys from 7 years on.

Throwing form clearly changes as a function of age at different rates for boys and girls, but these age and sex interactions are tempered by environmental and task factors. For example, Burton, Greer, and Wiese (1992) found that differences between males and females were minimised when ball diameter was less than the performer's hand width. Two task factors that have been manipulated in studies of throwing form include ball size (Burton *et al.*, 1992; Burton, Greer and Wiese-Bjornstal, 1993) and force-vs.-accuracy requirements (Langendorfer, 1987).

In their study on the effect of ball size on throwing patterns, Burton and colleagues asked second graders, fourth graders, sixth graders, eighth graders, and young adults to throw styrofoam balls, ranging in diameter from 4.8 to 29.5 cm, 'as hard as possible' at a curtain 6.7m away. They did not specify an overhand throw, which allowed them to document incidences of one- and two-hand throws, underhand and sidearm throws, as well as variations in overhand patterns. Burton *et al.* (1993) reported that only 16 per cent of all throws were made with two hands, but 98 per cent of the two-handed throws were made with ball diameters greater than the individual's hand widths. A significant age and sex effect, showing that younger children and females were more likely to throw with two hands even when ball size was scaled to hand size, supported the developmental progression from two- to one-handed throws. The most common two-hand patterns were over the shoulder (48 per cent) and directly over the head (36 per cent).

Next, Burton *et al.* (1992) addressed variations in one-hand throws, accounting for 84 per cent of all throws. First, they observed that almost all (98 per cent) of the one-hand throws for force were overhand. Then, they reported that the mean modal level of four of Roberton's (1984) five components (backswing, humerus, forearm, and trunk, but not feet) significantly decreased as relative ball size increased, but that this effect of relative ball size was significantly greater in younger children. The three components most proximal to the ball in the hand – forearm and backswing, followed by humerus – were most sensitive to ball-size manipulations.

The effect of different task goals – specifically, force vs. accuracy – was investigated by Langendorfer (1987). He had fourth-grade and young-adult males and females throw a tennis ball at a 2.4m-diameter target, with the centre marked with a red dot, from a distance of 6 to 10m in two task conditions: (a) hit the red dot, and (b) throw hard as possible. He found that the force condition yielded significantly higher levels on four of Roberton's (1984) five components (all except backswing) for the males, but that the force condition produced a higher component level for the females only on the feet component for fourth graders. The importance of considering task factors in evaluating throwing patterns was verified by Langendorfer's and Burton's studies.

One additional factor that has been shown to affect throwing form in adults is the time constraints on a throw. In a recent study, Barrett and Burton (in press) videotaped and analysed over 3,000 throws made by college-level baseball players in real games. They found that the highest-level combination of forearm, backswing, and feet components was used by pitchers and outfielders on 84 per cent and 85 per cent of the 'active' throws made in an attempt to get an opponent out, whereas the highest-level combination was used by catchers and infielders on only 4 per cent and 13 per cent of their active throws and only 1 per cent and 3 per cent of their inactive throws. They offered three possible explanations: (a) the limited amount of time available to catchers and infielders to relay the ball to another player on active throws; (b) the constraint of players' postures, particularly the catchers on both active and inactive throws; and (c) an adaptation of inactive throws to the pattern used most often on active throws. In their latest paper, two researchers who have studied throwing for almost 25 years, Langendorfer and Roberton (2000), acknowledged the importance of time constraints by specifying forceful throws made 'under unhurried conditions' (p. S67).

5. Future research and application

An area of developmental research usually begins with informal observations, then moves on to careful descriptive reports. Descriptive information leads to the formation of testable hypotheses, and finally culminates in experiments involving the manipulation of independent variables in a controlled setting. Research on the development of throwing over the past 70 years has been dominated by descriptive studies, with true experimental studies appearing only since the 1980s. We believe that future research on the development of throwing behaviour needs to take two paths: first, a continuation and extension of the recent experimental work and, second, a step back to informal observations.

Newell (1986), in his model of constraints on movement co-ordination, recognises that uniform progressions of fundamental movement skills such as throwing are 'due to the similarity of constraints imposed on the infant and young children rather than a consequence of a common set of genetic prescriptions for the human specifies' (p. 355). Accordingly, insight into the development of throwing behaviour in children requires a careful examination of performer, environmental, and task constraints in relation to variations in throwing behaviour. We believe that understanding the developmental process begins with understanding the throwing task or why the person is throwing. Just about all research on throwing development requires participants to throw balls for accuracy, force, or distance, but we believe that the reasons why children, particularly very young children, spontaneously throw, need to be investigated using informal observation methods. Specifically, we feel that observations by researchers and parents of why, what, and how children throw, even as early as 8 to 12 months of age, may offer some new ideas regarding the well-documented sex differences. Explanations for the consistent differences between males and females in just about all aspects of throwing – accuracy, velocity, distance, and form – have been sought in numerous studies, but few answers have been provided.

The implications of Newell's (1986) model are important for practitioners as well as researchers. We would encourage those who work with children to consider the centrality of the task in their assessment of children's throwing performance. Function recruits form, and as described by Barrett and Burton (in press), even highly skilled baseball players – acting under real time constraints – use many throwing forms to accomplish the task. Further, assessment tools that only observe children throwing for speed or distance miss the key ingredient in most throwing behaviour; that is, the active targeting of an object at some distance from the body. The subtle calibration of force and distance to effect accuracy suggests a range of possible throwing solutions to the functional problem of accuracy.

Differences in throwing behaviour between various age and sex groups have been described in the literature at least back to the 1930s. The importance of task and environmental factors, such as ball size and distance, have been acknowledged for many years, but experimental research and the application of this research to practical problems in movement behaviour is fairly recent. Clearly, Newell's (1986) model and Thelen's (1995) dynamic systems approach to motor development have been instrumental in directing more attention to the study of these factors. We believe that future work on the effect of performer, environmental, and task constraints on throwing behaviour need to consider not just a single dependent variable – such as accuracy, velocity, or form – but also to emphasise accuracy as well as velocity and form. Analyses of the relationships between the steps in this sequence of measures, from function to form (Oslin and Mitchell, 1998), as key variables are manipulated, should expand our understanding of throwing development.

References

Barrett, D. and Burton, A.W. (in press) Throwing patterns used by collegiate baseball players: implications for physical education curriculum. *Research Quarterly for Exercise and Sport.*

Bertenthal, B.I., Campos, J.J. and Barrett, K.C. (1984) Self-produced locomotion: An organizer of emotional, cognitive, and social development in infancy. In R.N. Emde and R.J. Harmon (eds), *Continuities and Discontinuities in Development* (pp. 175–210). New York: Plenum Press.

Branta, C., Haubenstricker, J. and Seefeldt, V. (1984) Age changes in motor skills during childhood and adolescence. *Exercise and Sport Sciences Reviews*, 12, 467–520.

Burton, A.W., Dancisak, M., Barrett, D. and Rodgerson, R.W. (2000) Effect of age, sex, and distance on throwing accuracy and velocity. Manuscript submitted for publication.

Burton, A.W., Greer, N.L. and Wiese, D.M. (1992) Changes in overhand throwing patterns as a function of ball size. *Pediatric Exercise Science*, 4, 50–67.

Burton, A.W., Greer, N.L. and Wiese-Bjornstal, D.M. (1993) Variations in grasping and throwing patterns as a function of ball size. *Pediatric Exercise Science*, 5, 25–41.

Burton, A.W. and Miller, D.E. (1998) *Movement Skill Assessment*. Champaign, IL: Human Kinetics.

Calvin, W.H. (1982) Did throwing stones shape hominid brain evolution? *Ethology and Sociobiology*, 3, 115–24.

Calvin, W.H. (1994) The emergence of intelligence: language, foresight, musical skills and other hallmarks of intelligence are connected through an underlying facility that enhances rapid movements. *Scientific American*, 271, 4, 101–7.

Churchill, S.E. and Trinkaus, E. (1990) Neanderthal scapular glenoid morphology. *American Journal of Physical Anthropology*, 83, 147–60.

Davis, W.E. and Burton, A.W. (1991) Ecological task analysis: translating movement behavior theory into practice. *Adapted Physical Activity Quarterly*, 8, 154–77.

Eibl-Eibesfeldt, I. (1989) *Human Ethology*. New York: Aldine de Gruyter.

Eliot, L. (1999) *What's Going on in There? How the Brain and Mind Develop in the First Five Years of Life*. New York: Bantam Books.

Fragaszy, D. (1998) How non-human primates use their hands. In K.J. Connolly (ed.), *The Psychobiology of the Hand* (pp. 76–96). Cambridge: MacKeith Press.

Gallahue, D.L. and Ozmun, J.C. (1998) *Understanding Motor Development: Infants, Children, Adolescents, Adults*, 4th edn. Boston, MA: McGraw-Hill.

Gardiner, E.N. (1930) *Athletics of the Ancient World*. Chicago: Ares.

Geary, D.C. (1998) *Male, Female: The Evolution of Human Sex Differences*. Washington, DC: American Psychological Association.

Goodall, J. (1986) *The Chimpanzees of Gombe*. Cambridge, MA: Belknap.

Groos, K. (1911) *The Play of Animals*. New York: Appleton.

Halverson, H.M. (1940) Motor development. In A. Gesell (ed.), *The First Five Years of Life: A Guide to the Study of the Preschool Child* (pp. 65–107). New York: Harper and Row.

Halverson, L.E., Roberton, M.A. and Langendorfer, S. (1982) Development of the overhand throw: movement and velocity changes by seventh grade. *Research Quarterly for Exercise and Sport*, 53, 198–205.

Hicks, J.A. (1931) *The Acquisition of Motor Skill in Young Children.* Iowa City, IA: University of Iowa.

Hoffman, S.J., Imwold, C.H. and Koller, J.A. (1983) Accuracy and prediction in throwing: a taxonomic analysis of children's performance. *Research Quarterly for Exercise and Sport,* 54, 33–40.

Indermill, C. and Husak, W.S. (1984) Relationship between speed and accuracy in an over-arm throw. *Perceptual and Motor Skills,* 59, 219–22.

Jardine, R. and Martin, N.G. (1983) Spatial ability and throwing accuracy. *Behavior Genetics,* 13, 331–40.

Keogh, J.F. (1969) Change in motor performance during early school years (Tech. Rep. No. 2-69, United States Public Health Service Grant HD 01059). Department of Physical Education, University of California, Los Angeles.

Kolakowski, D. and Malina, R.M. (1974) Spatial ability, throwing accuracy and man's hunting heritage. *Nature,* 251, 410–12.

Langendorfer, S. (1987) Motor-task goal as a constraint on developmental status. In J.E. Clark and J.H. Humphrey (eds), *Advances in Motor Development Research* (Vol. 1, pp. 16–28). New York: AMS Press.

Langendorfer, S.J. and Roberton, M.A. (2000) Does the backswing limit development of differentiated trunk rotation in throwing? *Journal of Sport and Exercise Psychology,* 22 , S67.

Lenneberg, E.H. (1967) Biological Foundations of Language. New York: Wiley.

Marzke, M., Longhill, J. and Rasmussen, S.A. (1988) Gluteus maximum muscle function and the origin of hominid bipedality. *American Journal of Physical Anthropology,* 77, 519–28.

National Federation of State High School Associations. (1997) Summary: 1996–97 athletics participation survey. Kansas City, MO: National Federation of State High School Associations.

Nelson, J.K., Thomas, J.R., Nelson, K.R. and Abraham, P.C. (1986) Gender differences in children's throwing performance: biology and environment. *Research Quarterly for Exercise and Sport,* 57, 280–7.

Newell, K M. (1986) Constraints on the development of coordination. In M.G. Wade and H.T.A. Whiting (eds), *Motor Development in Children: Aspects of Coordination and Control* (pp. 341–60) Dordrecht: Nijhoff.

Oslin, J.L. and Mitchell, S.A. (1998) Form follows function. *Journal of Physical Education, Recreation and Dance,* 69, 6, 46–9.

Payne, V.G. and Isaacs, L.D. (1999) *Human Motor Development: A Lifespan Approach,* 4th edn. Mountain View, CA: Mayfield.

Pulito, B.R., Roberton, M.A. and Langendorfer, S. (2000) Boys' and girls' throwing development: a comparison of two cohorts twenty years apart. *Journal of Sport and Exercise Psychology,* 22, S87.

Rippee, N.E., Pangrazi, R.P., Corbin, C.B., Borsdorf, L., Petersen, G. and Pangrazi, D. (1991) Throwing profiles of first and fourth grade boys and girls. *The Physical Educator,* 47, 180–5.

Roberton, M.A. (1977) Stability of stage categorizations across trials: Implications for the 'stage theory' of overarm throw development. *Journal of Human Movement Studies,* 3, 49–59.

Roberton, M.A. (1978) Longitudinal evidence for developmental stages in the forceful overarm throw. *Journal of Human Movement Studies,* 4, 167–75.

Roberton, M.A. (1984) Changing motor patterns during childhood. In J.R. Thomas (ed.), *Motor Development During Childhood and Adolescence* (pp. 48–90). Minneapolis: Burgess.

Roberton, M.A. and Langendorfer, S. (1993) Developmental profiles: evidence for constraints on action. *Journal of Sport and Exercise Psychology*, 15, S66.

Sakurai, S. and Miyashita, M. (1983) Developmental aspects of overarm throwing related to age and sex. *Human Movement Science*, 2, 67–76.

Seefeldt, V. and Haubenstricker, J. (1982) Patterns, phases, or stages: An analytical model for the study of developmental movement. In J.A.S. Kelso and J.E. Clark (eds), *The Development of Movement Control and Co-ordination* (pp. 309–18) Chichester: J. Wiley and Sons.

Thelen, E. (1995) Motor development: a new synthesis. *American Psychologist*, 50, 79–95.

Thomas, J.R. (2000) Children's control, learning, and performance of motor skills. *Research Quarterly for Exercise and Sport*, 71, 1–9.

Tiger, L. (1984) *Men in Groups*. New York: Marion Boyars.

Tokida, E., Tanaka, I., Takefushi, H. and Hagiwara, T. (1994) Tool-using in Japanese macaques: use of stones to obtain fruit from a pipe. *Animal Behaviour*, 47, 1023–30.

Tooby, J. and DeVore, I. (1987) The reconstruction of hominid behavioral evolution through strategic modeling. In W.G. Kinsey (ed.), *The Evolution of Human Behavior: Primate Models* (pp. 183–287). Albany, NY: State University of New York Press.

Trinkaus, E. (1986) Bodies, brawn, brains and noses: human ancestors and human predation. In M.H. Nitecki (ed.), *The Evolution of Human Hunting* (pp. 107–45). New York: Plenum Press.

Westergaard, G.C. and Suomi, S.J. (1994) Aimed throwing of stones by tufted capuchin monkeys (Cebus apella). *Human Evolution*, 9, 323–9.

Wild, M.R. (1938) The behavior pattern of throwing and some observations concerning its course of development in children. *Research Quarterly*, 9, 20–4.

Wilson, F.R. (1998) *The Hand: How Its Use Shapes the Brain, Language, and Human Culture*. New York: Pantheon.

15 The co-ordination of kicking techniques in children

Mark A. Scott, Mark A. Williams and Robert R. Horn

1. Introduction

Kicking has been described as 'a unique form of striking in which the foot is used to impart force to a ball' (Wickstrom, 1977, p. 177).[1] This description encompasses actions such as the instep kick, punt, side-footed pass, drop-kick and chip where the aim is to direct the ball towards a target with appropriate power and accuracy. McCrudden and Reilly (1993) observe that the action of kicking is pervasive throughout all sports that fall under the classification of football (e.g. American Football, Gaelic Football, Soccer). As kicking is a common feature of many sports, it is important to understand how the mature kicking action is acquired. However, regardless of the importance of kicking techniques to successful performance in various codes of football, there has been relatively little research into their acquisition in children. In this chapter we provide an overview of our current understanding of how various kicking techniques are acquired and co-ordinated in young performers. Where appropriate, recommendations for future research are highlighted and practical applications identified.

2. Co-ordination characteristics of a mature kicking pattern

Turvey (1990, p. 938) proposed that co-ordination, when considered at the macroscopic level, can be described as 'the patterning of body and limb motions relative to the patterning of environmental objects and events'. Consequently, when examining the co-ordination of the kicking action there needs to be a description of the patterns of movement within a limb (intra-limb co-ordination), between limbs (inter-limb co-ordination) and between the performer and the ball (Lees and Davids, 2002).

Plagenhoef (1971) provided an initial qualitative description of the co-ordination characteristics of the mature kick. He suggested that the trunk needs to rotate in order to draw the kicking thigh backwards so as to allow a full swing of the lower leg. Wickstrom (1977) expanded upon these basic considerations and suggested that various co-ordination and timing features were characteristic of the mature kicking pattern. These features are described in table 15.1 and presented pictorially in figure 15.1. It is clear from this description that in the mature kicking technique performers try to maximise their performance by exploiting the open kinetic chain.

Although these general features are representative of a mature kicking pattern, the specific requirements of the kick will determine the precise action (Wickstrom, 1977). The features described by Wickstrom are common to the majority of mature kicking techniques. The soccer instep kick, punt and place kick have very similar movement patterns (Roberts and Metcalf, 1968).

3. Co-ordination changes observed in kicking

The kicking action is 'essentially a variation of running' (Roberts and Metcalf, 1968, p. 315). Gessell (1940, cited in Wickstrom, 1977) reported that children are able to kick soon after they are able to run. More specifically, Wickstrom (1977) argued that the potential for being able to kick a stationary ball emerges around 18 months of age. Although the potential for kicking occurs relatively early, the initial movement pattern is far removed from the mature pattern previously described. One of the earliest attempts to identify developmental changes in kicking a stationary ball was carried out by Deach (1952, cited in Wickstrom, 1977). In this study, a four-stage developmental classification was identified based on observations of children ranging in age from 2 to 6 years. Based on Deach's stage model, Wickstrom (1977, p. 182) characterised the changes observed as 'a gradual change from a relatively straight pendular leg action with little body movement to a sweeping, whip like action with gross body movement'. Although this description provides a qualitative assessment of the changes, a more detailed quantitative assessment across a greater age range is required.

Bloomfield, Elliott and Davies (1979) examined developmental changes in the soccer instep kicking technique using 56 boys between 2 and 12 years of age. The boys were required to kick a ball hard towards a target situated four metres away; the more accurate of two attempts were used for two-dimensional kinematic analysis and a qualitative assessment. Bloomfield *et al.* (1979) identified six developmental groupings with regard to the kicking pattern. The different groups

Table 15.1 A descriptive analysis of the mature kicking pattern (taken from Wickstrom, 1977)

Step	Description
1	A preliminary step is included in the action. This step allows for backwards rotation of the pelvis on the kicking side so that the thigh of the kicking leg can be extended.
2	There is a forward swing of the kicking leg, with simultaneous flexion of the hip and knee.
3	The shank of the kicking leg undergoes vigorous extension.
4	The forward movement of the kicking thigh ceases prior to ball contact, but the shank continues to extend.
5	To counteract the vigorous extension of the shank, the arm on the non-kicking side is swung forwards.

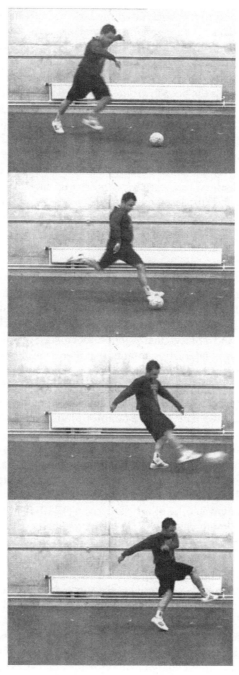

Figure 15.1 A pictorial representation of the skilled adult kicking pattern based on the work of Wickstrom (1977)

were based on a descriptive analysis of the kicking action and via comparison of some kinematic parameters and spatio-temporal measures. Those classified as group 1 had the most immature kicking action, whereas those placed in group 6 were perceived to have the most mature pattern.

The boys in groups 1 to 3 approached the ball with either no run-up or at most a single step, whereas the boys in groups 4, 5 and 6 utilised a multiple step run-up. The inclusion of the run-up into the action appeared initially to have a detrimental impact on other variables important for the production of a powerful kick. For example, maximal angular velocity and angular velocity of the kicking leg at ball contact increased steadily from groups 1 to 3, whilst these variables showed a decrease once a multiple step run-up was employed (i.e. group 4). However, as groups 5 and 6 learned to incorporate the run-up into the kicking action these values increased and surpassed those gained without a multiple step run-up. The boys in group 6 also started to employ an angled run-up, thereby increasing the potential range of pelvic rotation (Roberts and Metcalf, 1968). The distance between the support foot and the ball also provided an indication of how the boys' co-ordination pattern changed over the six groups. The boys in group 1 stood closest to the ball (10 cm), whilst those in groups 2 and 3 stood 25 cm and 22 cm away from the ball respectively. This finding suggests that boys with an immature kicking pattern tend to stand too close to the ball. Whilst using a multiple step run-up, the boys in group 4 planted their support foot 38 cm away from the ball, whereas the boys in groups 5 and 6 placed their support foot at a similar distance to the boys in groups 2 and 3. It is interesting to note that there was a gradual decrease in the between-subject standard deviation for foot placement from group 4 (26 cm) to group 6 (11 cm). This finding suggests that learning to place the foot an appropriate distance away from the ball is a key feature in learning the co-ordination between the performer and the ball. Some examples of an immature kicking pattern are shown in figure 15.2.

With regard to the co-ordination between the kicking leg and ball, Bloomfield *et al.* (1979) showed differences in the timing characteristics of the action. They found that the time between maximum angular velocity of the kicking leg and ball contact generally decreases, with a maximum difference of 60 ms for group 2 down to 17ms for group 6. Similarly, Luhtanen (1988) found that the average time between the maximum velocity of the shank and ball contact was 9 ms in skilled junior soccer players (age range of 9–18 years).

The importance of learning to co-ordinate the performer's kicking action with the ball is further highlighted when considering the punt kick. Although some elements of the punt kick are similar to the soccer instep kick, the co-ordination of the punt kick may be harder to acquire due to the increased spatial and temporal constraints (Haywood and Getchell, 2001). In punt kicking, kickers have to release the ball as they move forward and strike the ball as it falls. The increased difficulty of the punt kick is supported by the work of Elliott, Bloomfield and Davies (1980). They carried out a similar study to Bloomfield *et al.* (1979) where they examined developmental changes in the punt kicking technique of 51 boys aged between 2 and 12 years of age. The participants were required to kick a ball towards a target

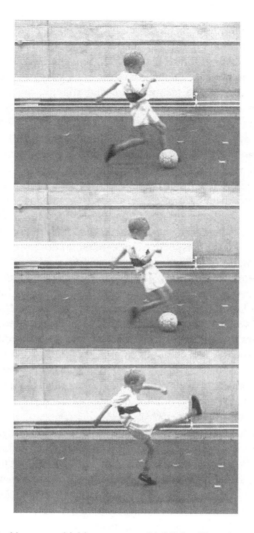

Figure 15.2 A typical immature kicking pattern as highlighted by a 6-year-old novice player

situated 4m in front of them. Six of the participants were unable to punt the ball before it hit the ground, highlighting the increased difficulty of this task compared to striking a stationary ball. Making appropriate contact with the ball was also difficult as only 80 per cent of the boys in the group with the highest level of technique maturity contacted the ball with the instep.

Some insight into the co-ordination between the kicker and the ball may be gained from the work of Bloomfield *et al.* (1979) and Elliott *et al.* (1980). From their qualitative descriptions of the instep and punt kicks, it is also possible to gain some indication of the changes in the intra-limb and inter-limb co-ordination. It is clear from both studies that as the mature kicking pattern develops there is an increase in the number of joints functionally involved in the action. As with other actions such as throwing, it is apparent that, when kicking, the participants initially used the legs only to impart force on to the ball. However, with increasing maturity the learners begin to increase the length of the back swing as well as flexion and extension at the knee. As the technique became mature, the boys increased the contribution of the open kinetic chain into the production of the movement. Also, the boys started to rotate the pelvis during the kick. In order to cope with the increased action of the kicking leg, Bloomfield *et al.* (1979) and Elliott *et al.* (1980) reported an increase in co-ordinated arm movement over the groups to oppose the action of the kicking leg and maintain balance.

Although the qualitative descriptions provided give an indication of the intra-limb and inter-limb co-ordination pattern, the kinematic analysis tends to focus on key parameters of the movement rather than examining the co-ordination of the action. This is not surprising, as the theoretical framework for the majority of this research was the stage perspective model of motor development (see Roberton, 1977; 1978). Using this approach, various developmental stages are identified for the movement being investigated. The focus of what movement characteristics need to be assessed when investigating skill acquisition and development has changed over the last 20 years with the emergence of the ecological perspective (for an overview, see Haywood and Getchell, 2001). From the ecological perspective, it is important to assess the intra-limb and inter-limb co-ordination patterns. The use of biomechanical techniques to assess co-ordination has become more prevalent in other aspects of motor development. For example, the shift from qualitative descriptions of walking patterns to detailed biomechanical analysis have provided valuable insight into the changes associated with the development of gait (e.g. Clark and Phillips, 1993).

There have been relatively few attempts to specifically assess intra-limb and inter-limb co-ordination in kicking using biomechanical techniques. Anderson and Sidaway (1994) examined the intra-limb co-ordination changes associated with practising an instep kick in six adult novices. The participants were required to specifically practise instep kicks for 10 minutes (15 to 20 kicks) twice a week at the start of a soccer class. Three trials recorded pre-practice were compared to three trials recorded post-practice. The novice players' pre and post-practice performances were also compared to those of expert soccer players.

Anderson and Sidaway (1994) found that there were distinct changes in co-ordination after practice that brought the novices' performance closer to that of the experts. The main aim was for the performers to maximise ball velocity, and after practice the maximum linear velocity of the foot was significantly higher than that recorded before practice. This increase was attributed to a change in the timing between hip and knee flexion. By quantifying changes in the timing and using qualitative assessments of the hip and knee joint represented in the form of angle-angle plots, Anderson and Sidaway (1994) suggested that improvement in speed at the foot were due to changes in the co-ordination pattern and not just due to an increase in the speed of the entire movement. As yet there are no similar investigations looking at intra-limb co-ordination changes in children. As the qualitative descriptions of the kicking action highlight, the rotation of the trunk and hips and the angle of approach are key features of the mature movement. This suggests that, when examining co-ordination of the kicking technique three-dimensional analysis should be used to gain a fuller understanding of the action (Davids *et al.*, 2000; Lees and Davids, 2002).

4. Considerations in aiding the acquisition of the kicking technique

It is clear from the investigations of Bloomfield *et al.* (1979) and Elliott *et al.* (1980) that performers need to learn to co-ordinate their own movements with the ball. In the case of the instep kick, learning the appropriate placement of the support foot in relation to the ball seems to be an important co-ordination characteristic. Therefore, providing guidance and feedback about foot placement is important when learning to incorporate a multi-step run-up into the action.

Although the studies of Bloomfield *et al.* (1979) and Elliott *et al.* (1980) are important in our understanding of the development of the kicking technique, further investigation needs to be undertaken. The role of practice, instruction and feedback in the acquisition of the mature kicking technique in children has not been considered. In the investigations of Bloomfield *et al.* (1979) and Elliott *et al.* (1980) the playing experience of the participants was not reported. The results showed that there is a general trend for the groupings to follow the mean ages of the groups. However, the age ranges show a considerable amount of overlap. Elliott *et al.* (1980) express that chronological age provided a poor indication of instep and punt kicking performance. The boys' experience at the task under various learning conditions could explain these large differences in performance between the different ages. The findings of Anderson and Sidaway (1994) show that in novice adults, practising kicking alone results in changes in the observed co-ordination pattern. Therefore, it is clear that kicking experience needs to be considered when examining cross-sectional data from children.

It is also possible that the acquisition of the mature pattern could be enhanced by practising the task under the influence of appropriate learning variables such as knowledge of performance and demonstration. Evidence for this suggestion may be found when considering studies that have investigated the acquisition of the kicking technique in novice adults. For example, Williams *et al.* (2001) examined the effect of practice and knowledge of performance on the acquisition of a soccer instep kick. Two groups of novice female players performed 60 practice trials of the instep kick once a week for four weeks. One group received feedback on movement form (knowledge of performance), whereas the other group received no knowledge of performance information. Kinematic data of the kicking leg was recorded pre-and post-practice. Kinematic data was also obtained from a third group of expert male soccer players to allow for comparison with the mature technique. Using angle–angle plots, Williams *et al.* (2001) found that the co-ordination patterns of both novice groups changed over practice, with post-practice angle–angle plots being closer to those of the experts. The main difference between the two novice groups after practice was not in the co-ordination of the movement but in the outcome. The group that received knowledge of performance had a significantly higher maximum ball velocity. Williams *et al.* (2001) concluded that the provision of information to the learner of movement form aided in the acquisition of a more effective kicking pattern.

With regard to movement outcome, the benefit of providing different types of feedback during the acquisition of a kicking technique can be seen in the findings of Wulf *et al.* (2002). They examined how the nature of feedback could enhance the acquisition of a lofted pass by comparing the provision of externally-focused feedback against providing internally-focused feedback. The internally focused feedback statements contained information related to the performers body movements (e.g. 'lock your ankle down and use the instep to strike the ball'), whereas the externally-focused statements predominately contained references to the movement effects (e.g. 'strike the ball below its midline to lift it; that is, kick underneath it'). Wulf *et al.* (2002) found that externally-focused feedback resulted in better shot accuracy for practice and retention than providing feedback that was internally focused. Whether similar effects are observed in children is yet to be determined. Although not a direct measure of co-ordination, Wulf *et al.* (2002) also examined the effects of providing externally-focused feedback against providing internally-focused feedback on the movement form observed in the volleyball 'tennis' serve. Externally-focused feedback was more beneficial during practice than an internal focus; however, there were no differences once feedback was removed in the retention test.

Horn, Williams and Scott (2002) investigated the role of observational learning on the acquisition of the soccer chip technique in adult females. The results indicated that participants who did not see a demonstration were as proficient in reducing error in the outcome of their kicks as those observing a model. However, for co-ordination, only those watching the demonstration changed their *global* movement pattern, modifying their approach to the ball by increasing the number of preparatory steps to match the model more closely. Interestingly, watching a demonstration did not facilitate the learning of intra-limb co-ordination. While further research is required to verify these findings, it appears that for novices (and therefore possibly children) watching a demonstration is not necessarily sufficient to influence *local* level co-ordination.

Although there is no specific research into the factors that may enhance acquisition of the appropriate co-ordination pattern for kicking in children, the research on novice adults clearly suggests that practice can bring the co-ordination pattern closer to that of the mature technique. Providing adult novices with feedback and demonstrations during acquisition improves the outcome of the kick. However, there is very limited evidence to suggest that they aid in the acquisition of the mature co-ordination pattern.

5. Conclusions

There have been relatively few attempts to assess biomechanically the co-ordination changes that occur when moving from an immature kicking pattern to a mature pattern. The research of Bloomfield *et al.* (1979) and Elliott *et al.* (1980) provides some indication of the changes in co-ordination between the performer and the ball. Learning to plant the support foot in an appropriate position and to strike the ball with the instep seem to be key factors in the acquisition of the instep kick and punt. However, further investigation is required to determine the intra- and inter-limb co-ordination changes. The studies performed on adults (e.g. Anderson and Sidaway, 1994) have assessed changes in co-ordination by quantifying the differences that occur in the timing of the kick and through qualitative assessment of the hip and knee joints via angle–angle plots. This approach still needs to be applied to children to assess their intra-limb co-ordination.

The work of Bloomfield *et al.* (1979) and Elliott *et al.* (1980) also suggest that age is a poor indicator of the maturational level of the kicking pattern. The wide variation in performance across the ages could be due to the different levels of experience that the children had in the action of kicking. Investigations using adults show that practice does result in changes in the co-ordination of the kicking technique (see Anderson and Sidaway, 1994; Williams *et al.*, 2001). Therefore, experience in the kicking action also needs to be considered when investigating children. Factors that can enhance the acquisition of the mature kicking pattern also need to be investigated. Thus far, evidence gained from studies using adult populations suggests that providing feedback and demonstrations does not aid in the acquisition of intra-limb co-ordination. However, such information may aid the global co-ordination and in the quality of the movement outcome.

Note

1 This definition excludes kicking techniques from martial arts and other combat sports.

References

Anderson, D.I. and Sidaway, B. (1994) Co-ordination changes associated with practice of a soccer kick. *Research Quarterly for Exercise and Sport*, 65, 93–9.

Bloomfield, J., Elliott, B.C. and Davies, C.M. (1979) Development of the soccer kick: a cinematographical analysis. *Journal of Human Movement Studies*, 5, 152–9.

Clark, J.E. and Phillips, S.J. (1993) A longtitudinal study of intralimb co-ordination in the first year of independent walking. *Child Development*, 64, 1143–57.

Davids, K., Lees, A. and Burwitz, L. (2000) Understanding and measuring co-ordination and control in kicking skills in soccer: Implications for talent identification and skill acquisition. *Journal of Sports Sciences*, 18, 703–14.

Elliott, B.C., Bloomfield, J. and Davies, C.M. (1980) Development of the punt kick: A cinematographic analysis. *Journal of Human Movement Studies*, 6, 142–50.

Haywood, K.M. and Getchell, N. (2001) *Life Span Motor Development*. Champaign, IL: Human Kinetics.

Horn, R.R., Williams, A.M. and Scott, M.A. (2002) Learning from demonstrations: the role of visual search during observational learning from video and point light models. *Journal of Sports Sciences*, 20, 253–69.

Lees, A. and Davids, K. (2002) Co-ordination and control of kicking in soccer. In K. Davids, G.J.P. Savelsbergh, S.J. Bennett and J. van der Kamp (eds), *Interceptive Actions in Sport: Information and Movement* (pp. 273–87). London: Routledge.

Luhtanen, P. (1988) Kinematics and kinetics of maximal in-step kicking in soccer. In T. Reilly, A. Lees, K. Davids and J.W. Murphy (eds), *Science and Football* (pp. 441–8). London: E and F.N. Spon.

McCrudden, M. and Reilly, T. (1993) A comparison of the punt and drop-kick. In T. Reilly, J. Clarys and A. Stibbe (eds), *Science and Football II* (pp. 362–8). London: E and F.N. Spon.

Plagenhoef, S. (1971) *Patterns of Human Motion*. Englewood Cliffs, NJ: Prentice-Hall.

Roberton, M.A. (1977) Stability of stage categorizations across trials: implications for the stage theory of overarm throw development. *Journal of Human Movement Studies*, 3, 49–59.

Roberton, M.A. (1978) Longitudinal evidence for developmental stages in the forceful overarm throw. *Journal of Human Movement Studies*, 4, 167–75.

Roberts, E.M. and Metcalf, A. (1968) Mechanical analysis of kicking. In J. Wartenweiller, E. Jokl and M. Hebbelink (eds), *Biomechanics I* (pp. 315–19). Basel: Karger.

Turvey, M.T. (1990) Coordination. *American Psychologist*, 45, 938–53.

Wickstrom, R.L. (1977) *Fundamental Motor Patterns*. Philadelphia: Lea and Febiger.

Williams, A.M., Alty, P. and Lees, A. (2001) Effects of practice and knowledge of performance on the kinematics of ball kicking. In T. Reilly, W. Spinks and A. Murphy (eds), *Science and Football IV* (pp. 320–5). London: E and F.N. Spon.

Wulf, G., McConnel, N., Gärtner, M. and Schwarz, A. (2002) Enhancing the learning of sport skills through external-focus feedback. *Journal of Motor Behavior*, 34, 171–82.

16 Development of locomotor co-ordination and control in children

Jill Whitall

1. Introduction

To accomplish the important task of upright locomotion, humans adopt one of five distinctive gait forms or skills: walking, running, galloping, hopping and skipping. The purpose of this chapter is to discuss the development of these skills in children aged 4 to 12 years. One might reasonably ask, to what end? There are already many chapters and textbooks in which evidence-based developmental changes in the quality/process and performance/product of these skills across childhood are described (e.g. Branta *et al.*, 1984; Gabbard, 1996; Haywood and Getchell, 2001; Payne and Isaacs, 1991; Roberton and Halverson; 1984). There are also chapters in which the discussion and analysis of locomotion is less descriptive and focuses on how these changes occur (e.g. Clark and Whitall, 1989a; Whitall, 1995). Why devote another chapter to this topic? In addition, although the rationale for understanding the development of walking, and to a lesser extent running, is self-evident, the other locomotor skills seem of little relevance to the study of motor behaviour (as indicated by the dearth of studies on them). Why discuss these other locomotor skills? Both of these questions can be easily answered. First, there are principles of (motor) development that can be illustrated with an analysis of previous locomotor studies of this age span and that complement rather than repeat previous writings. Second, there are several, albeit non-obvious, reasons why studying all the locomotor skills is important and, indeed, to be strongly encouraged. This chapter focuses primarily on discussing principles of motor development in ten sections, with the theme emerging that locomotor co-ordination has been studied more extensively than locomotor control. The three remaining sections address the importance of studying locomotor development and the specific need for research on locomotor control to provide a more complete understanding of how locomotor skills continue to develop over childhood.

2. Development is teleological in the sense that there is always a 'goal'

Motor development has been defined as the changes in motor behaviour *over the lifespan* and the process(es) that underlie these changes (Clark and Whitall, 1989b).

While few would quibble with this definition, many implicitly consider motor development as only worth studying during infancy either as a pre-verbal window into cognitive development or, more commonly, as a microcosm for studying developmental processes that occur as balance, gait and visually-directed reaching emerge in a functional state. For example, Thelen has provided elegant description and analysis of the developmental process that occurs when infants learn to reach (Thelen *et al.*, 1993) and in the lead-up stages to walking (Thelen and Ulrich, 1991); both processes occurring in the first year of life. Yet, is the emergence of the functional motor state all that is important about developmental processes? Consider the 4-year-old. There is substantial evidence that a typically developing 4-year-old can functionally perform all the locomotor skills mentioned above with the exception, for some, of skipping (Branta *et al.*, 1984; Roberton and Halverson, 1984; Sinclair, 1973). Thus, the developmental processes that underlie the emergence of these locomotor skills have come and gone. So what develops between 4 and 12 years? Clearly, the ability to perform each skill well also results from a developmental process. None would argue that the typical 4-year-old could perform any of the locomotor tasks as skilfully as a typical adolescent or adult. In other words, the goal of development in the skills discussed here has changed from emergence to skilfulness (later in the lifespan, the developmental goal will change to maintenance and lastly to functional adaptation to the ageing process). That the developmental process of acquiring motor skilfulness should be studied is obvious to physical educators or coaches whose goal it is to facilitate this process. Readers who question the importance of locomotor skilfulness should skip to section 11 before continuing through the principles! As will be argued later, the study of locomotor skilfulness or expertise has barely begun in a scientifically rigorous way. However, the developmental process of becoming skilful in locomotor activities does illustrate well the current 'dynamic' and perhaps 'post-dynamic' approaches to understanding development.

3. Development towards skilfulness consists of form/pattern and function/adaptation

For at least two decades, the scientific understanding and approach to studying development in general, and motor development in particular, has been strongly influenced by the idea that development is a 'dynamic' process. That is, development follows dynamic (and mathematical) principles of change that apply to all complex systems from atoms to weather patterns (e.g. Abraham *et al.*, 1989). One aspect of this approach is to distinguish between forms or patterns of a system and the action of that system (i.e. its function or adaptation to its surround). In mathematical and synergetic terms, the state of a system can be mapped via order parameters as an attractor in state space, while changes in the system's control parameters may or may not result in a change of the attractor state. That is, the attractor state is usually immune to minor changes of control parameters remaining stable in state space. However, at critical scaling values of a control parameter, the attractor will shift in state space and a new pattern self-organises. These abstract concepts have been translated into movement-related concepts by Kugler, Kelso and Turvey (1980; 1982).

Kugler *et al.* (1980) suggest first that a movement system is constrained to behave in a stable fashion (characterised by an equation of constraint) and that this 'constraint coordinates in the sense that it enforces (automatically) a relationship among several variables' (p.14). Put another way, a system is defined by its co-ordination (form or pattern) and this, in turn, can be defined as the relationship between limbs (segments) that comprise a particular form of locomotion (Kugler *et al.*, 1982). For example, running co-ordination can be described as alternating leg and arm movements with particular segmental relationships. Importantly, it is the prevailing constraints (of all types) that define the pattern of co-ordination, rather than a pre-determined programme. Second, it is argued that the co-ordinative relationship can be modified by variables that control the relationship in the sense that they can provoke qualitative (a recognisable change in co-ordination pattern e.g. running on ball of foot) or quantitative (little change in co-ordination but a change in absolute time, space, or effort; e.g. running faster) change or both. That is, locomotor control is the act by which the relationship (locomotor co-ordination) is modified in a flexible and precise manner (Kugler *et al.*, 1980; 1982). This act can be both consciously (intentional change of pace) and sub-consciously (adapting ground reaction forces on a new surface) enacted. Thus, locomotor co-ordination and locomotor control can be conceived of as two distinct (but related) entities, both of which contribute to locomotor skilfulness. Unfortunately, only one of these aspects of locomotion, co-ordination, has been studied in some detail.

4. Changing developmental constraints produce species-typical co-ordination changes

Just as typically developing children from 4 to 12 years pass through Piaget's later stages of cognitive development, so these same children go through 'stage-like' patterns of locomotor co-ordination development within each skill. For each of the five gait skills, there are published intra-skill developmental sequences of overt co-ordination. Two ways of describing these sequences have been proposed. In one type of sequence, early to late forms of co-ordination for a particular skill are described for the body as a composite whole. For example, the earliest form of running is described as arms held high, short stride, little knee flexion and foot contact with full sole (see Seefeldt and Haubenstricker, 1982 or Gallahue, 1989 for examples of this 'whole-body' approach). In the other form of sequence, each component of the body has its own developmental sequence for each skill. For example, an early form of running might be described as consisting of the legs showing a flat-footed run with minimal flight (the initial form) while spinal rotation swings the arms bilaterally to counterbalance rotation of the pelvis and swing leg (the second form) (see Roberton and Halverson, 1984 for examples of the 'component' approach). Regardless of the approach used, the important concept is that for each locomotor skill, early appearing forms of co-ordination are qualitatively different from later/advanced forms of co-ordination. Moreover, there is large agreement on how these early forms differ from later forms. For example, children begin walking with arms held in mid-guard, a wide base of support (Burnett and Johnson, 1971), limited and variable intralimb leg co-ordination (Clark and Phillips, 1993), and variable interlimb leg co-ordination (Clark *et al.*, 1988). By 4 years of age, most children have reached an advanced pattern of co-ordination for walking that includes reciprocal arm swinging, heel-to-toe walking and double knee extension (Sutherland *et al.*, 1980). For all skills, it is proposed that the early, intermediate and advanced co-ordination patterns appear to be 'attractive' states of muscle synergies (sometimes called co-ordinative structures) that are somewhat unchanged or stable for a period of time.

The fact that changes in locomotor co-ordination appear to be species-typical can be attributed to the prevailing constraints from which the co-ordination emerges. Following Newell (1986), constraints arise from the organism, the environment and the task. Organismic constraints consist of structural and functional body components. Therefore, if these components develop typically, all other constraints being equal, one child's co-ordination pattern will develop similarly to another. When this does not occur, for example in congenitally blind children, the pattern of walking may be qualitatively different (involving an asymmetric walking pattern). Similarly, if environmental and task constraints are the same for all, one would expect a similar course of co-ordination development.

5. Advanced co-ordination patterns are not necessarily indicative of maximal performance since covert (control) changes in underlying neuromuscular strategies will occur

There is an assumption that the most advanced co-ordination pattern will be the one resulting in the most biomechanically efficient performance. Theoretically, this is true, but a co-ordination pattern that looks adult-like in pattern to the observer may be undergoing covert changes in the underlying neuromuscular synergies. For example, if we consider walking again; between 4 and 6–8 years there are changes in muscle firing patterns, the use of non-muscular forces and anticipatory control of centre of pressure that enable the child to produce an adult-like, biomechanically efficient walk (Ledebt *et al.*, 1998; Sutherland *et al.*, 1980). Thus biomechanically efficient co-ordination can only be detected by sophisticated biomechanical analysis. The underlying changes that produce this efficient state can be considered as covert and sub-conscious changes in the control of locomotion. From about 7 to 12 years, further changes in walking typically occur only in the overtly (and mostly consciously) controlled aspects, such as range of speed as discussed later. A similar case can be made for running which, according to Fortney (1983) and Seefeldt and Haubenstricker (1982), can show an advanced co-ordination pattern by 4 to 6 years. However, a mechanical analysis of running across age demonstrates that the ability to produce mechanical power is not completely adult-like until 12 years (Schepens *et al.*, 1998). It should be noted that this latter study did not control for developmental co-ordination level.

Indeed the developmental co-ordination level can be considered a confound in the reported studies of maximal performance in children. For example, reports of maximum running speed or endurance could be biased if a child 'chose' to use a less advanced co-ordination pattern than that of which they were capable, or, for that matter, used a newly-acquired advanced co-ordination pattern that was not yet tuned (controlled) for maximal performance. Studies of running and hopping, the only skills documented for maximal performance, have not accounted for co-ordination level. However, the data are interesting because of the apparent influence of gender and cohort. Maximal running speed for short distances has been measured in many studies. These consistently show a linear increase for boys and girls (with boys about 0.5 SD faster) until about 12 years, when girls slow their rate of increase quite abruptly while boys carry on at a similar rate (Keogh and Sugden, 1985; Thomas and French, 1985). Interestingly, data from Europe around the same time do not show the girls rate of increase levelling off so abruptly, indicating an effect of cultural cohort (Eckert, 1987). A study of endurance in the 12-minute run test of 8- to 12-year-olds in Poland also found a slight advantage for boys, which increased across age (Drabik, 1989). On the other hand, times for the 50-foot continuous hop across 5 to 9 years of age found boys up to a year behind girls (Keogh, 1969). Since boys of this age range typically show a slight advantage for strength (Malina and Roche, 1983) and speed (see Keogh and Sugden, 1985 for review) it is not surprising that they run faster even though they are slightly shorter and less biologically mature than girls. Boys also tend to acquire the advanced levels of running co-ordination earlier, even though they are later in initial acquisition (Seefeldt and Haubenstricker, 1982). So why can girls hop faster, a task that would also require strength and speed?

The answer might be that hopping requires good balance, an ability in which girls have a small advantage (but less than 0.5 SD according to Thomas and French, 1985), possibly from greater practice. Not surprisingly, girls tend to acquire all co-ordination levels of hopping (and skipping) earlier (Seefeldt and Haubenstricker, 1982). Taken together, the above findings illustrate the important role of task and environmental constraints in influencing development of both co-ordination and control in the sense of maximum performance. Given that many of the quoted studies above are over 15 years old, however, they are not necessarily a true representation of gender differences today as sport has become relatively more popular for American girls. Conflicting gender differences found across skills can be largely attributed to practice effects because co-ordination changes within locomotor skills are very similar.

6. Co-ordination changes within each locomotor skill have similar developmental pathways

A child of 4 years who walks with a smooth, advanced co-ordination pattern is likely to have a skipping co-ordination pattern that looks as awkward and stiff as their early attempts at walking. That is, despite having a neuromuscular system that has 'matured' over 3 years, the demands of a more complex locomotor task result in an 'immature' co-ordination. This paradox is strong evidence for the effect of task constraints on movement as opposed to the effect of 'neuromaturation' alone. It accounts for the concept of 'reciprocal interweaving' where a child apparently regresses to an earlier 'stage' or form before becoming more advanced (Gesell, 1954). In fact, a brief review of the developmental co-ordination profiles indicates that each skill develops in a similar fashion that appears to involve mastery of one or both of two major components of movement: balance and bilateral co-ordination.

The following are key changes for locomotor skills that can be compared with walking and which illustrate a recurring adaptation to balance and bilateral co-ordination. Running progresses from a flat-foot toe-out landing, limited leg motion, stiff or reactive arms and variable interlimb co-ordination to heel–toe (jog) and/or toe (sprint) landing, full leg motion and reciprocal sagittal plane arm action (Roberton and Halverson, 1984). Galloping progresses from a flat footed landing, one-sided and overlapping trailing leg, stiff or reactive arms and variable interlimb co-ordination to heel–toe (lead) and toe–heel (trail) landing, either leg trailing behind the lead and arms assisting the motion (Sapp, 1980; Whitall, 1989; Whitall and Caldwell, 1992). Continuous hopping progresses from limited and one-sided support leg motion, swing leg and arms inactive or reactive to flexed and fully extended (either sided) support leg motion with active (leading) swing leg and reciprocal arm action (Halverson and Williams, 1985). Skipping progresses from a one-sided, jerky step-hop and inconsistent arm action to a two-sided smooth and rhythmic leg action with reciprocal arm action (Wickstrom, 1987). Taken together, the remarkable similarity of co-ordination progression for these very different locomotor skills demonstrates the importance of gaining the ability to balance and perform skills bilaterally under increasing task demands. In addition to these similarities, however, there is also individual variation.

7. Species-typical co-ordination changes are neither universal nor mandatory

The argument that common constraints result in common developmental pathways of locomotor co-ordination must be complemented with the realisation that constraints themselves are uniquely configured. Although typically developing children never demonstrate an advanced-to-early co-ordination pattern progression in any given skill, there is variability in how they actually progress and also whether they ever reach the advanced pattern. The very fact that alternative (whole-body and component) developmental sequences are proposed, coupled with the argument that component approaches describe children more accurately, indicate that children do not pass through identical progressions of a skill. For example, in the well-validated component hopping sequence (Halverson and Williams, 1985), one child might go through a phase of level three legs (projected takeoff; swing leg assists) and level three arms (bilateral assist) while another may be at level two for one component (swing leg inactive or bilateral reactive) and never actually be at level three for both components. Regardless of their individual pathways, both children could end up with the same advanced levels of hopping (projection delay; swing leg leads and arms assisting in opposition). A recent paper by Langendorfer and Roberton (2002) illustrates this point by following individual developmental level profiles for overarm throwing longitudinally. For locomotor co-ordination, only hopping has been reported in a longitudinal study, although individual profiles were not presented (Roberton and Halverson, 1988). Seven children were studied over fifteen years and the authors report that each child progressed at their own rate with at least two children showing regressions at some point, possibly owing to weight gain (a structural organism constraint) at that time. By 12 years the leg action was fully advanced for all seven children while the arm action was fully advanced for most but not all. By 18 years, all seven children were demonstrating the most advanced co-ordination patterns. This detailed longitudinal information is not available for any other locomotor skill.

According to Seefeldt and Haubenstricker (1982), 60 per cent of children show advanced co-ordination for running, hopping and skipping by 7 years of age, while a recent study reports over 95 per cent for skipping by 7 to 8 years (Loovis and Butterfield, 2000). The question is, do all typically developing children reach the most advanced co-ordination patterns or, like Piaget's Stages of Cognitive Development or Kohlberg's Stages of Moral Development, do some individuals never get to the most 'advanced' level? No studies directly evaluate this question but, from personal experience of over fifteen years of observing 20+-year-old college students perform locomotor skills, it is clear that a small minority do not progress to advanced levels of co-ordination in all of the locomotor skills, despite a largely full-grown neuromuscular system and years of practice with upright locomotion. Whether this fact is a reflection of a poor physical education experience or a regression due to lack of practice or some other constraint change is not known. What seems important, if we want to develop skilful children and adults, is that typically developing children accomplish the most advanced co-ordination patterns in all locomotor skills by somewhere around 7 years of age. If this could be accomplished, at the very least, we would know that children could perform close to, or at, their maximal possible performance given a particular level of control. An understanding of how the co-ordination changes occur would be useful to achieve this goal, because just growing older and (by default) acquiring a more 'mature' central nervous system is apparently not how the advanced form of co-ordination emerges.

8. Control and rate-limiting parameters induce changes of co-ordination pattern

If constraints shape a co-ordination pattern, then those constraints that become control parameters, as defined earlier, will organise a change of co-ordination pattern when scaled to a critical value. The well-known examples of increasing the rate of finger wagging to induce a change from antiphase to in-phase co-ordination (Kelso, 1984) or, more aptly for this discussion, increasing the speed of a treadmill to induce running from walking (Diedrich and Warren, 1995) are instructive but they reflect real-time rather than developmental-time change. Thelen (1986) argues that developmental change is more complicated because many co-operating systems (constraints) will contribute to the acquisition of a new co-ordination pattern (or skill) and that change will occur only when the slowest of the necessary systems for that new co-ordination pattern (skill) reaches a certain state. Any such system is called a rate limiting parameter because it limits an individual's rate of development at that time. Thus, as teachers (or therapists) involved in facilitating movement acquisition, we need to know which systems (potential rate-limiting parameters) in general are necessary for developmental change and, subsequently, for each individual, which of these parameters is likely to be playing the role of the rate-limiter. In the present context, we can ask two general questions. First, which systems assist a child of 4 years who has early co-ordination patterns for galloping, hopping and skipping to achieve an advanced co-ordination pattern for these skills by 7 years or older?

Although very little research addresses this question, given the earlier discussion, one might guess that balance and bilateral co-ordination abilities are key rate-limiting parameters at a global level of analysis. However, what underlies the growth of these abilities? For example, does balance ability rely on a level of muscular strength (or strength-to-weight ratio), the ability to produce specific neural firing patterns in anticipation of or response to a perturbation, and/or instantaneous control of the centre of pressure? Further, what would underlie or control these parameters? Would this be myelination of the CNS, growth of limbs/muscle, and/or synaptic changes caused by practice? Levels of analysis can go deeper still but we have little idea about how all of these factors (and many more) interact.

At the neuromuscular level, studies on anticipatory postural adjustments during locomotion show that 4- to 5-year-olds have sufficient anticipatory leg muscle activation for stability; however, the latency and sequence of activation is not adult-like until somewhere between 10 and 14 years old (Assaiante *et al.*, 2000; Hirschfield and Forssberg, 1992). Another study indicated that muscular response to a platform perturbation also had longer and more variable latencies around 4 to 6 years but again, the response itself was functional (Shumway-Cook and Woollacott, 1985). Relatedly, Ledebt and colleagues (Ledebt *et al.*, 1998) have demonstrated that anticipatory control of the centre of pressure during gait initiation, taken as a reflection of postural control, begins at 2.5 years and is in place by 6 to 8 years. No attempts to correlate the developing postural adjustment ability with locomotor co-ordination level exist at present. However, overall balance ability did not correlate with skipping level if one can really assess the former accurately with one-leg stance tests (Loovis and Butterfield, 2000). Perhaps balance ability is sufficient by 5 to 6 years and bilateral co-ordination becomes a more relevant (rate-limiting) constraint beyond these ages. An interesting study on hopping development supports this idea.

Using visual and verbal cues, Roberton, Halverson and Harper (1997) asked 5-year-olds, who exhibited earlier forms of hopping, to use their swing leg actively and their arms in reciprocal action. Most children appeared to focus on their knee and arms (showing attention to the task) but did not produce the next developmental co-ordination level of hopping. Instead they produced unique (and not functional) co-ordination patterns such as hopping twice on their landing leg while the swing leg moved forward and backward *independently*. In this case, the rate limiter for most children was not balance but the ability to 'co-ordinate' one leg with the other. That is, children were unable to use verbal cues to help them achieve a more advanced hopping co-ordination level because they had not yet learned how to control their own neuromuscular system bilaterally.

The fact that most children improve their developmental levels of hopping (or galloping/skipping) on one side prior to the other also indicates a difficulty of bilateral co-ordination within each gait form. This asymmetry of development was nicely used in a study by Getchell and Roberton (1989) who found children with a level two hopping on one side of the body and a level three on the other, thus allowing subjects to act as their own control. Instantaneous and estimated whole-body 'stiffness' proved to discriminate between the two levels of hopping; specifically, the level three hopping leg consistently had lower levels of stiffness allowing a softer ('more controlled') landing. How this regulation of stiffness is achieved is not clear but before considering alternative teaching approaches to changing co-ordination levels based on these findings, a second question needs to be asked. Which systems are involved in enabling a child of 4 years who walks or runs with an overt advanced co-ordination pattern to become a child of 7 or 12 years respectively who has a biomechanically efficient covert co-ordination pattern for these skills?

As this question is less obvious from the teaching perspective, even fewer relevant studies exist. In a mechanical analysis of running (Schepens *et al.*, 1998), children under 12 years showed similar mechanical characteristics as adults while their mass-specific power spent against gravity was smaller. Using a simple spring-mass model, Schepens *et al.* (1998) demonstrated that step frequency in children decreased with age because mass was increasing while stiffness remained constant. At 12 years and beyond, mass and stiffness increased at similar rates resulting in a constant step frequency and higher power against gravity. Whether training would alter the regulation of stiffness in younger children's legs in order to facilitate the production of more power is not known. Conceivably, muscle stiffness and power output are largely influenced by mass (growth) and would not respond to repetition per se, but this remains untested. Interestingly, as discussed in the previous paragraph, stiffness regulation has also been considered a factor in the advancement of hopping co-ordination level. If this ability can be viewed as a critical control or rate-limiting parameter for moving a child towards a particular level of locomotor skilfulness, when and how does one go about teaching a child to scale or regulate muscle stiffness?

One answer might be that the regulation of muscle stiffness cannot be directly taught but will self-organise towards appropriate critical values through repetition/practice (with or without increase in mass). Relatedly, muscle stiffness per se may be a by-product of a change in another constraint. Recall the study of 5-year-olds hopping with an inactive swing leg. Presumably, the children were unable to co-ordinate the extra degrees of freedom in that leg with the required control of the landing leg and, thus, responded by freezing the swing leg. Since drawing attention to the swing leg does not work in 5-year-olds for acquiring a more advanced co-ordination pattern, perhaps asking the child to change another parameter that *is* under their control would (e.g. speed or force of the landing leg movement). This might result, at a critical value, in an unintended but biomechanically advantageous increase in swing leg movement and a corresponding change in muscle stiffness of the landing leg. Of course, this speculation relies on the child having the ability to change speed or force of movement, thus bringing us to the concept of having overt control over one's co-ordination pattern and therefore adapting to changing task and environmental constraints as needed.

9. Being skilful requires the ability to assign optimal values to (control) co-ordination

As argued earlier, skilfulness is composed of optimal co-ordination *and* optimal control. How well does a child use a particular locomotor skill in adapting to the environment and to task parameters? Put another way, can a child optimally adapt spatial and temporal requirements of, say, running for the context in which these adaptations are required (either intentionally or reactively)? Clearly, it is important to acquire a degree of control over one's locomotor skills. Except for continuous hopping, which is used mainly when injury occurs to one leg, the other locomotor skills are rarely used without specific temporal/spatial requirements. For example, how often does one walk or even run on a flat surface at a preferred speed with no obstacles or people in sight? Running, of course, is an integral component of interactive sports and requires exquisite temporal/spatial accuracy performed alone (as in creating space) or in combination with other skills, implements and/or people. The importance of control is apparent if one observes a child who is a fast runner with a good co-ordination pattern but who cannot adjust his pace to receive a ball or break free from a covering opponent. Regarding the other locomotor skills, galloping and skipping steps are common components of dances that, while less commonly engaged in than sports, also require sophisticated control over timing (e.g. keeping to a beat) and spatial navigation (e.g. interacting with others, changing direction etc). Given the desirability of having control over locomotor skills, we now ask when and how this is accomplished.

There is little direct evidence about the developmental profile(s) of locomotor control. A few early studies reveal observations of locomotor control across childhood but suffer limitations regarding interpretation. For example, producing a range of walking speeds, and particularly a slow speed, has been shown to improve dramatically across childhood (Constantini *et al.*, 1973; Gipsman, 1973). However, these studies did not include controls for co-ordination pattern or biomechanical constraints. Varying the spatial direction of a run using a 'zigzag' pattern shows steady improvement across childhood (Johnson, 1962) but the directional change itself is not differentiated from the forward running progression. One study that did isolate the ability to turn focused only on 5-year-olds, thus providing no information regarding developmental change (Harper, 1975). Running to intercept a moving object is reported to change from being too late (under-estimation), to being too early (over-estimation) to being just right across age by Keogh and Sugden (1985) yet no ages, percentage rates of success or citation to the original work is given.

In sum, no researchers appear to have systematically looked at how the control of running (or other skills) is developed for use in a game (or dance) situation. Even studies that look at the development of game play (e.g. French and Thomas, 1987) tend to concentrate on changes in perceptual/cognitive strategy rather than on the changing interaction between running, available perceptual information and cognitive intention. For those who are interested in this area, there are a series of studies in the adult gait literature by Bonnard, Pailhous and colleagues (Bonnard and Pailhous, 1993; Bonnard, Pailhous and Danion, 2000; Danion, Bonnard and Pailhous, 1997; Varraine *et al.*, 2000) that have investigated the intentional modulation of walking. These studies could act as an adult template for comparable *developmental* studies in running as well as walking. Recently, a few researchers have provided information on the development of locomotor control not by looking at intentional modulation but by studying the sub-conscious interaction between perception and walking/running.

10. Perception–action coupling underlies locomotor control both unconsciously and consciously

In conjunction with the dynamic approach to motor development and control, and following Gibson (1979), the relationship between perception of and action in the environment is considered to be inseparable, bidirectional and fundamental to movement from the earliest age (Kugler *et al.*, 1982; Turvey and Fitzpatrick, 1993). In particular, the coupling of vision with locomotion has been explored through the concept of affordances or the properties of an object–environment interaction that directly (unconsciously) specify action for a particular individual. That is, locomotion is guided by information gained through transformations of the optic array on the retina. For example, Savelsbergh *et al.* (1998) investigated the ability of children to use body-scaled information to determine the passability of a doorway-like opening. Younger children (5 to 8 years) were less able to employ body-scaled information in judging aperture width than older children (9 to 13 years), but when performances in passing through the openings were adjusted for differences in body width, both groups had similar outcomes. This result suggests that even young children can use visual information well to adapt their walking to the environment. Another example of perception–action coupling is the ability to visually estimate distance to a target (5m away) and then walk without vision to that target as accurately as possible (Corlett *et al.*, 1985). In this case, 9-year-old children were less accurate estimators than adults and, unlike the adults, were heavily influenced by processing time, with greater scanning time and less delay between scanning and walking resulting in fewer errors. This study suggests that children need longer to process information and therefore their ability to adapt to new conditions may be far from adult-like or skilful.

For example, in a study where decisions had to be made on the run (no pun intended!), 4-year-olds were rather different from adults. Wann, Edgar and Blair (1993) investigated the approach and deceleration toward a target on the wall while 4-year-olds and adults ran and touched the wall as in a relay race. They found that both groups decelerated in two phases and contacted the surface with similar relative kinetic energy, suggesting that children use optical information to judge time to contact equally as well as adults. However, the children used an inappropriate 'reckless' strategy for time to contact in the first deceleration phase, compared to the adults, resulting in the necessity of a larger deceleration in the second deceleration phase. More importantly, when a stick was held in the hand when doing the same task, the children, unlike the adults, did not modify their deceleration strategy at all, resulting in a larger kinetic energy at surface contact. In addition to investigating direct perception, this study nicely demonstrates some limitations in the running control of young children and reinforces the appropriateness of teaching self-control in running before adding implements.

Studies such as Wann *et al.* (1993) and Corlett *et al.* (1985) are important indicators that children control locomotor activities differently from adults. Regrettably, however, both of these studies use children as a comparison group to adults rather than looking across a developmental landscape in order to ask developmental questions. How children actually learn to integrate perception of an object with perception of self and the production of motion across childhood (towards skilfulness) has not been systematically studied. Again, there is a series of bio-mechanically-based studies in the adult literature, this time by Patla and colleagues (e.g. Patla *et al.*, 1996; 2002) that investigate visual information-processing during walking in 'cluttered' environments. For example, in adults it is known that obstacle information provided by vision is used in a feed-forward rather than an on-line control mode to regulate locomotion (Patla and Vickers, 1997). How soon children use a similar feed-forward control, and whether this is amenable to training or determining the limits of a particular control system for a particular environment seem appropriate questions to ask. One study did assess the walking performance of children on three pathways of increasing complexity and found that children under 8 years of age made significantly more errors in the obstacle path and larger than necessary steps over obstacles (Pryde *et al.*, 1997). More systematic testing of the interaction between visual information and the environment is necessary, though, to understand how children become more skilful at walking (running, etc.) in a changing environment. One suggestion is to combine the methods of perception–action experiments such as Savelsbergh *et al.* (1998) with more traditional information-processing approaches to test, for example, whether there is a certain 'amount of information' that allows children to perceive affordances as accurately as adults and/or allows feed-forward processing. Put in the dynamic systems framework, one would see information (however defined) as a potential control parameter that could be manipulated (and possibly trained) to improve gait adaptation to tasks and environments. No such comprehensive studies of subconscious perception–action coupling in children's locomotion appear to have been investigated yet. What has begun to be investigated is a more conscious form of perception–action coupling; that is, the deliberate attempt to couple footsteps with a beat, such as galloping steps in dance.

From a dynamic perspective, coupling limb movements to a rhythmic beat is seen as a special case of coupling between non-linear limit-cycle oscillators. A key prediction from the coupled oscillator model, which is well-verified in adults, is that, within frequency boundaries, limbs should couple to an auditory beat either in-phase (usually easier) or antiphase with a fairly stable (limit-cycle) relationship (Kelso *et al.*, 1990). Research documenting children's ability to keep to a beat when tapping has suggested that intentional coupling to a beat is not a natural tendency but has to be learned. Unfortunately, few studies have looked at similar rhythmic ability with respect to locomotion. One early study reported that children of 5 years were only able to keep time with a beat when walking and clapping 48 per cent of the time, and this ability continued to develop across childhood (Jersild and Bienstock, 1935). More recently, Parker (1990) has shown that boys of 9 years can accomplish star jumping (jumping jacks) to a beat with similar accuracy as adults across a range of tempos, while 7-year-olds were as accurate as adults only at fast tempos. These studies suggest that children do indeed have difficulty in adapting to different frequencies of auditory information.

Other studies have looked at coupling between limbs without an external beat but providing one's own beat. When children were asked to combine clapping cymbals with walking or galloping they did not automatically co-ordinate the clap (which provided a strong auditory signal) with a footstep (or any part of the limb cycle) as would be predicted by an oscillator model (Getchell and Whitall, 2002). At 4 years, children primarily showed stable but frequency-unlocked relationships between the arms and the legs. Only by 10 years of age were the arms and legs (for walking in particular) mostly in a tight frequency-locked relationship. Since the children were not asked to intentionally couple their clap with a footstep, the intention of the child was a potential confound for interpreting the data. In fact, in the same paradigm, adults too sometimes showed a frequency-unlocked but stable relationship between clapping and walking, although less often than the children (Muzii *et al.* 1986; Whitall and Getchell, 1996). It is interesting to speculate whether the children's lack of frequency-locking across limb girdles was a result of an inability to couple with a beat (or another limb) while the adults' demonstration of a lack of frequency-locking was a function of an ability, albeit subconscious, to resist the absolute coupling relationship. Further work is necessary to understand this development. What is clear, however, is that children are able to produce stable and consistent coupled oscillator-like phasing relationships between their lower limbs (one girdle), at least in self-paced, uncluttered running and galloping, by 4 years if not earlier (Whitall, 1989). Therefore, as argued earlier, it is the superposition of task/environmental requirements that require additional cognitive processing that will provide further information about the development of locomotor skilfulness.

11. Cognitive aspects of development such as processing speed and attentional ability impact on locomotor skilfulness

In an interactive environment, be it sport, work or daily living, the ability to attend to more than one task and/or process perceptual information quickly is part of locomotor skilfulness. Studies mentioned earlier have indicated that information-processing is different or slower in children. Although no studies appear to have tested reaction time in children *while they locomoted*, it is very probable that this improves across childhood, as it does when children are sitting (Thomas *et al.*, 1981). Further, one might argue that combining reaction time with locomotion is bound to be more difficult for children since they have less ability to attend either to relevant information (Connolly 1970; Herkowitz, 1972) or to two tasks at once (Wickens and Benel, 1982). Combining locomotion with a cognitive task was investigated by Whitall (1991) who had children from 2 to 10 years and adults run or gallop while singing or memorising letters (the latter task was comparable in attentional demand for each age group). She found that children of 4 years and above were able to combine both tasks equally as well as adults in the sense that the co-ordination characteristics of running and galloping were unchanged under dual-task conditions. Likewise, under dual-task conditions, all age groups demonstrated a change in the control characteristics of locomotion, with singing tending to affect step-time and memorising tending to affect step-length. This study did not, however, test subjects under extreme task-demanding conditions such as moving as fast as possible, which is a more realistic test of attentional demands and skilful control and may have resulted in a qualitative change in co-ordination pattern. No such studies exist of running or other locomotor skills; however, one study has shown that young boys (6 to 8 years) who skated as fast as possible through pylons, with and without dribbling a hockey puck, showed a greater increase in time with the puck than older boys of 14 years (Leavitt, 1979). Again, this demonstrates the difficulty of combining an implement (and additional skill) with pure locomotion and reinforces the idea that key underlying constraint changes are connected with central processing systems. Unfortunately, no one has followed up with systematic investigations of the interaction between locomotion and cognitive processing that characterises locomotor control and ultimately skilfulness. Perhaps part of the reason for this lack of study is that locomotor skilfulness is not considered an important developmental goal.

12. The acquisition of locomotor skilfulness is a worthwhile research goal

One might argue that locomotor skilfulness should be studied because it enables perceptual/cognitive phenomena to be understood or because it is useful in clinical applications or even simply because it is not yet understood. These are all valid reasons. A fourth reason, however, is that locomotor skilfulness is an intrinsically worthwhile individual goal in most, if not all, societies. Technological advances may mean that advanced civilisations do not need to be skilful in order to hunt, gather, and adapt to user-unfriendly terrain, but, regardless of technology, the same Darwinian goal of survival remains. If individuals want to live a long and healthy life, then becoming skilful in locomotion could assist that goal in a number of ways. First, since regular physical activity is known to increase the quality and quantity of life and given that locomotion is a simple physical activity, it follows that locomotion is an easy choice for achieving a better, longer life. However, relatively few Westerners actually engage in regular physical activity and a good proportion of those who do choose fitness activities like weight-training, biking or treadmill training that hardly depend on locomotor skilfulness. One explanation for these facts, albeit speculative, is that children (and adults) give up many sporting physical activities precisely because they are not skilful in moving with implements and other people. Furthermore, these same people may not enjoy moving in crowded environments or uneven terrain and are less likely to walk when they need not. At a later stage of the lifespan, it is theoretically possible (but not yet investigated) that those who give up activities involving locomotor skills early also tend to lose walking mobility earlier, possibly (at least partially) through decreased confidence in their skills, resulting in a lower quality of life.

One could argue that the above sentiment justifies a goal of skilfulness in walking and running (and their study) but not in the other fundamental locomotor skills. There are four counter arguments to this viewpoint. First, as mentioned earlier, galloping and skipping steps (the latter including hopping) are fundamental to many forms of dance. Again, one reason why formal dancing is not a more popular form of physical activity may be that individuals feel uncomfortable with their ability to perform dance-like steps and need to be taught, early on, to be more skilful. Second, galloping steps, in particular, are used quite heavily in many sporting activities. For example, sports such as fencing and boxing consist primarily of gallop-type steps, whereas court games and other field games that require sideways and backwards locomotion promote sliding steps (a form of gallop). The argument again is that children would be better and more likely to continue with these types of sports if they were skilful in galloping. Third, rather surprisingly, hopping, galloping and skipping are used in daily life activities. For example, running downstairs, down a slope or around a sharp bend will often elicit a gallop, particularly at a faster pace, while stopping suddenly can result in hopping steps (De Clercq, 2000). These spontaneous gaits may occur relative to safety considerations while spontaneous skipping is related to feelings of happiness (Burton *et al.*, 1999). Whether being skilful in these activities would have any effect on the quality of everyday living is unknown but, at least, they can be considered from a safety and emotional viewpoint. Finally, there is recent recognition, outside the kinesiological arena, that the gait of galloping (and skipping) is of interest from an evolutionary perspective based, in part, from its prevalence in a non-gravitational environment as well as in other animals (Farley, 1998; Minetti, 1998; Verstappen *et al.*, 2000).

13. Future research should focus more on locomotor control and how co-ordination and control combine towards skilfulness.

Given the above discussion, what are important research questions to ask regarding the development of locomotor co-ordination and control in children? The following is a personal, general and nonexclusive list of relevant questions. What is the natural time-course of the development of locomotor control (i.e. which elements of control emerge first and when in each gait)? What is the relationship between co-ordination level and control (e.g. is control specific to one locomotor gait and co-ordination level, or is it generalised across all gaits regardless of co-ordination level)? What are the critical control parameters (and rate-limiters) that can be manipulated actively or passively (i.e. through repetitive practice alone) to improve a child's chance of gaining locomotor skilfulness (e.g. how are anticipatory units of action, that would allow adaptation, developed)? Specifically, how do underlying processing systems contribute to adaptive locomotion? Importantly, too, we also need to know if children's locomotor skilfulness is related to increased physical activity, quality of life and mobility later in life.

14. Concluding remarks on the development of locomotor skilfulness

In this chapter, principles of motor development have been illustrated by an analysis and description of what is presently known about locomotor co-ordination and control. It should be clear that, currently, far more is known about age-related changes in co-ordination than about age-related changes in control. To the extent that locomotor control is intimately bound with perceptual and cognitive processes, ensuring a complex entity to study, this is understandable. Nevertheless, if one accepts the premise that locomotor skilfulness is a desirable goal, understanding how the development of locomotor co-ordination *and control* interact to produce that skilfulness is critical. Achieving this understanding will not be easy, but the principles of development outlined above suggest that a combination of the dynamic systems, perception–action and cognitive/information–processing approaches is needed. Specifically lacking are longitudinal or even cross-sectional studies investigating the development of sub-conscious (cf. Wann *et al.*, 1993; Corlett *et al.*, 1985; Pryde *et al.*, 1997) or intentional modulation (cf. Danion *et al.*, 2000; Danion *et al.* 1997) of perception–action coupling in locomotion with task and environmental constraints.

References

Abraham, F.D., Abraham, R.H. and Shaw, C.D. (1989) *A Visual Introduction to Dynamical Systems Theory for Psychology*. Santa Cruz, CA: Aerial Press.

Assaiante, C., Woollacott, M. and Amblard, B. (2000) Development of postural adjustment during gait initiation: kinematic and EMG analysis. *Journal of Motor Behavior*, 23, 211–26.

Bonnard, M. and Pailhous J. (1993) Intentionality in human gait control: modifying the frequency-to-amplitude relationship. *Journal of Experimental Psychology: Human Perception and Performance*, 19, 429–43.

Bonnard, M., Pailhous, J. and Danion, F. (2000) Adaptation of neuromuscular synergies during intentional constraints of space–time relationships in human gait. *Journal of Motor Behavior*, 32, 200–8.

Branta, C.J., Haubenstricker, J. and Seefeldt, V. (1984) Age changes in motor skill during childhood and adolescence. *Exercise and Sport Science Reviews*, 12, 467–520.

Burnett, C.N. and Johnson, E.W. (1971) Development of gait in childhood: part II. *Developmental Medicine and Child Neurology*, 13, 207–15.

Burton, A.W., Garcia, L. and Garcia, C. (1999) Skipping and hopping of undergraduates: recollections of when and why. *Perceptual and Motor Skills*, 88, 401–6.

Clark, J.E. and Phillips, S.J. (1993) A longitudinal study of intralimb co-ordination in the 1st year of independent walking: a dynamical systems analysis. *Child Development*, 64, 1143–57.

Clark, J.E. and Whitall, J. (1989a) Changing patterns of locomotion: from walking to skipping. In M.H. Woollacott and H.G. Williams (eds), *Development of Posture and Gait Across the Lifespan* (pp. 128–51). Columbia, SC: University of South Carolina Press.

Clark, J.E. and Whitall, J. (1989b) What is motor development? The lessons of history. *Quest*, 41, 183–202.

Clark, J.E., Whitall, J. and Phillips, S.J. (1988) Human interlimb co-ordination: the first 6 months of independent walking. *Developmental Psychobiology*, 21, 445–56.

Connolly, K.J. (1970) Response speed, temporal sequencing and information processing in children. In K.J. Connolly (ed.), *Mechanisms of Motor Skill Development* (pp. 161–88). New York: Academic Press.

Constantini, A.F., Corsini, D.A. and Davis, J.E. (1973) Conceptual tempo, inhibition of movement and acceleration of movement in 4-, 7- and 9-year-old children. *Perceptual and Motor Skills*, 37, 779–84.

Corlett, J.T., Patla, A. and Williams, J.G. (1985) Locomotor estimation of distance after visual scanning by children and adults. *Perception*, 14, 237–63.

Danion, F., Bonnard, M. and Pailhous, J. (1997) Intentional on-line control of propulsive forces in human gait. *Experimental Brain Research*, 116, 525–38.

De Clercq, D. (2000) Personal communication.

Diedrich, F.J. and Warren, W.H. Jr. (1995) Why change gaits? Dynamics of the walk–run transition. *Journal of Experimental Psychology: Human Perception and Performance*, 21, 183–202.

Drabik, J. (1989) The general endurance of children aged 8–12 years in the 12 min run test. *Journal of Sports Medicine and Physical Fitness*, 29, 379–83.

Eckert, H.M. (1987) *Motor Development*, 3rd edn. Indianapolis, IN: Benchmark Press.

Farley, C.T. (1998) Locomotion. Just skip it. *Nature*, 394, 721–3.

Fortney, V.L. (1983) The kinematics and kinetics of the running pattern of two- four-, and six-year-old children. *Research Quarterly for Exercise and Sport*, 54, 126–35.

French, K.E. and Thomas, J.R. (1987) The relation of knowedge development to children's basketball performance. *Journal of Sports Psychology*, 9, 15–32.

Gabbard, C. (1996) *Lifelong Motor Development*. Dubuque, IA: Wm. C. Brown.

Gallahue, D.L. (1989) *Understanding Motor Development in Infants, Children and Adolescents*. Indianapolis, IN: Benchmark Press.

268   *Whitall*

Getchell, N. and Roberton, M.A. (1989) Whole body stiffness as a function of developmental level in children's hopping. *Developmental Psychology*, 25, 920–8.

Getchell, N. and Whitall, J. (2003) How do children coordinate simultaneous upper and lower extremity tasks? The development of dual task co-ordination. Manuscript in revision. *Journal of Experimental Child Psychology*.

Gesell, A. (1954) The ontogenesis of infant behavior. In L. Carmichael (ed.), *Manual of Child Psychology* (pp. 295–331). New York: Wiley.

Gibson, J.J. (1979) *An Ecological Approach to Visual Perception*. Boston: Houghton Mifflin.

Gipsman, S. (1973) Control of range of movement rate in primary school children. Unpublished, University of California, Los Angeles.

Halverson, L.E. and Williams, K. (1985) Developmental sequences for hopping over distance: a prelongitudinal screening. *Research Quarterly for Exercise and Sport*, 56, 37–44.

Harper, C.J. (1975) Movement responses of kindergarten children to a change of direction task – an analysis of selected measures. Unpublished, University of Wisconsin, Madison.

Haywood, K.M. and Getchell, N. (2001) *Lifespan Motor Development*. Champaign, IL: Human Kinetics.

Herkowitz, J. (1972) Moving embedded figures test. *Research Quarterly*, 43, 479–88.

Hirschfeld, H. and Forssberg, H. (1992) Development of anticipatory adjustments during locomotion in children. *Journal of Neurophysiology*, 68, 542–50.

Jersild, A.T. and Bienstock, S.F. (1935) Development of rhythm in young children. *Child Development Monographs* (no. 22).

Johnson, R. (1962) Measurements of achievement in fundamental skills of elementary school children. *Research Quarterly*, 33, 94.

Kelso, J.A.S. (1984) Phase transitions and critical behavior in the human bimanual co-ordination. *American Journal of Physiology*, 246, R1000–4.

Kelso, J.A.S., DelColle, J. and Schöner, G. (1990) Action–perception as a pattern formation process. In Jeannerod, M. (ed.), *Attention and Performance XIII* (pp. 139–69). Hillsdale: Erlbaum.

Keogh, J.F. (1969) *Analysis of Limb and Body Control Tasks* (Rep. No. Technical Report 1-69 (USPHS HD 01059)). Department of Physical Education, University of California.

Keogh, J. and Sugden, D. (1985) *Movement Skill Development*. London: Collier Macmillan Publishers.

Kugler, P.N., Kelso, J.A.S. and Turvey, M.T. (1980) On the concept of coordinative structures as dissapative structures. I. Theoretical lines of convergence. In G.E. Stelmach and J. Requin (eds), *Tutorials in Motor Behavior* (pp. 3–47). New York: North Holland.

Kugler, P.N., Kelso, J.A.S. and Turvey, M.T. (1982) On the control and co-ordination of naturally devoloping systems. In J.A.S. Kelso and J.E. Clark (eds), *The Development of Movement Control and Co-ordination* (pp. 5–78). Chichester: John Wiley and Sons.

Langendorfer, S. and Roberton, M.A. (2002) Developmental profiles in overarm throwing: searching for attractors, constraints, and stages. In J.E. Clark and J.H. Humphrey (eds), *Motor Development: Research and Reviews*, Volume 2 (pp. 1–25). Reston, VA: NASPE Publications.

Leavitt, J. L. (1979) Cognitive demands of skating and stickhandling in ice hockey. *Journal of Applied Sports Sciences*, 4, 46–55.

Ledebt, A., Bril, B. and Brenière, Y. (1998) The build-up of anticipatory behaviour: an analysis of the development of gait initiation in children. *Experimental Brain Research*, 120, 9–17.

Loovis, E.M. and Butterfield, S.A. (2000) Influence of age, sex and balance on mature skipping by children in grades K-8. *Perceptual and Motor Skills*, 90, 974–8.

Malina, R.M. and Roche, A.F. (1983) *Manual of Physical Status and Performance in Childhood: Vol. 2. Physical Performance*. New York: Plenum.

Minetti, A.E. (1998) The biomechanics of skipping gaits: a third locomotion paradigm? *Proceedings of Royal Society of London Biological Sciences*, 265, 1227–35.

Muzii, R.A., Lamm, C. and Gentile, A.M. (1984) Coordination of the upper and lower extremities. *Human Movement Science*, 3, 337–54.

Newell, K. M. (1986) Constraints on the development of coordination. In M.G. Wade and H.T.A. Whiting (eds), *Motor Development in Children: Aspects of Co-ordination and Control* (pp. 341–60). Boston: Martinus Nijhoff.

Parker, H.E. (1990) The development of coordination and timing in a rhythmic multi-limbed task. University of Western Australia, Perth.

Patla, A.E., Adkin, A., Martin, C. and Holden, R. (1996) Characteristics of voluntary visual sampling of the environment for safe locomotion over different terrains. *Experimental Brain Research*, 112, 513–22.

Patla, A.E., Niechwiej, E., Racco, V. and Goodale, M.A. (2002) Understanding the contribution of binocular vision to the control of adaptive locomotion. *Experimental Brain Research*, 142, 551–61.

Patla, A.E. and Vickers, J.N. (1997) Where and when do we look as we approach and step over an obstacle in the travel path? *Neuroreport*, 8, 3661–5.

Payne, V.G. and Isaacs, L.D. (1991) *Human Motor Development. A Lifespan Approach*. Mountain View, CA: Mayfield.

Pryde, K.M., Roy, E.A. and Patla, A.E. (1997) Age-related trends in locomotor ability and obstacle avoidance. *Human Movement Science*, 16, 507–16.

Roberton, M.A. and Halverson, L.E. (1984) *Developing children – Their Changing Movement*. Philadelphia: Lea and Febiger.

Roberton, M.A. and Halverson, L.E. (1988) The development of locomotor co-ordination: longitudinal change and invariance. *Journal of Motor Behavior*, 20, 197–241.

Roberton, M.A., Halverson, L.E. and Harper, C.J. (1997) Visual/verbal modeling as a function of children's developmental levels in hopping. In J.E. Clark and J.H. Humphrey (eds), *Motor Development: Research and Reviews*, Volume 1 (pp. 122–48). Reston, VA: NASPE Publications.

Sapp, M.M. (1980) The development of galloping in young children: a preliminary study. Master's project, Michigan State University.

Savelsbergh, G.J.P., Douwes-Dekker, L., Vermeer, A. and Hopkins, B. (1998) Locomoting through apertures of different width: a study of children with cerebral palsy. *Pediatric Rehabilitation*, 2, 5–13.

Schepens, B., Willems, P.A. and Cavagna, G.A. (1998) The mechanics of running in children. *Journal of Physiology*, 509, 927–40.

Seefeldt, V. and Haubenstricker, J. (1982) Patterns, phases, or stages: an analytical model for the study of developmental movement. In J.A.S. Kelso and J.E. Clark (eds), *The Development of Movement Control and Co-ordination* (pp. 309–18). New York: John Wiley and Sons.

Shumway-Cook, A. and Woollacott, M.H. (1985) The growth of stability: postural control from a developmental perspective. *Journal of Motor Behavior*, 17, 131–47.

Sinclair, C.B. (1973) *Movement of the Young Child. Ages Two to Six*. Columbus, OH: Charles E. Merrill.

Sutherland, D.H., Olshen, R., Cooper, L. and Woo, S.L.Y. (1980) The development of mature gait. *Journal of Bone and Joint Surgery*, 62A, 336–53.

Thelen, E. (1986) Development of coordinated movement: Implications for early human movement. In M.G. Wade and H.T.A. Whiting (eds), *Motor Development in Children: Aspects of Co-ordination and Control* (pp. 107–24). Boston: Martinus Nijhoff.

Thelen, E., Corbetta, D., Kamm, K., Spencer, J.P., Schneider, K. and Zernicke, R.F. (1993) The transition to reaching: mapping intention and intrinsic dynamics. *Child Development*, 64, 1058–98.

Thelen, E. and Ulrich, B.D. (1991) Hidden skills: a dynamic systems analysis of treadmill stepping during the first year. *Monograph Society Research Child Devevelopment*, 56, 1–98.

Thomas, J.R. and French, K.E. (1985) Gender differences across age in motor performance. *Psychological Bulletin*, 98, 260–82.

Thomas, J.R., Gallagher, J.D. and Purvis, G.J. (1981) Reaction time and anticipation time: effects of development. *Research Quarterly for Exercise and Sport*, 52, 359–67.

Turvey, M.T. and Fitzpatrick, P. (1993) Commentary: development of perception–action systems and general principles of pattern formation. *Child Development*, 64, 1175–90.

Varraine, E., Bonnard, M. and Pailhous, J. (2000) Intentional on-line adaptation of stride length in human walking. *Experimental Brain Research*, 130, 248–57.

Verstappen, M., Aerts, P. and Van Damme, R. (2000) Terrestrial locomotion in the black-billed magpie: kinematic analysis of walking, running and out-of-phase hopping. *Journal of Experimental Biology*, 203, 59–70.

Wann, J.P., Edgar, P. and Blair, D. (1993) Time-to-contact judgement in the locomotion of adults and preschool children. *Journal of Experimental Psychology: Human Perception and Performance*, 19, 1053–65.

Whitall, J. (1989) A developmental study of the interlimb co-ordination in running and galloping. *Journal of Motor Behavior*, 21, 409–28.

Whitall, J. (1991) The developmental effect of concurrent cognitive and locomotor skills–time-sharing from a dynamic perspective. *Journal of Experimental Child Psychology*, 51, 245–66.

Whitall, J. (1995) The evolution of research on motor development: new approaches bringing new insights. *Exercise and Sport Science Reviews*, 20, 243–73.

Whitall, J. and Caldwell, G.E. (1992) Co-ordination of symmetrical and asymmetrical human gait: kinematic patterns. *Journal of Motor Behavior*, 24, 339–54.

Whitall, J. and Getchell, N. (1996) Multilimb co-ordination patterns in simultaneous dissimilar upper and lower limb tasks. *Human Movement Science*, 15, 129–55.

Wickens, C.D. and Benel, D.C.R. (1982) The development of time-sharing. In J.A.S. Kelso and J.E. Clark (eds), *The Development of Movement Control and Co-ordination* (pp. 253–72). New York: John Wiley and Sons.

Wickstrom, R.L. (1987) Observations on motor pattern development in skipping. In J.E. Clark and J.H. Humphrey (eds), *Advance in Motor Development Research*, Volume 1 (pp. 49–60), New York: AMS Press.

Index

abnormal reflexes 97, 98–9
action–perception coupling 3–4, 51, 102, 261–3; with cerebral palsy 216
aerobic capacity 118
affordances 3–4; cerebral palsy and 216–17
allocentric constraints 158–9; on semi-circle; drawing with hemiplegic cerebral palsy 67–72
anaerobic capacity 118
anchoring 69–70
Attention Deficit Hyperactivity Disorder (ADHD) 113–14
attentional ability 264

balance, as constraint 119–21, 258
Basic Motor Ability Test – revised 110
bicycling behaviour 34–7; road crossing judgements 35–7
bimanual movements 156–7; allocentric constraints 158–9, 167–72; development 160–2; egocentric constraints 158–9, 167–72; healthy populations 157–60; temporal constraints 158; with hemiplegic cerebral palsy 162–72, see also grasping; movement co-ordination
Bruininks–Oseretsky Test of Motor Proficiency (BOTMP) 110, 111, 112

catching skills development 6–7, 123, 191–2, 207–9; constraints and 194–205; developmental movement disorder and 123–4; information–movement coupling 205–7; theoretical perspective 192–4, see also movement co-ordination development
cerebral palsy (CP) 85, 177–8, 213; affordances and 216–17; as an organismic constraint on movement co-ordination 215; bimanual co-ordination and 162–72; definition 162; gait abnormalities 178, 182–4; impact on spoon use learning 85–9; interceptive action 215–16, 217–20; motor impairments 178; perception–action coupling 216; sports activities and 220–2; walking prognosis 178–82

choice reaction time, with Down syndrome 140–4
closed-loop models 2
clumsiness 151
co-ordination see co-ordination difficulties; movement co-ordination; movement co-ordination development
co-ordination difficulties 107; cerebral palsy and 178; developmental co-ordination disorder (DCD) 108; interventions 124–7; reaction time and 114; timing and rhythm 115–17, see also developmental movement disorder; movement co-ordination; movement co-ordination development
co-ordinative structure theory 6–8
cognitive aspects of development 264
Cognitive Orientation to daily Occupational Performance (COOP) 126
constraints 6–8, 61–2, 75–6; balance and postural control 119–21; cerebral palsy and 217; in movement co-ordination development 6–8, 192–4, 214–15, 237, 253–60; interaction of 69–70, 117–21; on bimanual co-ordination 158–9, 167–72; on catching skills development 194–205; on drawing and writing skills 62, 64–7, 70–1, 167–72; on skill co-ordination 117–19; on spoon use learning 75–89; physical fitness as constraint 117–19, see also environmental constraints; organismic constraints; task constraints
corpus callosum maturation 161
crawling, prognostic significance with cerebral palsy 179–80

degrees of freedom 1, 201–2, 205, 214; cerebral palsy and 217, 218, see also constraints
development: bimanual movements 160–2; catching skills 191–2, 200–5; cognitive aspects 264; drawing and writing skills 56–8; grasping behaviour 3–4; grip 58–9, 82–4; information–movement coupling

Lightning Source UK Ltd.
Milton Keynes UK
24 July 2010

157404UK00003B/4/P